P9-CDB-757

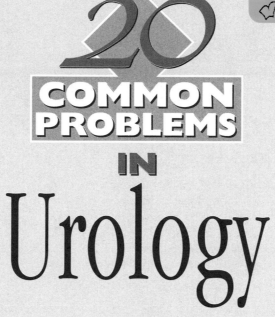

20 COMMON PROBLEMS IN Urology

EDITOR

JOEL M.H. TEICHMAN, M.D., F.R.C.S.C.

Associate Professor
Division of Urology
University of Texas Health Science Center in San Antonio
San Antonio, Texas

SERIES EDITOR

BARRY D. WEISS, M.D.

Professor of Clinical Family and Community Medicine
University of Arizona College of Medicine
Tucson, Arizona

McGraw-Hill
Medical Publishing Division

New York   St. Louis   San Francisco   Auckland   Bogotá   Caracas   Lisbon   London   Madrid
Mexico City   Milan   Montreal   New Delhi   San Juan   Singapore   Sydney   Tokyo   Toronto

McGraw-Hill

*A Division of The **McGraw·Hill** Companies*

20 COMMON PROBLEMS IN UROLOGY

Copyright © 2001 by **The McGraw-Hill Companies, Inc.** All rights reserved. Printed in the United States of America. Except as permitted under the United States Copyright Act of 1976, no part of this publication may be reproduced or distributed in any form or by any means, or stored in a data base or retrieval system, without the prior written permission of the publisher.

1 2 3 4 5 6 7 8 9 0 DOC/DOC 0 9 8 7 6 5 4 3 2 1 0

ISBN 0-07-063413-0

This book was set in Garamond by Circle Graphics.
The editors were Andrea Seils and Susan R. Noujaim.
The production supervisor was Phil Galea.
Project management was provided by Andover Publishing Services.
The cover designer was Marsha Cohen-Parallelogram.
R.R. Donnelley & Sons was printer and binder.

This book is printed on acid-free paper.

Library of Congress Cataloging-in-Publication Data

Teichman, Joel
    20 common problems in urology for primary care clinicians/author, Joel Teichman.
      p. ; cm.
    Includes bibliographical references and index.
    ISBN 0-07-063413-0
    1. Genitourinary organs—Diseases. 2. Urology. I. Title: Twenty common problems in urology for primary care clinicians. II. Title: Urology for primary care clinicians. III. Title.
    [DNLM: 1. 1. Urogenital Diseases—diagnosis. 2. Primary Health Care—methods. 3. Urogenital Diseases—therapy. WJ 140 T262z 2001]
RC871.T45 2001
616.6—dc21   00–033236

To Claire, Rachel, and Colleen

Contents

Part **3** Miscellaneous

A color insert falls between pages 240 and 241.

Contributors

M. David Bomalaski, M.D., F.A.A.P.
Chief, Pediatric Urology
Department of Urology
Wilford Hall Medical Center
Lackland AFB, Texas

R. Duane Cespedes, MD
Chief, Female Urology and Urodynamics
Wilford Hall Medical Center
Lackland AFB, Texas
Clinical Assistant Professor
University of Texas Health Science Center
San Antonio, Texas

Joseph Chin, M.D., F.R.C.S.C.
Chief of Urology
London Health Sciences Center
Professor and Chairman
Division of Urology
University of Western Ontario
London, Ontario, Canada

Sakti Das, M.D.
Professor of Urology
Department of Urology
University of California Davis Medical Center
Sacramento, California

LTC Dirk M. Elston, M.D., MC USA
Chairman
Department of Dermatology
Wilford Hall Medical Center
Brooke Army Medical Center
Lackland AFB, Texas

Peter D. Furness III, M.D
Assistant Professor of Surgery
Associate Chairman, Pediatric Urology
The Children's Hospital
University of Colorado Health Sciences Center
Denver, Colorado

James H. Gilbaugh III, M.D.
Wichita Urology Group
Wichita, Kansas

S. Larry Goldenberg, M.D., F.R.C.S.C.
Professor and Head
The Prostate Center at Vancouver Hospital
Division of Urology
Department of Surgery
University of British Columbia
Vancouver, British Columbia, Canada

Tomas L. Griebling, M.D.
Assistant Professor of Urology
Assistant Scientist--Center on Aging
The University of Kansas
Kansas City, Kansas

C. Darryl Jones, M.D.
Assistant Professor
Department of Radiology
University of California Davis Medical Center
Sacramento, California

George W. Kaplan, M.D.
Chief of Urology
Children's Hospital
Clinical Professor of Surgery and Pediatrics
University of California San Diego
San Diego, California

MAJ George Keough, M.D., MC USA
Department of Dermatology
Wilford Hall Medical Center
Brooke Army Medical Center
Lackland AFB, Texas

Barry A. Kogan, M.D.
Chief, Division of Urology
Professor of Surgery and Pediatrics
Albany Medical College
Albany, New York

Martin A. Koyle, M.D., F.A.C.S., F.A.A.P.
Professor of Surgery
Chairman of Pediatric Urology
The Children's Hospital
University of Colorado Health Sciences Center
Denver, Colorado

Lori Landau, M.D.
Urology Resident
Department of Urology
New York Medical College at Westchester County Medical Center
Valhalla, New York

MAJ Richard Laws, M.D., MC USA
Department of Dermatology
Wilford Hall Medical Center
Brooke Army Medical Center
Lackland AFB, Texas

Roger K. Low, M.D.
Assistant Professor of Urology
Department of Urology
University of California Davis Medical Center
Sacramento, California

Stephen Lynch, M.D.
Department of Urology
Wilford Hall Medical Center
Brooke Army Medical Center
Lackland AFB, Texas

J. Curtis Nickel, M.D., F.R.C.S.C.
Professor of Urology
Department of Urology
Queen's University
Kingston, Ontario, Canada

C. Lowell Parsons, M.D.
Professor of Surgery/Urology
Division of Urology
Department of Surgery
University of California San Diego Medical Center
San Diego, California

Ryan F. Paterson, M.D.
The Prostate Center at Vancouver Hospital
Division of Urology
Department of Surgery
University of British Columbia
Vancouver, British Columbia, Canada

Margaret S. Pearle, M.D., Ph.D.
Associate Professor
Department of Urology and The Center for Mineral Metabolism
University of Texas Southwestern Medical Center at Dallas
Dallas, Texas

Jon L. Pryor, M.D.
Associate Professor
Departments of Urologic Surgery and Obstetrics and Gynecology
Interim Chair
Department of Urologic Surgery
University of Minnesota Medical School
Minneapolis, Minnesota

J. Bruce Redmon, M.D.
Assistant Clinical Professor
Division of Endocrinology and Diabetes
Department of Medicine and
Department of Urologic Surgery
University of Minnesota Medical School
Minneapolis, Minnesota

Thomas A. Rozanski, M.D.
Urology Service
Brooke Army Medical Center
Lackland AFB, Texas
Assistant Professor of Surgery
Uniformed Services University of the Health Sciences
San Antonio, Texas

Edmund S. Sabanegh, Jr., M.D.
Chairman
Department of Urology
Wilford Hall Medical Center
Lackland AFB, Texas

Christopher K. Schreiber, M.D.
Resident in Urology
Department of Urology
University of California Davis Medical Center
Sacramento, California

Joel M.H. Teichman, M.D., F.R.S.C.
Associate Professor
Division of Urology
University of Texas Health Science Center
San Antonio, Texas

Ian M. Thompson, M.D.
Chief
Division of Urology
University of Texas Health Science Center
San Antonio, Texas

Edward Tieng, M.D.
Chief Resident in Urology
Department of Urology
Wilford Hall Medical Center
Lackland AFB, Texas

Dean Troyer, M.D.
Associate Professor
Department of Pathology
University of Texas Health Science Center
San Antonio, Texas

MAJ Joseph Wilde, M.D. MC USA
Department of Dermatology
Wilford Hall Medical Center
Brooke Army Medical Center
Lackland AFB, Texas

Edith D. Wilson, M.D., F.R.C.S.C.
Fellow, Pediatric Urology
The Children's Hospital
University of Colorado Health Sciences Center
Denver, Colorado

Introduction

This book is part of McGraw-Hill's 20 Common Problems series, which is geared towards primary care clinicians. The genitourinary problems discussed in this book are the reason for at least 6% of patient visits to primary care clinicians and 8% of emergency room visits. The need for primary care clinicians to manage genitourinary problems is therefore important. This book addresses this need. It is intended to be a resource for primary care clinicians who are managing common genitourinary problems at the primary care level. This approach is unique because most other urology textbooks are intended for urology specialists or medical students learning about urology.

Primary care clinicians have learning needs in the areas of genitourinary problems and pathology that are distinctly different from those of urologists. In a recent study, the topics and skills needed by primary care clinicians were assessed. Family practice residency directors throughout the United States were surveyed to rate how well family practice physicians should know various topics (Table A). Family practice residency program directors were also asked to rate the needed proficiency for various skills (Table B).

The results show that primary care clinicians need to know urinary tract infections, hematuria, and diagnostics extremely well. The skills needed are also geared towards diagnostics. Circumcision and vasectomy are relatively important skills for many primary care clinicians. Conversely, the staging and management of cancer are relatively unimportant. The ability of primary care clinicians to perform such technical procedures as urodynamics is relatively unimportant. We assume that the ability to perform standard urologic surgery is also of no importance to primary care clinicians.

In preparing this book, I have sought out contributing authors who can focus on problems of relevance to primary care clinicians. This focus is unique, as most urology textbooks are aimed at urologists, not primary care clinicians. Thus, I have solicited chapters on urologic infections and urologic diagnostics, the two problems that are most relevant at the primary care level. There are separate chapters for adult and pediatric urinary tract infections and sexually transmitted diseases (urethral discharge). There is a separate chapter for interstitial cystitis, which is commonly confused with bacterial cystitis or prostatitis. The chapter on genitourinary skin rash covers cutaneous infections of the genitals. In contrast, the only cancer-specific chapter focuses on prostate cancer screening, with no attempt to cover the topic of prostate cancer management. The chapters on hematuria, scrotal masses, and urologic imaging briefly reference other cancers, but in the context of the clinical approach to these patients.

The chapters are organized into pediatric and adult genitourinary problems. This division is admittedly arbitrary. Not all problems are exclusive to these domains. For example, children with nocturnal enuresis may become enuretic adults. Adults with interstitial cystitis may first develop voiding symptoms as a child. The chapters on genitourinary skin rash and urologic imaging affect both adults and children.

Table A.

"How well does a family practice physician need to know this topic?"

Topic	Mean response (mean ± standard deviation)
Urinary tract infections	1.0 ± 0.2
Sexually transmitted diseases	1.0 ± 0.2
Epididymitis	1.1 ± 0.3
Hematuria	1.1 ± 0.4
BPH diagnosis	1.1 ± 0.4
Prostate specific antigen screening	1.2 ± 0.5
Testis torsion	1.2 ± 0.5
Urolithiasis	1.2 ± 0.5
Prostate cancer diagnosis	1.2 ± 0.6
Impotence diagnosis	1.3 ± 0.5
Urinary incontinence diagnosis	1.3 ± 0.5
BPH management	1.3 ± 0.5
Scrotal masses	1.4 ± 0.5
Testis cancer diagnosis	1.4 ± 0.6
Bladder cancer diagnosis	1.6 ± 0.7
Renal cancer diagnosis	1.6 ± 0.8
Impotence management	1.8 ± 0.7
Urinary incontinence management	1.8 ± 0.7
Vesicoureteral reflux	1.9 ± 0.8
Neurogenic bladder diagnosis	1.9 ± 0.8
Male infertility	2.2 ± 0.9
Neurogenic bladder management	2.5 ± 1.1
Congenital urological abnormalities	2.6 ± 0.9
Prostate cancer management	3.0 ± 1.0
Prostate cancer staging	3.1 ± 1.0
Testis cancer staging	3.3 ± 1.0
Bladder cancer staging	3.4 ± 0.9
Bladder cancer management	3.5 ± 0.8
Renal cancer staging	3.5 ± 0.9
Testis cancer management	3.5 ± 0.9
Renal cancer management	3.6 ± 0.8

Responses were 1 = extremely well, 2 = moderately well, 3 = somewhat well, 4 = slightly well, or 5 = not well at all

Several chapters focus on common problems that may or may not be recognized as such. Geriatric urology and male menopause are under-recognized as problems. As the authors articulate, their chapters cover problems that affect a large number of patients likely to be seen in a primary care practice. I believe this textbook will serve as a useful resource for primary care clinicians, internists, family practice physicians, pediatricians, nurses, nurse practitioners, and medical and nursing students. The textbook is not intended to be a comprehensive coverage of urology or even a comprehensive treatment of the topics addressed. Nonetheless, it should serve as a user-

Table B.

"How proficient does a family practice physician need to be in performing these skills?"

SKILL	MEAN RESPONSE (MEAN ± STANDARD DEVIATION)
Abdominal exam	1.0 ± 0.2
Vaginal exam	1.0 ± 0.2
Digital rectal exam	1.1 ± 0.3
Testis exam	1.1 ± 0.3
Interpret urinalysis	1.2 ± 0.4
Neonatal circumcision	1.4 ± 0.9
Insert Foley catheter	1.6 ± 0.8
Interpret films of kidneys, ureters, and bladder	1.7 ± 0.7
Prostate massage	1.7 ± 0.9
Vasectomy	2.3 ± 1.3
Interpret semen analysis	2.8 ± 1.3
Interpret IVP	3.0 ± 1.0
Interpret abdominal CT	3.2 ± 1.2
Interpret abdominal MRI	3.5 ± 1.0
Interpret renal ultrasound	3.6 ± 1.0
Urodynamics (cystometry)	3.6 ± 1.1
Insert suprapubic catheter	3.9 ± 1.2
Insert percutaneous nephrostomy tube	4.8 ± 0.5

Responses were 1=highly proficient, 2=moderately proficient, 3=somewhat proficient, 4=mildly proficient, 5=not at all proficient.

friendly resource for primary care clinicians to address common genitourinary problems.

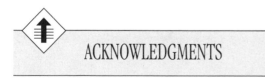

ACKNOWLEDGMENTS

I am indebted to my contributing authors. They have articulated their chapters superbly and concisely.

I wish to thank Barry Weiss, M.D., who serves as the executive editor for the 20 Common Problems series. Barry's suggestions and insights were invaluable and made my job much easier. He made me appreciate how primary care clinicians approach genitourinary problems differently than urologists.

I also wish to thank Susan Noujaim and the staff at McGraw-Hill for their assistance throughout this endeavor.

BIBLIOGRAPHY

Marsland DW, Wood M, Mayo F: A data bank for patient care, curriculum, and research in family practice: 526,196 patient problems. *J Fam Pract* 3:25, 1976.

Schappert SM: Ambulatory care visits to physician offices, hospital outpatient departments, and emergency departments: United States, 1996. *Vital Health Stat* 13: 11–19, 1998.

Teichman JMH, Weiss BD, Solomon D: Urologic needs assessment for primary care practice: implications for undergraduate medical education. *J Urol* 161: 1282–1285, 1999.

Part

1

Common Pediatric Genitourinary Problems

Lori Landau
Barry A. Kogan

Chapter

1

Fetal and Postnatal Hydronephrosis

How Common Is Fetal and Neonatal Hydronephrosis?

Hydronephrosis is one of most common fetal abnormal findings on a prenatal ultrasound examination. Although there are numerous causes of hydronephrosis, most result from obstruction at the ureteropelvic junction (UPJ). Most of the complications of hydronephrosis—including urinary tract infection, pain, hematuria, calculi, and subsequent renal injury—should be limited by the early diagnosis and treatment of this condition. However, in spite of the potential benefits of prenatal ultrasound, the most difficult clinical question regarding hydronephrosis is determining when the abnormality is serious enough to require operative intervention. The primary role of neonatal evaluation is to determine the etiology and natural history of the hydronephrosis, and to make appropriate recommendations for treatment or nontreatment. It is important to realize that not all patients require treatment.

The number of patients diagnosed with hydronephrosis has increased markedly in recent years. This is not so much due to a change in disease frequency but in its diagnosis. Whereas in the past, children with hydronephrosis would come to a physician's attention only when symptomatic, the overwhelming majority are now diagnosed by prenatal sonography and are asymptomatic. In Europe, where virtually all pregnant women undergo prenatal sonography, the incidence of neonatal GU abnormalities is 0.2 to 1.0 per thousand, and most of these are cases of hydronephrosis.

Definitions

Hydronephrosis refers to a dilated renal collecting system. *Hydroureteronephrosis* refers to a dilated renal collecting system and ureter. *Ureteronephrosis* refers to a dilated ureter.

Not all cases of hydronephrosis have a dilated ureter. Similarly, not all cases of hydroureter have a dilated renal collecting system. Dilation of the kidney or ureter may be partial and not involve all segments.

Differential Diagnosis

The differential diagnosis of a dilated collecting system in a neonate is extensive (Table 1–1), and the treatments vary widely by category. The general categories include obstructive uropathy (generally at the ureteropelvic junction, ureterovesical junction, or posterior urethra); vesicoureteral reflux (primary or secondary); or nonobstructive lesions caused by developmental abnormalities (megacalycosis, ureteroceles, or polycystic kidney disease). Because the majority of cases of hydronephrosis are related to a partial obstruction of the UPJ, most of the discussion in this chapter will focus on that problem.

Anatomy

Unilateral hydronephrosis is caused most commonly by ureteropelvic junction (UPJ) obstruction. The postulated etiologies of UPJ obstruction

Table 1–1

Differential Diagnosis of a Dilated Collecting System in a Neonate

- Obstructive uropathy (UPJ, UVJ, or posterior urethra)
- Vesicoureteral reflux (primary or secondary)
- Megacalycosis
- Ureteroceles
- Polycystic kidney disease
- Normal variant (based on maternal progesterones causing reduced peristalsis and increased neonatal urine flow due to limited tubular reabsorption)
- *Note:* Resolving obstruction may also give this appearance.

in infants include intrinsic abnormalities such as fetal folds or an adynamic (aperistaltic) ureteral segment, or extrinsic abnormalities such as fibrosis or anomalous crossing of a lower-pole blood vessel that either intermittently or continuously blocks the free flow of urine. Independent of the primary cause, there is invariably a secondary kink of the UPJ, and often a secondary high insertion of the ureter into the pelvis.

Pathophysiology

Congenital hydronephrosis due to a UPJ obstruction is a manifestation of an abnormality that hinders urine from adequately clearing the renal pelvis. This defect in urine flow is nearly always partial and compensated. In essence, the renal pelvis dilates in response to an increase in pressure that results from the lack of urine flow. Once dilated, an equilibrium is reached; renal pelvic pressure returns to normal and renal injury is limited. However, a new fluid challenge or a change in conformation of the renal pelvis can result in another pressure increase, renewed dilation of the renal pelvis, and potential renal injury, until an equilibrium is reached again. In this way, progressive renal injury may occur. Furthermore, even in the absence of direct renal injury, the stasis that results both from the hindered drainage and the large pelvis and calyces makes infection more likely. Infection will result in much more rapid renal injury. The stasis may also result in renal calculi, hematuria, and pain.

Diagnosis

Prenatal Evaluation

Each year there are over 3 million prenatal ultrasounds performed throughout the United States. The advent and widespread use of ultrasound dur-

ing pregnancy has changed both the clinical course and outcome of hydronephrosis and UPJ obstruction in children. Most cases are now diagnosed prenatally and in neonates who are totally asymptomatic. There are specific indications for genitourinary evaluation in utero (Table 1–2). These indications include (1) a history or physical exam (e.g., decreased fundal height) suggesting a small uterus or oligohydramnios; (2) a significant family history of renal disease (e.g., polycystic kidney disease, medullary cystic kidney disease, prune belly syndrome, or vesicoureteral reflux); or (3) elevated alpha-fetoprotein (a marker for renal agenesis, congenital nephrotic syndrome, or neural tube defect). However, in practice, most prenatal ultrasound studies are performed for relatively minimal or nonspecific indications, such as to confirm pregnancy or determine the date of pregnancy. The incidence of congenital anomalies detected by ultrasound is almost 2%. Of these, as many as 50% are associated with malformations of the genitourinary system, hydronephrosis being the most common.

The ultrasonographic finding of hydronephrosis is made easily in the fetus because of the contrast between the fluid-filled renal pelvis and the surrounding tissues, particularly as there is no fetal bowel gas to obscure the echoes. Hydronephrosis has been reported as early as the 12th week of gestation, but it is generally not until the 15th week of gestation that the kidney is visualized clearly. In community practice, the hydronephrotic kidney is seen most often at 16 to 18 weeks. Amniotic fluid also should be visible at 18 weeks. Because amniotic fluid production is determined largely by fetal urine production, oligohydramnios after week 16 is indicative of disorders of urine production or amniotic fluid leak.

Table 1–2

Indications for GU Evaluation in Utero

- History/family history (vesicoureteral reflux or polycystic kidney disease)
- Physical exam (abnormal fundal height, due to oligohydramnios or polyhydramnios)
- Elevated alpha-fetoprotein

When hydronephrosis is discovered, it is important to determine the grade of the hydronephrosis, as well the exact size of the renal pelvis and the amount and type of renal parenchyma. The most commonly used grading system is that of the Society for Fetal Urology, which grades the hydronephrosis on a scale of 1 to 4 (Fig. 1–1). The AP diameter of the renal pelvis should also be measured, taking the gestational age into consideration (Table 1–3). When evaluating the parenchyma, severe thinning, loss of corticomedullary differentiation, increased cortical echogenicity, and/or cysts

Table 1–3

Assessment of Prenatal Hydronephrosis

OBJECTIVE CRITERIA (SOCIETY FOR FETAL UROLOGY)	
GRADE	DESCRIPTION
0	Normal echogenic renal complex
1	Dilated renal pelvis splitting central renal complex
2	Dilated renal pelvis confined to the sinus and no dilated calyces
3	Renal pelvis dilated beyond the sinus and dilated calyces with no parenchymal thinning
4	Dilated renal pelvis and calyces as well as parenchymal thinning ($\frac{1}{2}$ of normal side)

SUBJECTIVE CRITERIA (BASED ON GESTATIONAL AGE)		
DATE OF DETECTION	SEVERITY	RENAL PELVIS AP DIAMETER
2nd Trimester	Mild	5–8 mm
	Moderate	8–10 mm
	Severe	>10 mm
3rd Trimester	Mild	10 mm
	Moderate	10–15 mm
	Severe	>15 mm

Figure 1–1

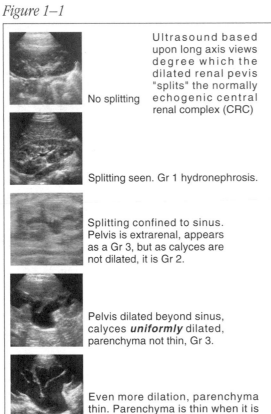

No splitting — Ultrasound based upon long axis views degree which the dilated renal pevis "splits" the normally echogenic central renal complex (CRC)

Splitting seen. Gr 1 hydronephrosis.

Splitting confined to sinus. Pelvis is extrarenal, appears as a Gr 3, but as calyces are not dilated, it is Gr 2.

Pelvis dilated beyond sinus, calyces *uniformly* dilated, parenchyma not thin, Gr 3.

Even more dilation, parenchyma thin. Parenchyma is thin when it is <1/2 opposite normal side, Gr 4.

Grading of hydronephrosis. Grading system based on Society for Fetal Urology recommendations. (Palmer LS, Maizels M, Cartwright PC, et al. Surgery versus observation for managing obstructive grade 3 to 4 unilateral hydronephrosis: A report from the Society for Fetal Urology. *J Urol* 159: 228, 1998).

are all prognostic signs of poor renal function. The clinician also should be concerned with the presence or absence of ureteral dilation or bladder distension, both of which would suggest a diagnosis other than UPJ obstruction. Obviously the state of the contralateral kidney should be evaluated as well as the volume of amniotic fluid, because oligohydramnios is a very poor prognostic sign. When hydronephrosis is unilateral and there is no oligohydramnios, no further prenatal evaluation is needed.

Postnatal Evaluation

Infants in whom hydronephrosis is detected prenatally should be evaluated postnatally to confirm the diagnosis, even if asymptomatic. A postnatal ultrasound should be done, but not until at least the third day of life, as the limited neonatal urine output in the first several days of life may lead to an underestimation of the degree of hydronephrosis. Because vesicoureteral reflux is found in one third of these neonates, most centers recommend that a voiding cystourethrogram also be performed in the neonatal period (Fig. 1–2).

Although previously the "gold standard," intravenous urography is difficult to perform in infants, adds radiation exposure, and generally does not provide additional information. Therefore, it is needed only rarely, such as when imaging studies suggest an upper tract obstruction and intravenous urography would assist in localizing the anatomic site of obstruction.

Ancillary Tests

Voiding Cystourethrogram

The voiding cystourethrogram (VCUG) is an important study to obtain after the postnatal ultrasound confirms hydronephrosis. The VCUG is done with a small-caliber catheter placed into the bladder. Contrast is instilled by gravity into the bladder while fluoroscopic and radiographic images are taken. Because the test is designed to identify vesicoureteral reflux, the VCUG should not be performed in children who have infected urine until urine studies normalize. Thus a urinalysis and/or urine culture should be done prior to the VCUG to verify that the risk of iatrogenic introduction of bacteria into the upper tract is minimized.

Diuretic Renal Scan

A diuretic renal scan is indicated in cases of upper tract obstruction, such as when ultrasound shows hydronephrosis and the voiding cystourethrogram is normal. In such cases, the most likely diagnosis would be ureteropelvic junction obstruction but may also include ureterovesical junction obstruction or ureterocele (Table 1–1). The amount of any

functional impairment and the degree of restriction to flow are assessed primarily by diuretic renography. This involves intravenous injection of Tc99m-DTPA or -MAG-3 (radionuclides that are excreted rapidly by the kidney), followed by a diuretic. Using this technique, the relative renal function of the two kidneys and the rapidity of "washout" of radioisotope can be quantitatively assessed. In particular, the use of the diuretic allows for differentiation of the dilated obstructed from the nonobstructed kidney (Fig. 1–3). Calculation of the time until half the radioisotope has left the kidney is thought to correlate with the degree of obstruction. This noninvasive test is valuable, but has many pitfalls and should performed in a standardized manner by experts in the technique. Even then, the actual rapidity of washout depends not only on the degree of obstruction but on the size of the renal pelvis and the volume of urine output from the hydronephrotic kidney. In many cases it is not possible to distinguish obstruction with certainty.

Whitaker Test

An alternative study to the diuretic renal scan is the antegrade pressure–flow perfusion (Whitaker) test. This test is performed by antegrade perfusion of the urinary collecting system using a percutaneous nephrostomy tube. Although popular in the past, it is invasive and seldom helpful, and so should not be considered a part of the standard evaluation. Indications for performing a Whitaker test are cases of hydronephrosis and normal voiding cystourethrogram where a prior diuretic renal scan was nondiagnostic or (false) negative; or in cases where a percutaneous nephrostomy tube has already been placed.

Algorithm

An algorithm is shown in Fig. 1–4. The key points are that a voiding cystourethrogram is done to identify vesicoureteral reflux, and that hydronephrosis

Figure 1–2

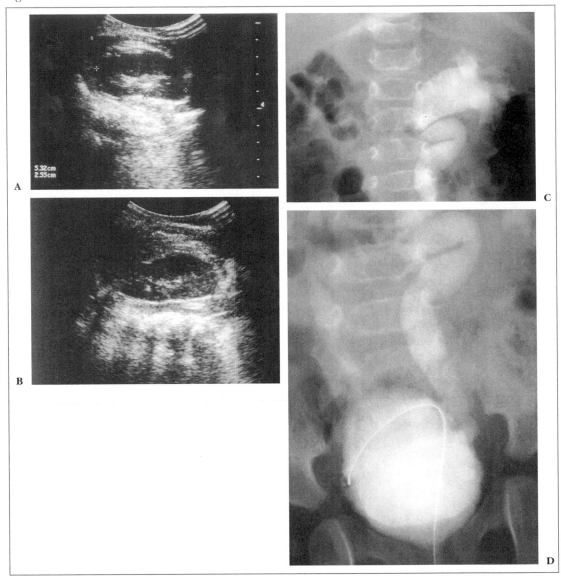

Significant postnatal reflux despite resolution of prenatal hydronephrosis. **A, B.** Normal postnatal renal ultrasound.
C, D. Significant reflux on VCUG.

without vesicoureteral reflux does not necessarily imply obstruction. Further, when obstruction is identified, only certain children are candidates for surgical intervention. Also, long-term observation and repeat imaging are often required.

It is important to remember that hydronephrosis (even in the absence of reflux) is not diagnostic of obstruction, even in severe cases. The best definition of obstruction is "a restriction of urinary flow that results in renal injury." Unfortunately,

Figure 1–3

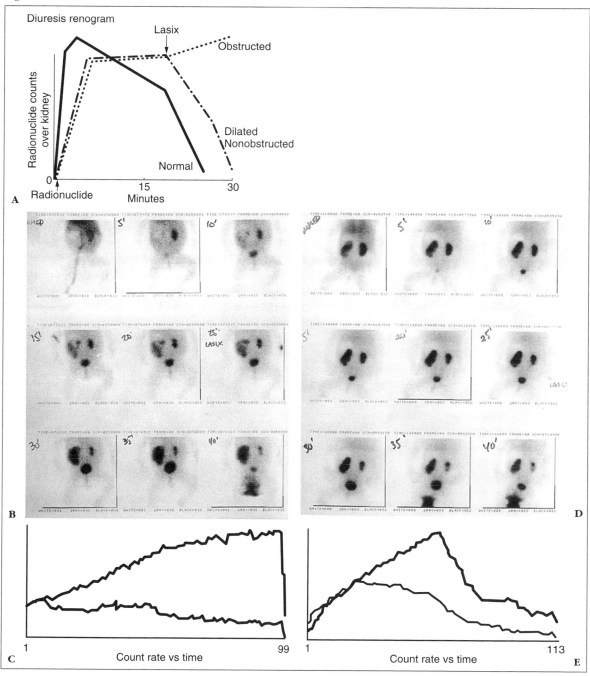

Diuretic renography. **A.** Hand-drawn example of the time–activity curve from a diuretic renogram. **B, C.** Images and time–activity curve from a diuretic renogram in an infant with a left UPJ obstruction. Note that the amount of radioisotopic activity increases with time. **D, E.** Same studies in the same patient after surgical repair. Note that after administration of the diuretic, the amount of radioisotopic activity decreases. (Reprinted with permission from Aslan A, Kogan B, Mandell J: Neonatal hydronephrosis. *Curr Opin Urol* 8:495–500, 1998.)

Figure 1–4

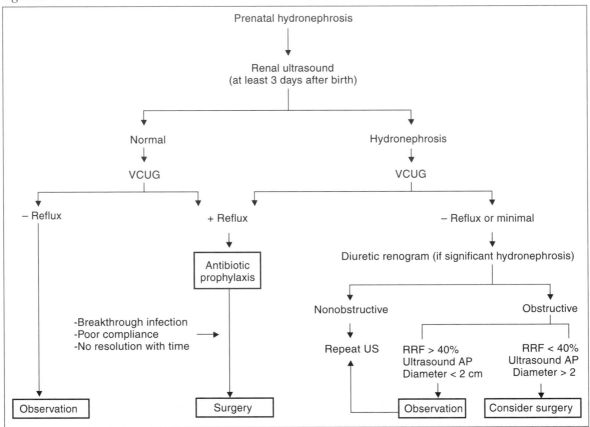

Algorithm for evaluation of neonatal hydronephrosis.

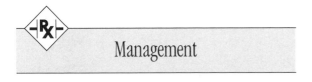

Management

The real dilemma is to predict the natural history of each individual case. The scenario of renal infection, stones, pain, and hematuria occurs in some uncorrected cases of UPJ obstruction and can be prevented by early surgical repair of neonatal hydronephrosis. However, it is a well-accepted observation that the hydronephrosis in many children will either resolve spontaneously or stabilize, and therefore surgical intervention may be unnecessary. Hence the real issue lies in distinguishing those patients with hydronephrosis in which the condition is likely to progress, from those whose hydronephrosis will stabilize and not trouble them. As in many areas of medicine, there are two schools of thought, those in favor of early surgical intervention and those in favor of observation with selective surgery as needed. In general, there is only a limited consensus on this subject.

this definition is suboptimal from a patient care standpoint in that it necessitates renal damage prior to diagnosis.

Ureteropelvic Junction Obstruction

INDICATIONS FOR SURGICAL INTERVENTION

After a number of years of retrospective review, several points are now clear. Fetuses with hydronephrosis and a renal pelvic diameter greater than 2 cm are much more likely to ultimately need surgical correction than those with a renal pelvic diameter that is smaller. Conversely, those less than 1 cm rarely have clinically significant hydronephrosis. In addition, even among patients with large renal pelves (grade 3 to 4 hydronephrosis) followed nonoperatively, only about 25% will eventually require surgical correction for reduced renal function, urinary infection, renal calculi, or similar abnormalities. Because it is not yet possible to predict these patients with certainty, they should be followed closely.

When the relative renal function is reduced on a diuretic renogram performed shortly after birth, there is less margin for error and hence earlier surgical intervention is appropriate. Conversely, when the relative renal function of a hydronephrotic kidney is normal, it is reasonable to give an asymptomatic patient an opportunity for observation. In those instances when it is unclear whether an operation is needed, generally it is best to observe the child with serial sonography.

A significant increase in renal pelvic size or thinning of renal parenchyma should trigger a repeat diuretic renogram and often surgical intervention.

SURGERY

Surgical correction of UPJ obstruction in the neonate is highly successful (>95%). In most centers this can be achieved with a minimum of morbidity and only a 1- to 2-day hospital stay.

The procedure involves resecting the area of obstruction and designing a flap of healthy renal pelvis that can be sewn that funnels in a dependent manner down into the healthy ureter below the area of the obstruction (Fig. 1–5). In some cases a nephrostomy and stenting catheter are used, but this is no longer considered mandatory. New techniques of endoscopic incision of the ureteropelvic junction offer reduced morbidity (although somewhat lower success rates) to older children and adults, but are not practical in young children.

Postoperative radiographic follow-up, with ultrasonography and sometimes diuretic renography, is essential, but most patients do extremely well. Although older children with a UPJ obstruction may be cared for by general urologists, young children, and especially neonates, are best managed by pediatric urologic specialists.

Figure 1–5

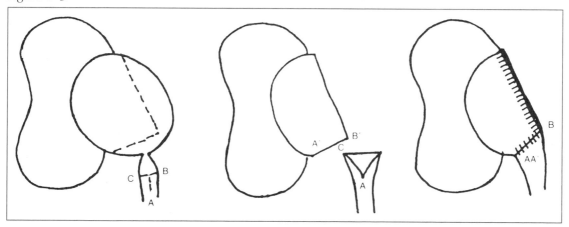

Pyeloplasty. Schematic illustration of surgical repair of a UPJ obstruction. (Reprinted with permission from Borhan A, Kogan B, Mandell J: Upper ureteral reconstructive surgery. In: Atal A (ed): Reconstructive urology. *Urol Clin North Am* 26:175–181, 1999.)

Other Diagnoses

URETEROVESICAL JUNCTION OBSTRUCTION

Although UPJ obstruction is by far the most common cause of hydronephrosis in infants, other causes are occasionally seen (Table 1–1). When ultrasound reveals a dilated ureter, in addition to hydronephrosis, the diagnosis is most likely vesicoureteral reflux or a ureterovesical obstruction. Reflux is covered in Chapter 2.

Prenatal ultrasound has dramatically changed the approach to ureterovesical obstruction. The condition is fascinating as in most cases no narrowing or stenosis can be found. Generally, there is an aperistaltic segment in the distal ureter, and fluoroscopic imaging with contrast demonstrates good ureteral peristalsis down to the aperistaltic segment, followed by retrograde peristalsis back-up, with the resultant classic picture of a very dilated distal ureter, less dilated proximal ureter and pelvis, and blunted calyces (Fig. 1–6).

The radiographic findings can be impressive and initially, surgery was recommended in nearly all cases. However, it has become apparent that as many as 50% of cases showed substantial improvement over time. Hence, observation has become the treatment of choice in asymptomatic neonates. There is a high rate of urinary infection in these patients, so it is best to keep them on prophylactic antibiotics until the natural history is clear (often about 2 years). Follow-up is recommended with ultrasound every 6 months or so. Infection or progression of hydronephrosis are the principal indications for surgical intervention.

DUPLICATIONS, URETEROCELES, AND ECTOPIC URETERS

Because hydronephrosis is easily diagnosed in utero, most cases of duplication anomalies resulting in ureteroceles or ectopic ureters will be discovered by prenatal sonography (Fig. 1–7). After birth, confirmatory ultrasound should be performed, as well as a VCUG and a diuretic nuclear renal scan to determine the relative renal function

Figure 1–6

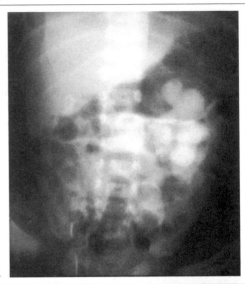

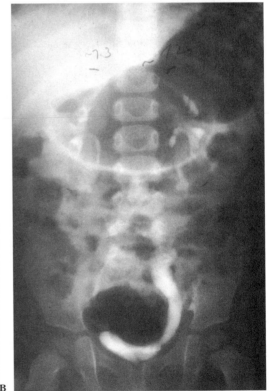

Megaureter. **A.** IVP from an infant with a functionally obstructed megaureter on the left. Note the massively dilated calyces and ureter. **B.** IVP on the same infant at 1 year of age. There has been dramatic spontaneous resolution.

Figure 1–7

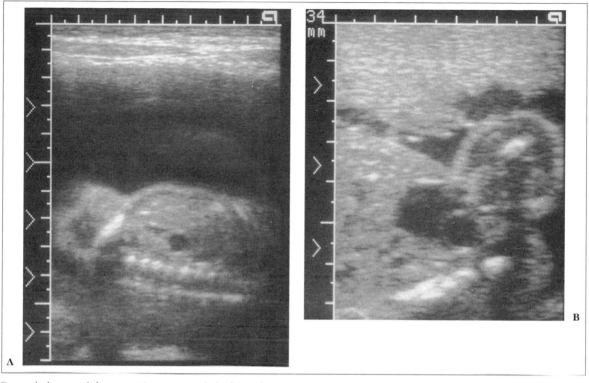

Prenatal ultrasound demonstrating upper pole hydronephrosis **A.** and a ureterocele in the bladder **B.**

and degree of obstruction where present. Surgical intervention is nearly always needed, but not immediately. Recently it has been shown that many of the ureteroceles can be punctured endoscopically, but all should be treated with prophylactic antimicrobials prior to definitive therapy. It should also be noted that generally, duplication anomalies are not identified prenatally unless associated with hydronephrosis, usually from a ureterocele, ectopic ureter, or reflux.

Urethral Valves

Although rare, bladder outlet obstruction, most often from posterior urethral valves, has received tremendous attention in both the scientific literature and the lay press. As in other cases of hydronephrosis, the diagnosis is easily made based on antenatal sonography.

An assessment of renal parenchyma (as described earlier) is mandatory. The fetal renal function can be crudely estimated by the amount of amniotic fluid, but in severe cases, percutaneous aspiration of fetal urinary electrolytes can provide additional prognostic information.

Once bladder outlet obstruction is detected, the mother and fetus are best followed in a high-risk obstetrical facility, not so much because prenatal intervention will be needed, but because early neonatal evaluation and treatment are important. Furthermore, the potential for pulmonary hypoplasia related to oligohydramnios and likelihood of neonatal surgery make delivery in a specialized center beneficial.

After birth, urethral catheter drainage is advisable in most cases, but the type of catheter is critical. Foley catheters are to be avoided in these cases, because of their relatively small internal lumen as well as the fact that these patients tend to have very spastic bladders and a tight contraction around the balloon may result in ureteral obstruction. A 5 or 8 FR feeding tube is best.

Serum creatinine should be monitored regularly, although it will be normal immediately after birth (a reflection of the mother's renal function, due to the placenta). Electrolytes should also be followed closely, as many of these infants will have significant salt wasting. A VCUG is important for diagnostic purposes.

When the infant is stable, primary endoscopic valve ablation is the next step. If the infant is too small or the correct equipment is not available, a vesicostomy is an acceptable alternative. Upper urinary tract drainage (either ureterostomies or pyelostomies) is indicated only rarely. The prognosis varies widely from neonatal demise due to pulmonary hypoplasia in severe cases, to chronic renal failure in as many as a quarter, to virtually normal renal function. Early diagnosis and treatment are important, especially in preventing urinary infection.

Patient Education

The advent of prenatal ultrasound has allowed for the early diagnosis of hydronephrosis. On the other hand, it has resulted in considerably increased anxiety on the part of parents. Few if any patients benefit from prenatal treatment, and most can be observed postnatally. Even those who require surgical intervention rarely need it immediately after birth. Although the conditions should not be ignored and postnatal evaluation is important, it is important to reassure a family that is anxious about the prenatal diagnosis. In many cases, there is no need subsequently for postnatal intervention. In most cases where postnatal intervention is required a successful outcome can be achieved.

Future Directions

The morbidity of surgery for UPJ obstruction has been markedly reduced in recent years, with the majority of children discharged within 2 days of the operation. Although open surgical correction of UPJ obstruction is standard treatment, endopyelotomy, a minimally invasive option, is an alternative treatment. Endopyelotomy involves an endoscopic incision of the stenotic UPJ segment, and the incised stricture heals with less obstruction. Endopyelotomy is a well-accepted treatment in adults but is not feasible in infants. Moreover, the success rate in adults drops from 98% for open surgical correction to approximately 82% for endopyelotomy.

Several groups are now studying the benefits of laparoscopic pyeloplasty and have shown good results. However, the technology for laparoscopic suturing continues to make this cumbersome and the procedure is long and tedious. In the future, as technology improves, this may be an excellent option.

Perhaps the most promising and, at the same time, disappointing work in the last decade has been on the prenatal treatment of posterior urethral valves. It is clear that the technology to allow this to happen is available currently. The diagnosis of bladder outlet obstruction can be made by 20 weeks gestation in most centers. An assessment of fetal renal function can be made (described earlier), and percutaneous drainage of the bladder can be performed. Moreover, a catheter can be placed between the bladder and the amniotic cavity and left in place. Unfortunately, there are very limited data demonstrating that this helps in limiting renal injury in the long term. Mostly this is because the attempts to drain the urinary tract have been done in patients whose kidneys are so severely damaged that they are unsalvageable. The technique is more likely to be effective in less severe cases. On the other hand there is the ethical issue of whether to treat less severe cases prenatally, as they tend to do reasonably well with postnatal treatment. Hopefully further data will be forthcoming.

Bibliography

Baskin LS, Zderic SA, Snyder HM, Duckett JW: Primary dilated megaureter: Long-term follow-up. *J Urol* 152: 618–621, 1994.

Bogart GA, Kogan BA, Mevorach RA, et al: Efficacy of retrograde endopyelotomy in children. *J Urol* 156: 734, 1996.

Davey MS, Zerin JM, Reilly C, Ambrosius WT: Mild renal pelvic dilatation is not predictive of vesicoureteral reflux in children. *Pediatr Radiol* 27:908–911, 1997.

Dhillon HK: Prenatally diagnosed hydronephronsis: The Great Ormond Street experience. *Br J Urol* 81:39–44, 1998.

Dremsek PA, Gindl K, Voitl P, et al: Renal pyelectasis in fetuses and neonates: Diagnostic value of renal pelvis diameter in pre- and postnatal sonographic screening. *AJR* 168:1017–1019, 1997.

Helin I, Persson PH: Prenatal diagnosis of urinary tract abnormalities by ultrasound. *Pediatrics* 78:879–883, 1986.

Mikkelson SS, Rasmussen BS, Jensen TM, et al: Long-term follow-up of patients with hydronephrosis treated by Anderson–Hynes pyeloplasty. *Br J Urol* 79:121, 1992.

Palmer LS, Maizels M, Cartwright PC, et al: Surgery versus observation for managing obstructive grade 3 to 4 unilateral hydronephrosis: A report from the Society for Fetal Urology. *J Urol* 159:222–228, 1998.

Woo HH, Farnsworth RH: Dismembered pyeloplasty in infants under the age of 12 months. *Br J Urol* 77: 449, 1996.

M. David Bomalaski

Urinary Tract Infections in Children

Introduction

Initial Evaluation

The UTI Dilemma

Urinary tract infection (UTI) in children is common, but the ideal method for radiologically evaluating UTIs remains controversial. Children, parents, and physicians can be distressed by the need for urethral catheterization involved in some clinical tests. Fear of the transitory discomfort of urethral catheterization causes many children to be underevaluated. Nonetheless, the cornerstones of management are prompt diagnosis, effective treatment, and prevention of future morbidity. Although patient discomfort needs to be minimized, the concept of watchful waiting should not be used to disguise neglect. Over 40 years ago, the urologist Hugh Cabot proposed the Doctrine of the Prepared Soil:

> *It is not rare to find in the active, devoted young hospital surgeon a state of mind in which he almost believes that bacteria are the cause of infection. He appears to forget that infection is a result, and that bacteria in and of themselves can do nothing except in contact with living tissue and then, often, only under highly specialized conditions.*[1]

This doctrine is as true today as it was 40 years ago. Successful management includes a search for why a patient has become infected.

Adding to the controversy of evaluation is an uncertainty about what to do about abnormalities that are detected. Aggressive surgical treatment of radiographic abnormalities, such as vesicoureteral reflux (VUR) or hydronephrosis, has always been thought to have a beneficial effect on patients. However, the interaction of patient anatomy and physiology as well as host factors is only beginning to be understood, and the significance and ideal management of VUR continues to be debated.

UTIs Present Cryptically

The symptoms of urinary tract infection in children may be nonspecific and incorrectly attributed to other entities (Table 2–1). In infants and small children the leading symptoms are fever, irritability, poor feeding, or vomiting. Frequently, the physician may assume that acute gastroenteritis, "early" otitis media, viral syndromes, or teething may be the explanation for these symptoms. Increased awareness and adequate urine collection is critical to establishing the diagnosis of UTI.

Adequate Urine Analysis

Properly collected urine for analysis and culture should be obtained in all children with the aforementioned symptoms. In the very young child, the urine is often collected by a bag placed over the perineum. A bagged urine collection is useful only if it is negative. If positive, it should be confirmed by a properly collected catheterized specimen to exclude the possibility that genitourinary skin flora have contaminated the specimen. Without proper urine analysis and culture, logical treatment of the patient cannot begin.

Table 2–1

Initial Symptoms of UTI in Children

Fever
Irritability
Poor feeding
Vomiting
Pain
Dysuria
Change in urine color and/or odor

Delay in Diagnosis

Smellie and associates published a review of children with renal scarring.[2] There was a delay in diagnosis or effective treatment of infection in 50 of 52 children with a history of symptomatic UTI and renal scarring. The severity of scarring was directly and significantly related to the delay in diagnosis. Renal scarring has been found in 12% of all children who have had a UTI.[3] This number jumps to 25% in children with a history of recurrent UTI. Delay in therapy is a common but preventable factor in the development of renal scarring, and the rapid introduction of antibacterial treatment can arrest or prevent the development of scars.[4,5] Greater than 24-hour delay in treatment results in localized inflammation, cellular derangement, and cell death with subsequent fibrosis and scar formation. Extrapolation of these findings into clinical situations suggests prompt treatment may diminish later renal scarring, hypertension, and chronic renal insufficiency.

Initial Treatment

UTI treatment should begin before culture results are available, and culture-specific antimicrobial therapy should be confirmed as soon as possible. Some studies have suggested that management of febrile children with UTI as outpatients receiving oral antibiotics can be as efficacious as inpatient intravenous therapy.[6] However, good family compliance and follow-up is mandatory. The recommended practice in toxic children with febrile UTI or with associated symptoms of costovertebral angle tenderness or vomiting is treatment with parenteral antibiotics and intravenous hydration until the patient is afebrile for at least 24 hours. Oral antibiotics can then be prescribed based on bacterial sensitivity profiles to complete a 10-day course of therapy (Table 2–2).

Johnson and colleagues evaluated the efficacy of a 3-day versus 10-day treatment with a combination of oral amoxicillin and clavulanate potassium for children with uncomplicated UTI.[7] The

Table 2–2

Initial Treatment of Febrile UTIs

1. Urine culture and sensitivity
2. Parenteral broad-spectrum antibiotics (ampicillin and aminoglycoside) and IV hydration until afebrile for ≥ 24 hours
3. When afebrile for ≥ 24 hours, and culture and sensitivities are known, oral antibiotics may be given (instead of parenteral) based on sensitivities, for 10 days
4. Imaging

success rate for the 10-day course was 82% compared to only 55% for the 3-day treatment. They concluded that 3-day treatment with oral antibiotics was insufficient for afebrile childhood UTI, and bacterial adhesion positive isolates and host VUR adversely affected treatment. This study points out the need for appropriate diagnosis, treatment, and radiologic evaluation of any child with signs of UTI.

Why Image the Patient?

Altered Host Anatomy

VESICOURETERAL REFLUX AND RENAL SCARRING

Urinary tract infection has a prevalence of 3% to 5% in girls and 1% in boys. Vesicoureteral reflux has been found in 35% to 50% of children with UTI and in 25% of those with asymptomatic bacteriuria.[8,9] Renal scarring is present in 12% of those with a history of UTI. If one includes reflux and a history of UTI, the incidence of renal scarring jumps to 33%. Clinical and experimental evidence has shown that renal scarring is directly related to the combination of UTI and VUR, and that the damage may be most severe early in life with the initial infection.[10]

HYDRONEPHROSIS

UTI may also be the first signal of anomalous pathology. UTI may be the first indication of upper tract obstruction such as UPJ obstruction, uretero-cele, primary obstructed megaureter, or nephro-lithiasis. It may also be a sign of lower urinary obstruction such as posterior urethral valves. All of these entities can be diagnosed with proper radio-graphic imaging. Furthermore, each of these dis-eases can cause progressive renal damage if left untreated.

Hydronephrosis on renal sonography man-dates further imaging. Although hydronephrosis does not equate with obstruction, it must be ruled out in each case.[11] Most clinicians depend upon the Lasix Tc 99m-diethylenetriamine pentaacetic acid (DTPA) or Lasix Tc 99m-mercaptoacetyl-triglycine (MAG3) renal scan to determine ob-struction. If the radiographic evaluation shows obstruction, renal damage can be progressive regardless of infection. These children should be referred to a pediatric urologist for further man-agement and possible surgery.

Standard Radiographic Evaluation

Methods of Cystography

FLUOROSCOPIC VOIDING CYSTOURETHROGRAM AND NUCLEAR VOIDING CYSTOURETHROGRAM

Two types of cystograms are available, a stan-dard fluoroscopic voiding cystourethrogram (VCUG) and a nuclear medicine voiding cys-tourethrogram (nVCUG). Both methods require catheterization of the child with instillation of either radiographic contrast or radionuclide.

The fluoroscopic VCUG allows anatomic eval-uation of the bladder, ureters, and urethra. This provides precise grading of the severity of the re-flux (important for prognosis) as well as detection of other pathology such as ureterocele or poste-rior urethral valves. Because fluoroscopic imaging is periodic, not continuous, low grade, intermittent reflux can be missed.

Alternatively, the nVCUG allows continuous imaging with a gamma camera (which may be more sensitive than a fluoroscopic VCUG) and ex-poses the child to approximately 1/50th of the ra-diation dose as a fluoroscopic exam.[12] However, the nVCUG is not anatomically precise in grading reflux and is limited in its ability to diagnose other genitourinary conditions associated with UTI (e.g., posterior urethral valves, bladder diverticula). Pediatric urologists often favor the fluoroscopic VCUG as the initial study of choice in the workup of UTI. Subsequently, follow-up exams in the known reflux patient may then be done with an nVCUG. When screening asymptomatic siblings it is reasonable to get an nVCUG as the initial study.

Renal Sonography and DMSA Scintigraphy

A renal ultrasound (including sonography of the bladder) should be done to exclude obstructive disease in any child presenting with a UTI. It can also detect **gross** renal scarring and allows evalu-ation of renal size.[13] Tasker and associates evalu-ated the ability of renal sonography to detect renal scarring by prospectively evaluating 100 children with proven UTI with both renal sonography and Tc 99m-dimercaptosuccinic acid (DMSA) scintig-raphy.[14] DMSA detected 19 scarred kidneys in 17 patients, but sonography was only able to detect the 7 most severely scarred kidneys. Sonographic evaluation missed 8 out of 19 scarred kidneys. A similar study by MacKenzie and co-workers in 112 children with UTI showed ultrasound to be par-ticularly effective in detecting the presence of di-lation, renal swelling, and parenchymal changes consistent with pyelonephritis.[15] However, ultra-sound failed to pick up half of those kidneys with scarring on DMSA scan. If accurate detection of renal scarring is important, DMSA renal scan is the most accurate study, with 90% sensitivity and 100% specificity.[16]

DMSA scan may also be useful to differenti-ate acute pyelonephritis from lower urinary tract infection.[17] DMSA can localize pyelonephritic changes in children with clinical symptoms of UTI but a nondiagnostic urine analysis. DMSA scintigraphy may show acute changes superimposed upon chronic scarring. It can be used to follow these patients to show either resolution or worsening of these changes.[18] However, the additional expense, radiation exposure (cortical imaging agent), and limited availability in all locations may make DMSA scintigraphy impractical to use in all patients.

Controversies

Screening Asymptomatic Siblings

Many children presenting with UTI will prove to have vesicoureteral reflux (VUR) and because VUR is often familial, it might make sense that siblings of children with VUR may have VUR, too. However, the screening of asymptomatic siblings of children with VUR is controversial. A sibling of a reflux patient has a one in three chance of VUR, and a child of a reflux patient has a two in three chance of having VUR.[19,20] Up to 75% of siblings with reflux will be asymptomatic, and in a series screening 354 siblings and 275 index cases, the early discovery of sibling reflux significantly lowered the rate of renal damage compared to index patients.[21] Based on this information, it is recommended that the siblings and children of known reflux patients be screened for reflux.

A cystogram is the only reliable method of detecting VUR. Because a cystogram requires the discomfort of urethral catheterization, some physicians limit their evaluation to a renal ultrasound. However, Blane and associates found that up to 75% of children with VUR will have a normal ultrasound, including up to half of patients with moderate to severe grades of reflux.[22] If the sibling being screened is a boy under the age of 5, a boy over the age of 5 but with a history of UTI, or a girl of any age, a cystogram as well as a renal ultrasound should be performed. Because development of new renal scars is uncommon in children over the age of 5, it can be argued that *clinically significant* reflux is unlikely to be missed in a *boy* older than 5 who has never had a UTI and has a normal renal sonogram or DMSA scan.

Do All Children Need Imaging?

AGE-RELATED SCARRING

The most significant concern in children with UTI is that they will develop renal scarring and the potential sequel of hypertension and renal insufficiency. It has been proposed that most renal scarring occurs with the initial infection and that the kidneys become more resistant to scarring with maturation (the "Big Bang" theory). Veron and associates studied 429 children aged 3 and 4 years with DMSA scan at the time of initial infection and 2 to 11 years later after further infections.[23] They found that children after the third birthday have only a 1 in 40 risk of developing new scars, and that after the fourth birthday, the rate of new scar development drops to nearly zero. In contrast, Greenfield and Wan evaluated over 1000 patients with reflux and showed that scarring with infection can occur at any age throughout adolescence.[24] These papers point out that although scarring may occur at any age, the infant kidney is most susceptible.

HYPERTENSIVE RISK

To evaluate the significance of renal scarring and hypertension, Wolfish and co-workers studied 146 children with VUR.[25] Renal scarring was seen in 34% of patients on renal sonography or intravenous pyelography. At a mean follow-up of 10 years, mean systolic and diastolic blood pressures were at the 42nd percentile and 19th percentile, respectively. They concluded that primary, uncomplicated VUR was not associated with hypertension, regardless of the number of documented UTIs, modality of treatment, presence of renal scarring, or duration of follow-up.

FUTURE PREGNANCY CONCERNS

Vesicoureteral reflux may lead to pyelonephritis. Pyelonephritis during pregnancy can contribute to fetal complications such as premature delivery and spontaneous abortion. Ramero and associates published a meta-analysis of pregnant women with asymptomatic bacteriuria and found that when untreated, there was a greater risk for preterm delivery.[26]

Williams and colleagues found a 21% incidence of VUR in women with bacteriuria during pregnancy. They found that the association of bacteriuria and VUR was more likely to result in acute pyelonephritis during the pregnancy and that the UTI was more difficult to treat.[27] Because of these studies and others, diagnosis and treatment of VUR has been assumed to be of great importance in females of childbearing years. Routine correction of VUR was recommended if it had not resolved by puberty.

Mansfield and associates evaluated a large group of adult women with an average follow-up of 25 years since their childhood diagnosis of VUR.[28] Sixty-seven women had undergone ureteral reimplantation surgery and 37 were followed without correction. They concluded that women with VUR as children have high rates of UTI with sexual activity and pregnancy whether or not they underwent ureteral reimplantation as a child. Furthermore, although the rate of UTI during pregnancy was high, the women were not at higher risk of miscarriage than the general population. In this study, the tendency towards infections was important, not the finding of VUR. The impact of VUR upon pregnancy continues to be debated.

FREQUENCY OF FOLLOW-UP STUDIES

Many providers obtain follow-up renal sonography and VCUG on an annual basis on reflux patients. The International Reflux Study showed a resolution rate approaching 80% for unilateral low-grade VUR over 5 years.[29] Other studies have shown the resolution rate of low to moderate VUR to be 20% to 30% over a 2-year period.[30] These studies show that VUR can resolve, but often over several years. It is our preference to obtain follow-up studies every 18 months instead of annually unless the child is having further infections, in which case the child should be referred for surgical correction (Table 2–3). This imaging schedule allows for fewer catheterizations, less radiation exposure, and lower overall costs.

What If the Studies Are Normal?

Host–Pathogen Interactions

BACTERIAL ADHESION

Physicians and families can easily grasp the significance of anatomic abnormalities. The child with recurrent UTI and a normal radiographic evaluation is a quandary. In these cases, the clinician may look for other factors that might predispose to infection. These host and bacterial factors include cell-surface antigens, bacterial adhesions, introital colonization, and dysfunctional voiding.

Table 2–3

Indications for Surgical Correction of VUR

INDICATIONS
Breakthrough UTIs despite prophylactic antibiotics
Poor tolerance or compliance with prophylaxis
High-grade VUR (grades IV or V)
Progression of renal scarring
RELATIVE INDICATIONS
Persistent VUR into adolescence
Poor renal growth
Parental preference

Blood group antigens are genetically controlled carbohydrate molecules, many of which are expressed on urothelial cells. These cell-surface antigens may play a role in bacterial adherence and host susceptibility to UTI. Jantausch and colleagues have shown that patients with UTI have a higher than expected frequency of blood group antigen Lewis (Le)(a–b–) and a lower than expected frequency of Le(a+b+).[31] It has also been suggested that enteropathic *Escherichia coli* adhere to epithelial cells via filaments termed bundle-forming pili or adhesins.[32] Adhesin-positive isolates are also more resistant to antibiotic treatment.[33]

Colonization

INTROITAL COLONIZATION

Because the female urethra is very short, it poses only a minimum barrier between the bladder and perineal bacterial flora. This means that introital colonization with enteropathic bacteria may play a role in UTI development in females. The makeup of the introital bacteria may shift with puberty and its associated hormonal changes. This may account for the spontaneous resolution of recurrent infections in some girls at the time of puberty. Alternately, in older females, the act of sexual intercourse may mechanically introduce enteropathic bacteria from the perineum into the bladder and thereby increase the incidence of UTI with the onset of sexual activity.

PREPUTIAL COLONIZATION

In a similar fashion, preputial bacteria may have a role in UTI development in boys. Although the pros and cons of circumcision are beyond the scope of this chapter, circumcision has been shown to decrease the risk of UTI. Meta-analysis of 10 published studies on the relationship of circumcision and UTI shows a 12-fold increase in UTI in uncircumcised infants.[34] This protective effect may decrease the risk of symptomatic UTI in preschool boys.[35] An uncircumcised male infant with UTI should be considered for circumcision if no anatomic abnormalities are discovered on radiographic evaluation.

Dysfunctional Voiding

PATHOPHYSIOLOGY

The bladder is a complex, dynamic organ with distinct anatomic and functional regions. It should store urine at a low pressure, and maintain continence until a socially acceptable time, when it should fully empty. These dynamic phases require the detrusor muscle and bladder neck to work in harmony. During storage, the bladder must stay relaxed, maintaining low detrusor pressures, despite increasing bladder volumes. At the same time, the bladder neck/internal sphincter maintains sufficient tone to preserve continence. The external sphincter is normally passive during storage. It serves to counteract socially inappropriate bladder contractions by temporarily increasing outlet resistance and by reflexively relaxing the detrusor contraction. It is the voluntary "on/off" switch for the bladder. During voiding, the detrusor contracts while the bladder outlet relaxes.

Detrusor sphincter dyssynergia is manifested by disruption of the coordinated, reciprocal action of the detrusor muscle and bladder outlet. The detrusor muscle may contract during attempted storage or the bladder outlet may fail to relax during voiding. This dyssynergy produces elevated storage pressures and incomplete emptying with increased postvoid residuals. Like any muscle that is forced to work against increased resistance, it can hypertrophy, leading to decreased compliance and VUR. This dyssynergy may be neurological in origin but is more commonly a behavioral or functional problem in a neurologically normal child.

EVALUATION

Just as a child must learn the socially important skills of walking and talking, so too the child must learn bladder and bowel control. Children may go through a period of bladder dyssynergy during this learning process. The responsible physician needs to thoroughly examine the voiding habits of any child with a UTI and pay special attention to infrequent voiding. Symptoms of urgency, diurnal enuresis, and constipation are common in these children. Children are busy exploring their world and may attempt to postpone bladder emptying until the last possible moment, at which a crisis is reached.

The history in dysfunctionally voiding children may reveal infrequent voiding. Urgency may be a sign of resultant detrusor instability that occurs at bladder capacity. When this unwanted contraction occurs, the external sphincter is used in an attempt to shut off the detrusor contraction. Vincent's curtsy is considered pathognomonic; the child squats and places the heel of the foot into the perineum to help augment the external sphincter, often in a failed attempt to maintain continence.

TREATMENT

Treatment needs to be directed at improving voiding dynamics. This involves the work and cooperation of both the child and parent. Without the cooperation of both, behavioral treatment is doomed to failure. The child should be instructed to attempt to void every 2 hours during the day. This requires a responsible adult to remind the child. Relaxation of the pelvic muscles should be stressed, and straining to void discouraged. Double voiding is the technique of attempting a second void several seconds after initial bladder emptying. Double voiding decreases postvoid residual and reinforces the concept of complete bladder emptying. Anticholinergic medication may help with detrusor instability. Finally, constipation needs to be addressed. There may be a global dysfunction of both bladder and bowel elimination. Treatment of voiding dysfunction and constipation has been shown to decrease the frequency of UTI.[36]

Asymptomatic Bacteriuria

Treatment of asymptomatic bacteriuria (ABU) remains controversial. The first priority is to establish that it is truly asymptomatic. There may be associated symptoms such as enuresis or infrequent voiding. Studies have shown that antibiotic treatment of ABU often has little impact on the rate of reinfection and that the risk of renal damage is low.[37] Theoretically, antibiotic treatment may alter the bacterial colonization to a more virulent strain of *E. coli*. In such cases, follow-up without antimicrobial treatment may be preferred.[38]

Antibiotic Prophylaxis

The ideal antibiotic for urinary prophylaxis should be safe, effective, inexpensive, and have no side effects. Although no antimicrobial is ideal, some are preferable in children. Prophylactic dosage is usually one quarter of the therapeutic dose given once per day. Too high a dose will increase side effects such as gastrointestinal upset and may alter fecal flora. The quinolones are commonly used for prophylaxis and treatment in adults, but they are inappropriate in children due to potential arthropathic effect upon active growth plates. More appropriate antibiotics in children include trimethoprim, sulfamethoxazole, Macrodantin, and amoxicillin.

Trimethoprim alone or in combination with sulfamethoxazole is the most commonly used antibiotic for both treatment and prophylaxis of UTI. It is inexpensive and has minimal adverse effects on the bowel and vaginal flora because it is excreted and concentrated in the urine. It may cause a hypersensitivity rash and gastrointestinal upset. It may rarely cause a megaloblastic anemia through folate antagonism and should be used with caution in patients with G6PD deficiency. It is not appropriate during the first month of life due to the risk of jaundice and hemolytic anemia in the newborn.

Another common prophylactic antimicrobial is nitrofurantoin (or Macrodantin). It is excreted in the urine, which allows urinary levels to be high while having few effects on fecal flora. It is inexpensive and comes in both a liquid and tablet preparation. It may also cause gastrointestinal upset. Rarely, it is associated with a peripheral neuropathy and pulmonary hypersensitivity. It should not be used in patients with impaired renal function or during the first month of life.

Amoxicillin is the prophylactic antibiotic of choice for the newborn because it can be safely metabolized in the first month of life. Its primary side effect is a hypersensitivity reaction in some pa-

tients. It also can alter gastrointestinal flora, which can lead to diarrhea and rarely pseudomembranous colitis. The liquid preparation requires refrigeration, which may be inconvenient. The cephalosporins have similar properties to amoxicillin but are more expensive.

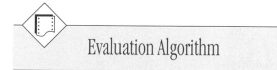

Evaluation Algorithm

The evaluation algorithm shown in Fig. 2–1 provides a rational basis for the basic evaluation of any child with the diagnosis of UTI. Using such a treatment plan should minimize the risk of missing significant genitourinary pathology and preventable renal damage.

Figure 2–1

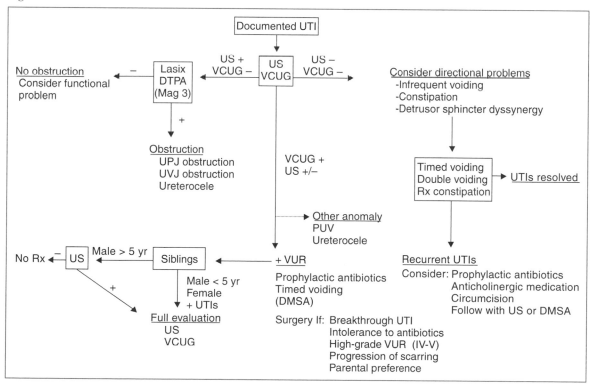

Evaluation algorithm.

Note: The author is a full-time federal employee. This work is in the public domain. The views expressed are those of the author, and are not to be construed as official or as reflecting those of the Department of Defense, the Army Medical Department or the U.S. Air Force.

References

1. Bloom DA, Faerber G, Bomalaski MD: Urinary incontinence in girls. *Urol Clin North Am* 22:521, 1995.

2. Smellie JM, Poulton A, Prescod NP: Retrospective study of children with renal scarring associated with reflux and urinary infection. *BMJ* 308:1193, 1994.

3. Newcastle Asymptomatic Bacteriuria Research Group: Asymptomatic bacteriuria in schoolchildren in Newcastle upon Tyne. *Arch Dis Child* 50:90, 1975.

4. Miller T, Phillips S: Pyelonephritis: The relationship between infection, renal scarring and antimicrobial therapy. *Kidney Int* 19:654, 1981.

5. Ransley PG, Risdon RA: Reflux nephropathy: Effects of antimicrobial therapy on the evolution of the early pyelonephritic scar. *Kidney Int* 20:733, 1981.

6. Hoberman A, Wald ER: Urinary tract infections in young febrile children. *Pediatr Infect Dis J* 16:11, 1997.

7. Johnson CE, Maslow JN, Fattlar DC, et al: The role of bacterial adhesins in the outcome of childhood urinary tract infections. *Am J Dis Child* 147:1090, 1993.

8. Smellie JM, Edwards D, Hunter N, et al: Vesicoureteric reflux and renal scarring. *Kidney Int* 8:s65, 1975.

9. Newcastle Asymptomatic Bacteriuria Research Group: Asymptomatic bacteriuria in schoolchildren in Newcastle upon Tyne. *Arch Dis Child* 50:90, 1975.

10. Ransley PG, Risdon RA: Reflux and renal scarring. *Br J Radiol Suppl* 14:1, 1978.

11. Ransley PG, Dhillon HK, Gordon PG, et al: The postnatal management of hydronephrosis diagnosed by prenatal ultrasound. *J Urol* 144:584, 1990.

12. Lebowitz, RL: The detection and characterization of vesicoureteral reflux in the child. *J Urol* 148:1640, 1992

13. Dinkel E, Ertel M, Dittrich M, et al: Kidney size in childhood: Sonographic growth charts for kidney length and volume. *Pediatr Radiol* 15:38, 1985.

14. Tasker AD, Lindsell DR, Moncrieff M: Can ultrasound reliably detect renal scarring in children with urinary tract infection? *Clin Radiol* 47:177, 1993.

15. MacKenzie JR, Fowler K, Hollman AS, et al: The value of ultrasound in the child with an acute urinary tract infection. *BJU* 74:240, 1994.

16. Rushton HG, Majd M: Dimercaptosuccinic acid renal scintigraphy for the evaluation of pyelonephritis and scarring: A review of experimental and clinical studies. *J Urol* 148:1726, 1992

17. Landau D, Turner ME, Brennan J, et al: The value of urinalysis in differentiating acute pyelonephritis from lower urinary tract infection in febrile infants. *Pediatr Infect Dis J* 13:777, 1994.

18. Jakobsson, B, Svensson L: Transient pyelonephritic changes on 99mTechnetium-dimercaptosuccinic acid scan for at least 5 months after infection. *Acta Paediatr* 86:803, 1997.

19. Noe HN: The long-term results of prospective sibling reflux screening. *J Urol* 148:1739, 1992.

20. Noe HN, Wyatt RJ, Peeden JR, et al: The transmission of vesicoureteral reflux from parent to child. *J Urol* 148:1869, 1992.

21. Noe HN: The current status of screening for vesicoureteral reflux. *Pediatr Nephrol* 9:638, 1995. Review.

22. Blane CE, DiPietro MA, Zerin JM, et al: Renal sonography is not a reliable screening examination for vesicoureteral reflux. *J Urol* 150:752, 1993.

23. Veron SJ, Coulthard MG, Lambert HJ, et al: New renal scarring in children who at age 3 and 4 years had normal scans with dimercaptosuccinic acid: Follow-up study. *BMJ* 315:905, 1997.

24. Greenfield SP, Wan J: Experience with vesicoureteral reflux in children: Clinical characteristics. *J Urol* 158: 574, 1997.

25. Wolfish NM, Delbrouck NF, Shanon A, et al: Prevalence of hypertension in children with primary vesicoureteral reflux. *J Pediatr* 123:559, 1993.

26. Ramero R, Oyarzun E, Mazor M, et al: Meta-analysis of the relationship between asymptomatic bacteriuria and preterm delivery/low birth weight. *Obstet Gynecol* 73:576, 1989.

27. Williams BL, Davies DKL, Evans KT, et al: Vesicoureteral reflux in patients with bacteriuria in pregnancy. *Lancet* 2:1202, 1968.

28. Mansfield JT, Snow BW, Cartwright PC, et al: Complications of pregnancy in women after childhood reimplantation for vesicoureteral reflux: An

update with 25 years of followup. *J Urol* 154: 787,1995.

29. Obling H, Claesson I, Ebel KD, et al: Renal scars and parenchymal thinning in children with vesicoureteral reflux: A 5-year report of the International Reflux Study in Children (European branch). *J Urol* 148:1653, 1992.

30. Report of the International Reflux Study Committee: Medical versus surgical treatment of primary vesicoureteral reflux: A prospective international reflux study in children. *J Urol* 125:277, 1981.

31. Jantausch BA, Criss VR, O'Donnell R, et al: Association of Lewis blood group phenotypes with urinary tract infection in children. *J Pediatr* 124: 863, 1994.

32. Giron JA, Ho AS, Schoolnik GK: Characterization of fimbriae produced by enteropathogenic *Escherichia coli. J Bacteriol* 175:7391, 1993.

33. Johnson CE, Maslow JN, Fattlar DC, et al: The role of bacterial adhesins in the outcome of childhood urinary tract infections. *Am J Dis Child* 147:1090, 1993.

34. Wiswell TE, Hachey WE: Urinary tract infections and the uncircumcised state: An update. *Clin Pediatr* 32:130, 1993.

35. Craig JC, Knight JF, Sureshkumar P, et al: Effect of circumcision on incidence of urinary tract infection in preschool boys. *J Pediatr* 128:23, 1996.

36. Koff SA: Bladder-sphincter dysfunction in childhood. *Urology* 19:457, 1982.

37. Jodal U: The natural history of bacteriuria in childhood. *Infect Dis Clin North Am* 1:713, 1987.

38. Shortliffe, LMD: The management of urinary tract infections in children without urinary tract abnormalities. *Urol Clin North Am* 22:67, 1995.

Edith D. Wilson
Martin A. Koyle
Peter D. Furness III

Chapter

3

Cryptorchidism

How Common Is the Undescended Testicle?

The empty scrotum is one of the most common genitourinary problems encountered in pediatrics. The term *cryptorchidism,* which literally means hidden testis, originated from the Greek words kryptos ("hidden") and orchis ("testis"). It was first described centuries ago by Galen and Vesalius.

Generically cryptorchidism encompasses all abnormalities of testicular descent in which the testis does not reach the dependent part of the scrotum. Today, abnormalities of the testicular descent are more commonly referred to as undescended testis (UDT). They are further classified by testicular location as intra-abdominal, intracannicular, gliding, retractile, or vanishing testis. Despite the apparent simplicity of this anatomic condition, the management of the UDT remains a source of controversy.

The UDT is one of the more common disorders of the male infant. Other than circumcision, disorders of the testis and processus vaginalis (hernia, hydrocele) account for the most common surgeries performed upon young male boys. The incidence in a full-term male infant is 3%, while in premature infants the incidence can be as high as 30%. Spontaneous descent is usually the rule, with descent usually occurring in the first 3 months of life, so that the overall incidence at 1 year of age and thereafter is about 1%. The right side is involved twice as often as the left side. In 20% to 30% of cases, the UDTs are bilateral.

Why Is the Undescended Testicle Important?

The UDT is considered to be at risk for a number of histologic and ultrastructural changes that provide rationale for our current management. These changes result in an increased incidence of testicular malignancy and decreased fertility.

Malignancy

It is well known that the UDT can undergo malignant transformation. In fact, of all the risk factors for developing testicular cancer, cryptorchidism is the most important, with 10% of all testicular cancer patients having a history of a UDT. This translates into a 20 to 40 times greater incidence of testicular cancer in patients with a UDT than the normal population.[2] An increase in malignancy also affects the contralateral descended testis, with an incidence four times that of a normal testis. Testes that are found higher along the pathway of descent, such as intra-abdominal testes, are more likely to undergo malignant transformation.

The most common histologic testicular tumor pattern is seminoma, with the majority of tumors presenting in the third decade of life. Further evidence of the potential malignant nature of the UDT is the high incidence of carcinoma in situ (1.7%) in biopsied testes at orchidopexy.[25] Carcinoma in situ has also been found in the contralateral descended testes.

Unfortunately, the current management of placing the testes into the dependent scrotum offers no protection against developing future malignancy. Placing the testis into the scrotum simply allows a more accurate examination. Teaching lifelong self-testicular examination should also be an important goal in the care of the patient with UDT.

Infertility

Infertility can also be a consequence of the UDT, and this appears to be related to abnormalities of the semen. Kogan reported that 41% of treated unilateral UDT patients will demonstrate a sperm count less than normal (i.e., 20 million/mL).[2] Men who had unilateral palpable UDT seem to have normal or acceptable semen while men with bilateral nonpalpable testis had worse semen quality.[26] Puri and O'Donnell found that all bilateral cryptorchid patients were azospermic in their study cohort.[27] It should be pointed out that most boys with cryptorchid testis will have a reasonable chance of being fertile, but fertility appears more likely in patients with unilateral palpable testis than in those with bilateral nonpalpable testes.

The testes of infants in the neonatal period histologically shows very little difference between the UDT and the normal testis. However, various ultrastructural changes occur with time in the UDT, and by the second to third year of life the UDT is clearly different from the normal testis. During the first year of life the normal testis has an increase in spermatogonia but in the UDT, the number of spermatogonia stays the same. Hadziselimovic has reported that one-third of UDTs show evidence of lost germ cells by 2 years of age and this deficit persists.[28]

These facts argue for early intervention in patients with UDT to allow for the best chance of fertility. The current practice among pediatric urologists is to achieve scrotal placement ideally by 6 months of age and by 1 year of age at the latest.[29] However, routine orchidopexy at this age is a fairly new concept, and the outcome of early orchidopexy in terms of fertility has not yet been adequately evaluated in follow-up. Indeed, the ultimate fate of fertility may already be affected prior to surgical correction when one observes the altered histology in the contralateral descended testis in patients with unilateral UDT.[30]

Principal Diagnoses

Undescended testes are classified clinically as (a) palpable or nonpalpable, and (b) either unilateral or bilateral, and subdivided into retractile, gliding, truly undescended, and ectopic.[3] The majority of UDTs are palpable and unilateral (66%). Most nonpalpable testes (unilateral or bilateral) are anatomically present but are located such that clinical identification is difficult. Truly nonpalpable testes (intra-abdominal or vanishing) comprise only 20% of UDTs.

Retractile testes are testes in a suprascrotal position, which on physical exam can be milked into a dependent part of the scrotum. Retractile testes constitute about one third of the testes suspected to be undescended in the pediatric urologist's office. Frequently, they will slowly return to a suprascrotal position due to an active cremasteric reflex, and hence are termed retractile. These testes do not require surgical intervention because normal histologic and maturational development takes place and most patients have normal fertility. These testes however, should be monitored on routine physical exam for the rare condition of testicular ascent, in which case orchidopexy is needed.[6]

A *gliding testis* is similar to the retractile testis in that it too can be manipulated into the scrotum from a suprascrotal position. However, the gliding testis, in contrast to the retractile testis, immediately returns to a suprascrotal position after release of manual tension. The return to its original position appears to be independent of the cremasteric reflex. Distinguishing a retractile from a gliding testis is important, because a gliding testis is thought to develop the same pathologic and functional changes as a true undescended testis.[7]

A true *undescended testis* refers to any testis in which migration arrests along the normal pathway of descent. The most common location of the UDT is between the internal and external rings of the inguinal canal (intracannicular) or just outside the external inguinal ring. These testes are commonly associated with a patent processus vaginalis or potential hernia. By definition, these testes cannot be pulled into a dependent scrotal position.

Ectopic testes refer to those palpable testes that do not follow the normal pathway of descent after exiting the external ring. The testicle may be located in the superficial skin of the groin or perineum, in the femoral canal, or in the opposite hemiscrotum. The most common site for an ectopic testis is the superficial inguinal space located between the external oblique fascia and the subcutaneous tissues medial to the external inguinal ring (the pouch of Denis Browne).

The *nonpalpable testis,* which is either absent (anorchia) or has an intra-abdominal location, comprises 20% of UDTs. Most nonpalpable testes, especially if bilateral, are actually present and located in the inguinal canal, but can only be identified on examination under anesthesia or at surgical exploration. Occasionally the testis cannot be surgically identified, even intra-abdominally, and these testes are thought to be lost to an antenatal or neonatal vascular accident (vanishing testis syndrome). Finding blind-ending gonadal vessels and a vas deferens either laparoscopically or at retroperitoneal exploration is the hallmark of testicular absence. The incidence of monorchidism and anorchidism among cryptorchid patients is 4% and 0.6%, respectively. Additionally, the finding of either (1) bilateral cryptorchidism or (2) unilateral cryptorchidism and hypospadias should prompt consideration of an intersex disorder.

Testicular reascent is a rare but reported condition.[8] Ascent is thought to occur in childhood secondary to disproportion of somatic growth resulting in an extrascrotal position of the testis, so that an initially descended testis ascends above the scrotum. As a result, the testis is subject to histologic changes similar to the true UDT.

Embryology of Testicular Descent

The mechanism of normal testicular descent is theorized to be multifactorial and involves hormonal, neural, and mechanical influences on the gubernaculum and testis itself.[4] The mechanism of testicular maldescent is probably an interplay of problems involving more than one of these factors of normal descent and is beyond the scope of this discussion. The embryology of testicular descent is generally considered to occur in three stages: germ-cell migration, transabdominal migration, and transinguinal descent into the scrotum.[3] Scrotal placement provides a cool environment, which is thought to be essential for normal spermatogenesis. The scrotum may be as much as 4°C cooler than the abdominal core temperature.

Germ-cell migration occurs at 7 weeks of gestation when the primordial germ cells travel from the yolk sac to the mesodermal ridge. The primitive gonad differentiates into a testis under the influence of testicular determining factor (a Y chromosome gene product). Testicular hormone activity occurs by the eighth week of gestation and produces both testosterone and Müllerian-inhibiting substance, which are responsible for the development of male internal ducts and regression of the potential female structures.

Transabdominal migration occurs between the seventh and twelfth weeks of gestation, as the testis descends from the kidney level to the level of the internal ring of the abdominal wall. A dormant period of testicular migration then occurs from the third to the seventh months of gestation. Transinguinal descent occurs when the testis further descends through the abdominal wall in the inguinal canal, exits the external ring, and finally rests in the scrotal location. The epididymis and vas deferens, a Wolffian derivative, join the tests in the first trimester and precede the descent of the testis proper. The transinquinal and scrotal descent of these structures occurs with a peritoneal evagination (patent processes vaginalis) and can predispose to a potential hernia.

Key History

The history should seek evidence of several risk factors or exposures that increase the likelihood of UDT. Infants at risk for undescended testis include low-birthweight infants, premature infants, and twins. Fortunately, most UDTs spontaneously descend, with 95% of the premature infants and 75% of the term infants descending into the scrotum within the first 3 months of life. Testicles that have had a history on previous exam of being in the scrotum suggest retractile rather than true UDTs. Maternal drug or toxin exposure may be relevant, particularly if the mother took a virilizing drug (e.g., anabolic steroids).

It is important to determine if the child or adult with UDT has had any inguinal surgery such as a hernia repair. Consultation with the operating surgeon or operative records may yield details on a testis previously brought to the scrotum or one that was surgically removed.

Physical Examination

The physical exam plays an essential role in the diagnosis of the UDT as it allows classification that is essential for management. It is important that a scrotal examination take place in a warm and nonthreatening environment. The physician should systematically examine the scrotum as well as the remainder of the genitalia. Evaluation should include the overall size of the scrotum (flat versus full and rugated) as well as the contents of each hemiscrotum. Discrepancies in size, shape, and consistency between the right and left testes should be noted. Additionally, any hernias, hydroceles, or genital anomalies should be noted.

If the child has an empty scrotum, then palpation along the inguinal canal should be done. This is best performed beginning at the internal ring and palpating medially along the inguinal canal toward the pubic tubercle. A helpful technique is to slide the second and third finger over the inguinal canal while the index finger of the opposite hand brushes up and down, like a painter's brush, just in front of the oncoming fingers. If a testis is palpated, an attempt should be made to milk it into the scrotum.

A maneuver that facilitates palpation involves placing liquid soap or K-Y Jelly over the inguinal canal.[5] This allows the examiner's fingers to slide over the skin and better identify any underlying structures, especially in obese patients. Another useful technique is to place the child in a cross-

legged position. This relaxes the cremasteric muscle and may allow the testis to fall into the scrotum.

Failure to palpate a testicle on physical examination can occur for several reasons. The testis can be absent, intra-abdominal, ectopic, or concealed by obesity. The true anatomic position of the testis may not be identified until surgical exploration. Nonetheless, the examiner should note if the testis is palpable or nonpalpable, as this information is useful in initial management of the patient.

Ancillary Tests

Ultrasound, CT, and MRI

An inguinal testis can be located accurately with ultrasound when performed by an experienced examiner with a small-parts scanner. There is, however, no therapeutic advantage, as the same information can usually be obtained from the physical exam.[17] Although ultrasound may be helpful in an obese patient with an inguinal testis, it has not been found reliable for localization of an intra-abdominal testis.[18]

Similar to ultrasound, the value of using CT and MRI is limited in identifying the undescended testicle. Correlations with operative findings of the undescended testis with CT and MRI were 33% and 0%, respectively.[19] The disadvantage of CT is radiation exposure, and both CT and MRI are expensive and require sedation in young children.

These imaging techniques (ultrasound, CT, and MRI) have been described in assisting in localizing the UDT.[18–22] Unfortunately, each of these studies has its drawbacks and no test has been found to be accurate enough for routine clinical use. The overall accuracy of ultrasound, CT, and MRI is no better than about 44%. When compared to the accuracy of the physical exam (54% of referring physical exams and 84% of pediatric urologists), these ancillary tests add little to the overall management of the UDT.[19] In the past, arteriography and venography have been used to localize the undescended testis. These tests have been abandoned because of the invasive nature, technical difficulty, and the superior alternative of diagnostic laparoscopy.

Diagnostic Laparoscopy

Laparoscopy has an important role in the localization and management of the cryptorchid testes, and in modern pediatric urologic practice, it has replaced other imaging studies for evaluating patients with a nonpalpable UDT. The findings on laparoscopy allow the surgeon to plan the remainder of the surgical procedure under the same anesthetic.

The technique of laparoscopy involves placing an umbilical transabdominal port through which a viewing telescope is passed. This provides direct visualization and localization of the testes if intra-abdominal, or may show blind-ending gonadal blood vessels and vas deferens in the case of the vanishing testis. If gonadal vessels are seen entering the internal ring, groin exploration is warranted. The laparoscope can also provide an operating element to perform the clipping of gonadal vessels in a staged procedure called a Fowler–Stevens orchidopexy. Additionally, this port can facilitate the removal of an atrophic nubbin in the case of the vanishing testis.[9]

Laparoscopic techniques have been developed to place an intra-abdominal testis into the scrotum in a single procedure without open surgery. The new procedure, laparoscopic orchidopexy, is taking on popularity and has been performed successfully and safely and with minimal morbidity.[10–13] Overall, laparoscopic procedures used to locate the nonpalpable testis have been found to be the most sensitive and specific means available.[14–15] Combining this with the surgical options available at the time of laparoscopy, as well as the low complication rate, accounts for the new popularity among pediatric urologists.[16]

Laparoscopy is also useful to confirm testicular absence. Finding blind-ending gonadal vessels and a vas deferens is the hallmark of testicular ab-

sence. A blind-ending vas deferens alone is not evidence of testicular absence and mandates that retroperitoneal and, if necessary, intraperitoneal exploration be performed until blind-ending gonadal vessels are identified. Again, laparoscopy may be useful in this setting.

Management

Once the diagnosis of cryptorchidism has been recognized, the goal of management is to have both testes rest in a dependent scrotal position. In 1903, Bevan performed the first successful surgical repositioning of a UDT into the scrotum (orchidopexy) and suggested that the UDT be brought down into this location before the teenage years. Usually, this occurs spontaneously. However, if descent does not occur spontaneously, surgical or hormonal treatment should be instituted to avoid potential testicular changes.

Surgical Therapies

PALPABLE UDT

An orchidopexy is a surgical procedure to bring the gonad into the scrotum and represents the gold standard in therapy. This involves a transverse inguinal incision with mobilizing of the testis and cord. Testicular cord lengthening is achieved by division and high ligation of the hernia sac (tunica vaginalis), as well as division of tethering cremasteric muscle and spermatic fascia. The testis is then brought down into the scrotum and fixed in a sub-dartos pouch. Recently, Bianchi has popularized a single high scrotal incision rather than the traditional two-incision approach for the palpable gonad.[36]

Success of surgery is related to location of the testis and the type of procedure performed to relocate the testis. A review of the literature by Docimo revealed that the surgical success rates by anatomic position of the testis at the time of surgery are 74%

intra-abdominal, 82% emergent, 87% intracannic-ular, and 92% for testes located below the exter-nal ring.[31] Excellent results from surgery include an adequate-sized testicle in a scrotal position. Sometimes the testicle remains in a high yet pal-pable location in the scrotum, which is acceptable. Complications related to surgery include injuries to the vas, testicular atrophy, and wound infec-tions, and occur in less than 4% of patients.

NONPALPABLE UDT

All newborns with bilateral nonpalpable testes or unilateral UDT with hypospadias warrant en-docrinologic and karyotypic evaluation to rule out intersex problems. Neonatal electrolytes should be monitored to identify salt-wasting congenital adrenal hyperplasia, which mandates early salt, fluid, and mineral-corticoid replacement.

Only 20% of UDTs are clinically found to be nonpalpable, and in only 0.6% of patients with bi-lateral nonpalpable testes are the testes absent. The condition of bilateral nonpalpable testes needs to be further investigated either hormonally or surgically to identify the presence or absence of testicular tissue.

Baseline elevation of FSH in conjunction with the inability to increase the low-baseline testos-terone level with a short course of hCG stimulation has been suggested to confirm absence of testicu-lar tissue. However, there have been reported ex-ceptions to this hormonal diagnosis of anorchia. Recently, laparoscopy has become the preferred modality to diagnose the absence or presence of a testis (bilateral or unilateral). When a testicle is identified at laparoscopy, the decision as to the best surgical approach to orchidopexy is made. The technique of orchidopexy chosen is governed by the length of the spermatic vessels and the sur-geon's individual expertise. Types of orchidopexy techniques vary from a routine inguinal incision to division of the spermatic vessels (Fowler–Stevens) and testicular autotransplantation.

An orchidopexy is performed for all viable tes-ticular tissue up until puberty. After puberty, an or-chiectomy is recommended secondary to the poor spermatogenic potential and the known incidence of malignant degeneration. After 32 years of age, it is felt that the risk of surgery to remove the testis outweighs the risk of mortality in germ-cell tumor development, and observation is recommended.

If a child is found to have no testicular tissue (anorchia), he will require hormone supplementa-tion at puberty and should be considered a candi-date for testicular prostheses (implant). Patients with unilateral testicular absence should also be of-fered the option of a testicular implant regardless of the underlying etiology. The testicular prosthe-sis that is available today is made of a silicone shell with an expandable saline interior. The timing of insertion is controversial, but the psychological benefit of having both testicles in the scrotum should not be underestimated, especially in an adolescent. If the family chose to have the implant placed prepubertally, then the implant will have to be changed to a larger size after puberty. The po-tential complications of a testicular implant are minimal in a healthy child, with the most common being infection, hematoma, and (rarely) erosion. If a complication should occur, the prostheses may have to be removed, but can be reinserted in a few months. The monorchid child should be instructed to wear a protective cup when participating in sports for protection of his remaining testis.

Medical Therapies

Hormonal treatment involves administering human chorionic gonadotropin, and/or gonadotropin-releasing hormone (GnRH). Human chorionic gonadotropin (hCG) is administered as an intra-muscular injection and works by stimulating testic-ular Leydig cell production of testosterone with the hopes of inducing subsequent testicular descent. Results with this treatment are variable, with some reporting successful descent in 30% of unilateral and 40% of bilateral UDTs.[32] Many of the initial studies supporting the use of hCG included not only truly undescended testes but also patients with retractile testes. Misleading results were con-strued from these studies because retractile testes usually will descend on their own. Rajfer's study suggested that true UDTs benefit little from hormonal therapy as a stimulus for descent when compared to placebo.[33]

Thus, the effectiveness of hCG in patients with UDT may be limited and at best may promote only partial descent of a true UDT. This in and of itself, however, may facilitate orchidopexy at the time of surgery.[34] The International Health Foundation has recommended that hCG be given by injection biweekly for a total of 5 weeks. For a young infant, the dose is 250 international units (IU); for children up to 6 years, 500 IU; and for older children, 1000 IU. Potential side effects with larger doses include premature closure of the epiphyseal plate and accelerated growth of secondary sex characteristics, which usually resolves with stopping the injections.

GnRH stimulates the release of follicle-stimulating hormone and leutinizing hormone from the pituitary gland and is administered as an intranasal spay (1.2 mg/day for 4 weeks). Recently, attention has focused on treatment of UDT with both hCG and GnRH with encouraging results.[35] Studies support the use of GnRH in promoting the development of germ cells as well as causing testicular

Figure 3–1

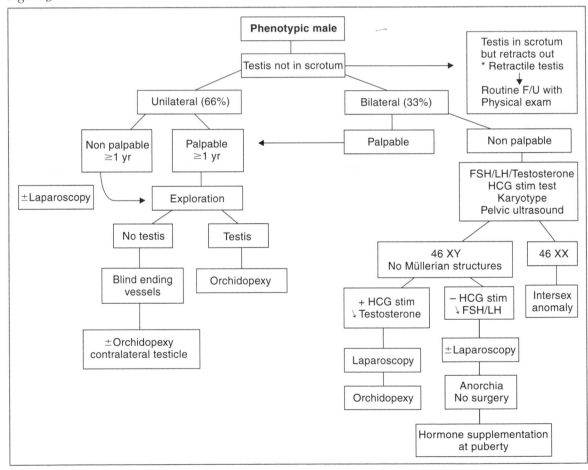

Management algorithm for the undescended testicle.

descent. The results are variable, but the side effects are fewer than with hCG. It is important to note that GnRH is not approved for this use by the United States Food and Drug Administration.

Algorithm

Our approach to management of the UDT is outlined in Fig. 3–1. A few points are worth clarification. All of our patients found to have UDT have identification of blind-ending vessels, rudimentary testis, or an orchidopexy of viable testicular structures. The palpable UDT undergoes an inguinal exploration with a scrotal orchidopexy. The truly nonpalpable UDT undergoes either an inguinal exploration or laparoscopy and inguinal exploration. If blind ending vessels are identified (vanishing testis), exploration is terminated and the contralateral descended testis is pexed to prevent possible torsion of the remaining testis. Some of our patients with laparoscopically identified high unilateral intra-abdominal testes have a course of hCG stimulation prior to inguinal exploration, as we feel this facilities orchidopexy from a vasal and spermatic vascular supply standpoint.

All newborns born with bilateral nonpalpable testes or unilateral UDT with hypospadias warrant endocrinologic and karyotypic evaluation to rule out intersex anomalies. Patients with bilateral anorchia will require hormonal supplementation at puberty. All patients with an absent testicle (vanishing or surgically removed) are offered a prosthetic insert.

References

1. Bevan AD: Operation for undescended testicle and congenital inguinal correction. The surgical treatment of undescended testicle. *JAMA* 41:718, 1903.
2. Kogan S: Cryptorchidism. In Kelais P, King L, Belman A (eds): *Clinical Pediatric Urology,* ed 3. Philadelphia, Saunders, 1992, pp 1050–1083.
3. Rajfer J: Congenital anomalies of the testis and scrotum. In Walsh PC, Retik AB, Vaughn ED, Wein AJ (eds): *Campbell's Urology,* ed 7. Philadelphia, Saunders, 1998, pp 2172–2192.
4. Walker RD: Cryptorchidism.
5. Hurwitz R: Society for Pediatric Urology Newsletter.
6. Docimo SG: Testicular descent and ascent in the first year of life. *Urology* 48:458–460, 1996.
7. Hadziselimovic F, Herzog M, Buser M: Development of cryptorchid testes. *Eur J Pediatr* 146(suppl):8–121, 1987.
8. Docimo SG: Testicular descent and ascent in the first year of life. *Urology* 50:826, 1997. Comment.
9. Rajfer J, Walsh PC: The incidence of intersexuality in patients with hypospadias and cryptorchidism. *J Urol* 116:769–770, 1976.
10. Bogaert GA, Kogan BA, Mevorach RA: Therapeutic laparoscopy for intra-abdominal testes. *Urology* 42:182–188, 1993.
11. Poppas DP, Lemack GE, Mininberg DT: Laparoscopic orchidopexy: Clinical experience and description of technique. *J Urol* 155:708–711, 1996.
12. Docimo SG, Moore RG, Adams J, et al: Laparoscopic orchidopexy for the high palpable undescended testis: Preliminary experience. *J Urol* 154:1513–1515, 1995.
13. Guat DD, Agarwal DK, Purohit KC, et al: Laparoscopic orchidopexy for the intra-abdominal testis. *J Urol* 153:479–481, 1995.
14. Moore RG, Peters CAM, Bauer SB, et al: Laparoscopic evaluation of the nonpalpable testes: A prospective assessment of accuracy. *J Urol* 151:728–731, 1994.
15. Caldamone A: Laparoscopy for the impalpable testis. *Dialog Pediatr Urol* 15:5–6, 1992.
16. Tennenbaum SY, Lerner SE, McAleer IM, et al: Preoperative laparoscopic localization of the nonpalpable testis: A critical analysis of a 10-year experience. *J Urol* 151:732–734, 1994.
17. Madrazo B, Klugo R, Parks J, et al: Ultrasonographic demonstration of undescended testis. *Radiology* 133:181–183, 1979.
18. Weiss RM, Carter, Rosenfield AT: High resolution real-time ultrasonography in the localization of the undescended testis. *J Urol* 13:936–938, 1986.
19. Hrebinko R, Bellinger M: The limited role of imaging techniques in managing children with undescended testes. *J Urol* 150:458–460, 1993.
20. Wolverson MK, Houttuin E, Heiberg, et al: Comparison of computer tomography with high-resolution real-

time ultrasound in the localization of the impalpable undescended testis. *Radiology* 146:133–136, 1983.

21. Miyano T, Kobryash H, Shimomura H, et al: Magnetic resonance imaging for localizing the nonpalpable undescended testes. *J Pediatr Surg* 26:607–609, 1991.

22. Green R: Computer axial tomography vs spermatic venography in localization of cryptorchid testes. *Urology* 26:513–517, 1985.

23. Levitt S, Kogan S, Engel R, et al: The impalpable testis: A rational approach to management. *J Urol* 120:515–520, 1978.

24. Martin DC: Malignancy in the cryptorchid testis. *Urol Clin North Am* 9:371–376, 1982.

25. Giwercman A, Bruun E, Frimodt-Moller C, et al: Prevalance of carcinoma in situ and other histopathological abnormalities in testes of men with a history of cryptorchidism. *J Urol* 142:998–1002, 1989.

26. Puri P, O'Donnell B: Semen analysis of patients who had orchidopexy at or after seven years of age. *Lancet* 2:1051–1052, 1988.

27. Puri P, O'Donnell B: Semen analysis in patients operated on for impalpable testes. *Br J Urol* 66: 646–647, 1990.

28. Hadziselimovic F: Cryptorchidism. In Gillenwater J, Grayhack J, Howards SS, et al. (eds): *Adult and Pediatric Urology*. Chicago, Year Book, 1987.

29. Kogan SJ, Tennenbaum S, Gill B, et al: Efficacy of orchidopexy by patient age 1 year for cryptorchidism. *J Urol* 144:508–509, 1990.

30. Lipshultz L, Caminos-Torres R, Greenspan C, et al: Undescended testis. *N Engl J Med* 295:15–18, 1976.

31. Docimo SG: The results of surgical therapy for cryptorchidism: A literature review and analysis. *J Urol* 154:1148–1152, 1995.

32. Bergada C: Clinical treatment of cryptorchidism. In Bjerich JR, Giarola A: *Cryptorchidism*. London, Academic Press, 1979.

33. Rajfer J, Handelsman DJ, Swerdloff RS, et al: Hormonal therapy for cryptorchidism. *N Engl J Med* 312:466, 1986.

34. Polascik TJ, Chan-Tack KM, Jeffs RD: Reappraisal of the role of human chorionic gonadotropin in the diagnosis and treatment of the nonpalpable testis: A 10-year experience. *Urology* 156:804–806, 1996.

35. Nane I, Ziylan O, Esen T, et al: Primary gonadotropin-releasing hormone and adjunctive human chorionic gonadotropin treatment in cryptorchidism: A clinical trial. *J Urol* 49:108–111, 1997.

36. Caruso AP, Walsh RA, Wolach JW, Koyle MA: Single scrotal orchipexy for the palpable undescended testicle. *J Urol* 164:156–159, 2000.

George W. Kaplan

Circumcision

How Common Is Circumcision?

Male circumcision is probably the most commonly performed operation in the United States. According to the National Center for Health Statistics, 64% of American male infants were circumcised in 1995.[1] The rate of male circumcision in other countries varies considerably. The rate is 48% in Canada, but circumcision is quite uncommon in most European countries, Central and South America, and Asia.[2] The rate of circumcision in the United States has declined over the past few years as a debate has raged over the indications for a neonatal circumcision.[3,4]

Conflicting Thoughts on Circumcision

In 1975, the American Academy of Pediatrics Committee on the Fetus and Newborn stated that "there are no valid medical indications for circumcision in the newborn period. This stance has been revisited, and current recommendations state that there are medical benefits to circumcision.[1] Nevertheless, a number of lay anti-circumcision groups (e.g., the National Organization of Circumcision Resource Centers [NOCIRC]) have attempted to discourage circumcision by applying pressure to third-party payers and by using lawsuits to intimidate physicians.[4]

Historical Aspects of Circumcision

Circumcision is one of the three oldest operations known (circumcision, lithotomy, and trephina-

tion).[5] One of the first records of circumcision is a bas relief on the tomb of Ankh-Mahor at Saqqara near Cairo, which is thought to depict circumcision (Fig. 4–1).[6] Male Jewish infants have been circumcised on the eighth day of life as a religious ritual for over 4000 years. The origin of this rite is found in the Bible, with the injunction "every male among you shall be circumcised."[5] Ritual circumcision is also practiced by Muslims, Africans, Australian aborigines, and several other groups in disparate parts of the world.[5] The origin of most of these practices is obscure.

Embryology

In order to understand both the circumcised and uncircumcised state, it is necessary to review normal phallic development. In the third intrauterine month, a fold of skin develops at the base of the glans penis and grows distally.[7] This fold ultimately becomes the prepuce but initially the dorsal aspect of the fold grows more rapidly than the ventral. However, when the glanular urethra is closed, the ventral aspect of the prepuce forms. Fusion of the ventral aspect of the prepuce is marked by the frenulum. Preputial formation is generally complete by the fifth intrauterine month. Initially, the inner preputial epithelium and the epithelium of the glans are fused, but late in gestation (presumably under the influence of androgen), squamous cells begin to keratinize and arrange themselves into whorls.[8,9] Desquamated cells (smegma) between the prepuce and the glans form little cystic spaces that gradually increase in size and coalesce, thereby resulting in separation of the inner preputial epithelium from the glans. This process is incomplete at birth and continues through childhood at varying rates.[10] Some infants and toddlers may experience a mild transient inflammatory reaction at some stage of the separation process, presumably because the smegma becomes infected. Organisms can be grown from encysted smegma.[11]

Figure 4–1

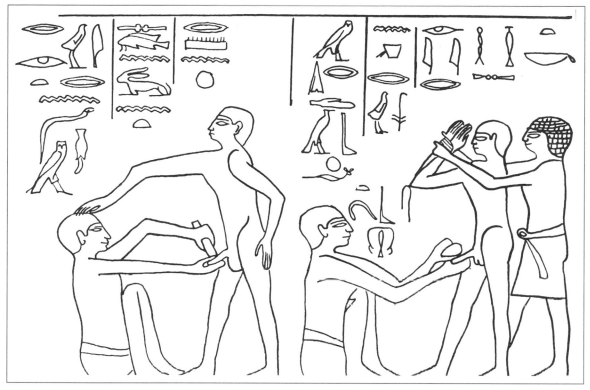

Line drawing of bas relief from Egyptian tomb thought to depict circumcision. (Reprinted from Bitschal J, Brodney ML: *A History of Urology in Egypt.* Cambridge, MA, Riverside Press, 1956.)

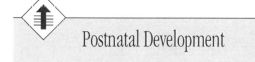

Postnatal Development

At birth, the prepuce is retractable in only 4% of boys and in most, it cannot be retracted sufficiently to even visualize the urethral meatus.[10] The prepuce gradually and spontaneously becomes retractable so that by age 6 years, one third of boys will have a completely retractable prepuce.[12] By age 17 years, the foreskin is completely retractable in almost all.[12]

Because the majority of males in the United States are circumcised, there has been little opportunity for practitioners to observe the natural history of the uncircumcised penis. If one defines phimosis only as the inability to retract the foreskin, then almost all males initially have phimosis. However, this is physiologic and not pathologic, and when phimosis is defined as the inability to retract the foreskin resulting in balanoposthitis or obstructive uropathy, the incidence of phimosis is quite low. When one attempts to determine the presence of phimosis by drawing the skin of the shaft proximally (toward the penile base), there often is what appears to be a pinpoint opening for the preputial orifice, leading to the conclusion that phimosis is present. However, if in the same individual the prepuce was pulled away from the body, it would be seen that the preputial opening is quite wide and could in no way interfere with voiding.

Some physicians and parents are convinced that the prepuce must be retractable at an early age so that the preputial sac can be washed and, for this reason, forcibly free the prepuce from the glans in infancy. This maneuver results in pain, bleeding, and occasionally paraphimosis. It is my opinion that this is unnecessary, because spontaneous separation will eventually occur without such maneuvers, and, if these maneuvers are repeated, they may produce scarring of the preputial orifice such that true pathologic phimosis is indeed produced. It is unnecessary to retract the foreskin to clean under it until such time as physiologic separation has occurred, at which point the child should be encouraged to wash the area under the prepuce.[13]

Indications

There are some true medical indications for circumcision but none of these pertain to the newborn. In the newborn, circumcision is performed for a number of reasons. There are certain medical benefits that accrue to newborn circumcision. Boys who have been circumcised experience fewer urinary infections, especially in the first year of life, than do boys who are not circumcised.[14] Adults who have been circumcised only rarely develop carcinoma of the penis.[15] Additionally, boys and men who have been circumcised avoid problems with balanoposthitis, phimosis, and paraphimosis.[5]

The increased incidence of urinary infections in boys who have not been circumcised presumably occurs because pathologic bacteria can adhere to the epithelium of the inner prepuce,[16] leading to periurethral colonization and eventual urinary infection.[14] In boys who have had problems with recurring urinary infections, especially those who have structural abnormalities of the urinary tract, circumcision often is beneficial in management.

Recurring episodes of balanoposthitis, pathologic phimosis (i.e., phimosis that interferes with voiding or persists beyond the point that would be considered physiologic and would resolve spontaneously), and paraphimosis are other indications for circumcision.[5]

Contraindications

There are certain contraindications to circumcision.[5] Circumcision is contraindicated in premature infants, those with blood dyscrasias, and those with a penile abnormality in which the foreskin may be needed for a later reconstruction. These abnormalities include hypospadias, epispadias, megalourethra, webbed penis, and chordee (Fig. 4–2).

Methods of Circumcision

General Concerns

There are a number of methods by which circumcision may be accomplished. They all share the common goal of removing enough inner preputial epithelium and shaft skin such that the glans is sufficiently uncovered to prevent or treat phimosis and to render the development of paraphimosis impossible.[11] In newborn infants, clamp methods are usually employed, whereas in older children and adults, excisional methods are generally utilized. Each method has its individual pitfalls and there are some complications that are relatively unique to each. Four principles are common to all forms of circumcision: asepsis, adequate excision of skin, hemostasis, and protection of the glans penis.[11] In theory, there is strict adherence to aseptic principles. In practice, however, this principle is probably frequently violated, especially in newborn circumcision. Fortunately, inoculated wounds infrequently become frankly infected and violating this principle only rarely results in harm.

Circumcision methods can be classified into one of four types or combinations of the four: dorsal slit, shield, clamp, and excision.[11]

Figure 4–2

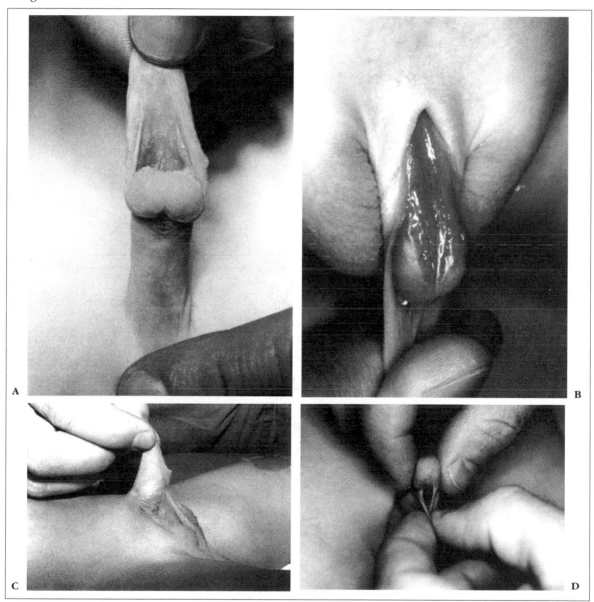

Lesions in which neonatal circumcision is contraindicated. **A.** Hypospadias. **B.** Epispadias. **C.** Webbed penis. **D.** Megalourethra. (Reprinted with permission from Ehrlich R, Alter G (eds): *Reconstructive and Plastic Surgery of the External Genitalia.* Philadelphia, Saunders, 1988, p 406.)

Dorsal Slit

Dorsal slit is actually common to many techniques and sometimes is used alone, especially in the presence of acute inflammation. An incision is made on the dorsum of the penis extending from the preputial orifice to the coronal sulcus through the inner and outer preputial layers (Fig. 4–3). A dorsal slit prevents both phimosis and paraphimosis, but the end result is usually cos-

Figure 4–3

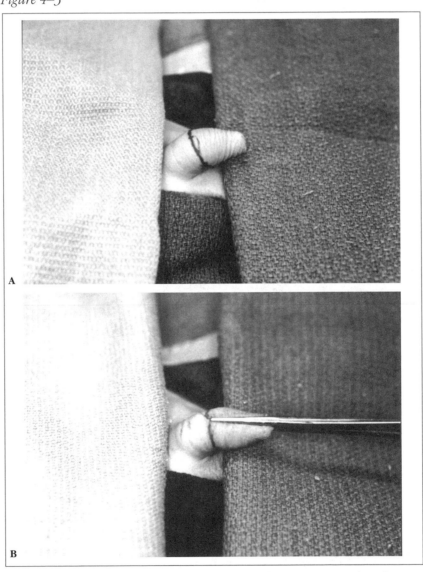

A. The penile skin has been marked to show the level of the corona. **B.** A clamp has been applied to the dorsal midline. (Reprinted with permission from Ehrlich R, Alter G (eds): *Reconstructive and Plastic Surgery of the External Genitalia*. Philadelphia, Saunders, 1988, p 407.)

Figure 4–3 (Continued)

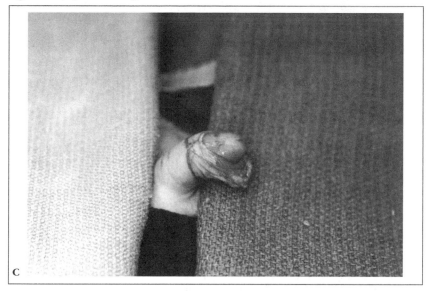

C. The dorsal slit has been completed.

metically unacceptable if the preputial tissue is not also excised because it leaves the prepuce as a ventral apron.

Shield

A shield is used routinely in ritual circumcisions and in certain clamp devices. In this technique, the glans is forced down by a grooved shield that is placed over the stretched prepuce. The excess prepuce is excised and hemostasis is secured. The inner preputial layer must be folded back off the glans either prior to or after excision to ensure full exposure of the glans after healing. The Mogen and the Lawton clamps utilize this principle (Fig. 4–4).

Clamp

There are other clamps that have been developed for use in newborn circumcision. The Gomco clamp (Fig. 4–5) and the Plastibell (Fig. 4–6) are probably the most widely utilized. After separation

of the inner preputial epithelium from the glans, a dorsal slit is made to facilitate placing the bell of the device over the glans. The outer prepuce is marked with ink at the level of the coronal sulcus before a dorsal slit is made. This mark is helpful in determining the amount of tissue to be excised. When using the Gomco clamp, the bell is placed

Figure 4–4

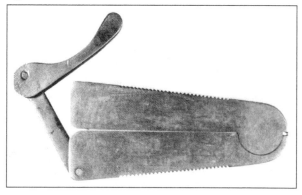

A Mogen clamp. (Reprinted from Grossman EA: *Circumcision: A pictorial history*. Great Neck, NY, Todd & Honeywell, 1982.)

Figure 4–5

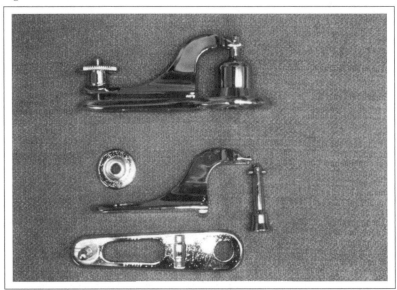

A Gomco clamp assembled and disassembled. (Reprinted with permission from Ehrlich R, Alter G (eds): *Reconstructive and Plastic Surgery of the External Genitalia.* Philadelphia, Saunders, 1988, p 407.)

Figure 4–6

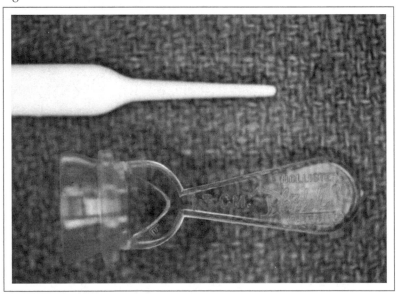

Plastibell device and probe. (Reprinted with permission from Ehrlich R, Alter G (eds): *Reconstructive and Plastic Surgery of the External Genitalia.* Philadelphia, Saunders, 1988, p 408.)

over the glans and the prepuce is drawn over the bell and held in place while the clamp is assembled and tightened, following which the previously marked area of skin is excised. When using the Plastibell, the previously marked area of skin comes to lie over a groove in the Plastibell, which is then tied down and the foreskin is excised past the outermost groove. The bell of the Plastibell device is then snapped off, leaving a ring of plastic to slough off several days later.

Excision

Surgical excision is best accomplished after marking the area of the outer penile shaft with ink where the coronal ridge is seen through the shaft skin. The outer shaft skin is then incised along this mark. A dorsal or both a dorsal and ventral slit are made down to the mark on the shaft skin, and the tissue distal to the coronal sulcus is excised by incising the inner prepuce, leaving a small cuff to be anastomosed to the shaft skin. At times, a sleeve of tissue is excised without a prior dorsal or ventral slit. With surgical excision, hemostasis is secured generally with electrocautery, and sutures are routinely used to coapt the skin edges to produce primary wound healing.

Anesthesia

Although in the past anesthesia was not routinely used with newborn circumcisions, it has been well demonstrated that newborn infants do experience pain and, for this reason, the American Academy of Pediatrics is now recommending that anesthesia routinely be employed with newborn circumcision.[1] A number of methods are available. An oral sucrose solution is preferable to placebo but really does not adequately block pain.[17] EMLA cream has been used and does afford some definite pain relief,[18] but the best pain relief is afforded by local anesthetic injected either as a dorsal block or as a ring block about the base of the penis.[19] In older children, general anesthesia is generally used for circumcision; in adolescents and adults, local anesthesia is possible and often preferable.

Complications

The true incidence of complications after circumcision is unknown, but in one large series, the rate was found to be between 0.2% and 0.6%.[20] There have been isolated reports of death following circumcision, generally as a result of anesthetic complications or overwhelming sepsis.[5] As is true with any surgical procedure, the risks and benefits of the operation should be discussed with the patient or with the parents before the operation is performed.

Bleeding

Bleeding is the most common of the complications associated with circumcision. This occurs in approximately 0.1% of cases, although there are reports as high as 35%.[11] Most of these bleeding episodes are quite minor and respond to wound pressure alone. It is extremely rare that bleeding would be significant enough to require a blood transfusion. Thrombin, silver nitrate, epinephrine, and fibrin have all been used to control post-circumcision bleeding, as have electrocautery and suture.

Infection

Infection is the second most common complication of circumcision, but most of the infections are minor in nature and are nothing more than some redness and purulent exudate at the circumcision site. Wound infections are a bit more common with the Plastibell device than with the Gomco clamp.[20] There have been rare reports of necrotizing fascitis, sepsis, and meningitis as a result of infected circumcision wounds.[5]

Recurrent Phimosis

When inadequate shaft skin is excised, there can be a recurrence of phimosis. During healing, the wound contracts, so that there is now a ring of scar that prevents retraction of the foreskin.[15]

Wound Separation

Surgical wounds occasionally will separate and in the adult, following circumcision, this often is produced by erections in the postoperative period. Inhalation of amyl nitrite aromatic capsules will often induce dilation of the corporeal smooth muscle and abort the erection. Ketoconazole can be utilized to block testosterone production and thereby prevent erection.[21]

Concealed Penis

When an excessive amount of skin has been removed from the shaft and yet an inadequate amount of inner preputial epithelium is excised, the penile shaft often is forced into the suprapubic fat and a stenotic preputial ring forms at the level of the skin of the abdominal wall, thereby forcing the penis into the suprapubic fat pad. The treatment of this complication again is repeat circumcision, but because there is inadequate shaft skin, the incision is best made at the former circumcision line; the shaft of the penis should be freed from the overlying skin, the stenotic ring excised, and the inner preputial epithelium folded back over the shaft of the penis to be used as skin cover. The suture line then lies in the mid- to proximal penile shaft but the need for skin graft for coverage is minimized.[5]

Synechia

Another complication is the formation of skin bridges between the penile shaft and the glans. These sometimes result in tethering of the erect penis and thereby produce pain or even penile curvature. In addition, smegma may accumulate under these bridges. It is unclear exactly how this problem arises, but some have suggested that there is injury to the glans at the time of circumcision with fusion of the circumcision wound to the glans.[5] In any event, the treatment of this is simple surgical division, and this can often be accomplished in the office utilizing EMLA cream as anesthesia.

Urinary Retention

Urinary retention occasionally is produced by either a tight circular bandage or occlusion of the meatus by dressing material (e.g., tincture of benzoin).[5] In some patients, pain and fear may lead to urinary retention.

Meatal Stenosis, Hypospadias, and Epispadias

Meatal stenosis is more common in circumcised than in uncircumcised males.[5] It is thought that meatitis or meatal ulcer, which are also more common following circumcision, leads to stenosis in these patients. The meatitis seems to develop in the child while still in diapers, because the glans is no longer protected by the prepuce and the urethral meatus is injured by bacterial-produced ammonia in urine-soaked diapers.

Hypospadias and epispadias may both result if the glans is split at the time of a dorsal or ventral incision in preparation for excision of the prepuce.[5]

Chordee

Chordee can rarely occur following circumcision, especially if the circumcision is performed during an acute episode of balanoposthitis. This may lead to a dense band of scar in the area of the frenulum and cause chordee on erection.[5]

Inclusion Cysts

Inclusion cysts have been reported to occur in the circumcision line. These may be caused by implantation of smegma in the circumcision wound or perhaps by surgically rolling in epidermis at the time of the circumcision. These cysts can become quite large and sometimes become infected. They are distinguished from penile epidermoid cysts only by their location.[5] Penile lymphedema occasionally occurs, especially if the wound separates after circumcision. This generally will resolve with treatment of the infection.[5]

Urethrocutaneous Fistula

Urethrocutaneous fistulas have been reported after circumcision.[5] These are usually associated with the use of a clamp device or placing sutures in the area of the frenulum to control bleeding. They are produced by injury to the urethra. Urethrocutaneous fistulas have also been reported in patients with unrecognized congenital megalourethra who underwent circumcision.

Penile Amputation and Necrosis

Amputation of a portion of the penis has been reported after circumcision.[11] This is especially true when the Mogen, Sheldon, or Lawton clamps are utilized. If this is recognized at the time, microsurgical reimplantation of the amputated part can be employed with good results.[11]

Tissue necrosis has been reported on rare occasions.[5] If cautery is applied to a metal clamp, the entire penis may slough. There also can be loss of tissue due to injections of epinephrine into the tissue or the employment of a tourniquet. When the Plastibell device is utilized, because the plastic ring is designed to remain in place for a number of days and then slough, there occasionally is migration of the ring onto the distal shaft with prolonged retention of the ring and secondary erosion of tissue by pressure necrosis.[11]

Conclusions

As the American Academy of Pediatrics Task Force on Circumcision has indicated, there are some potential medical benefits to circumcision; however, these benefits do not warrant recommending routine newborn circumcision for everyone. If circumcision is to be performed, pain control should be afforded the patient regardless of the patient's age. Lastly, if circumcision is to be performed, there should be informed consent provided either by the patient or the parents.

References

1. Lannon CM, Bailey AGD, Fleischman AR, et al: Circumcision policy statement. *Pediatrics* 103:686, 1999.
2. Leitch IO: Circumcision: A continuing enigma. *Aust Pediatr J* 6:59, 1970.
3. Schoen EJ: The status of circumcision of newborns. *N Engl J Med* 322:1308, 1990.
4. Thompson AC, King LR, Knox E, et al: Report of the Ad Hoc Task Force on Circumcision. *Pediatrics* 56:610, 1975.
5. Kaplan GW: Circumcision: An overview. *Curr Probl Pedtr* 7:1, 1977.
6. Bitschal J, Brodney ML: *A History of Urology in Egypt*. Cambridge, MA, Riverside Press, 1956.
7. Grey LB: *Developmental Anatomy,* ed 6. Philadelphia, Saunders, 1954.
8. Burrows H: The union and separation of living tissues as influenced by cellular differentiation. *Yale J Biol Med* 17:397, 1944.
9. Delbert GA: The separation of the prepuce in the human penis. *Penis Anat Rec* 57:387, 1933.
10. Gairdner D: Fate of the Foreskin: A study of circumcision. *Br Med J* 2:1433, 1944.

11. Cilento BG Jr, Kaplan GW: Circumcision. In Ehrich RM, Alter G (eds): *Reconstructive and Plastic Surgery of the External Genitalia.* Philadelphia, Saunders, 1988, pp 402–413.
12. Oster J: Further fate of the foreskin. *Arch Dis Child* 43:200, 1968.
13. Osborn LM, Metcalf TJ, Mariani EM: Hygienic care in uncircumcised infants. *Pediatrics* 67:365, 1981.
14. Wiswell TE, Hackey WE: Urinary tract infection and the uncircumcised state: An update. *Clin Pediatr* 32:130, 1993.
15. Persky L, deKernion J: Carcinoma of the penis. *CA Cancer J Clin* 36:258, 1986.
16. Fussell EN, Kaack B, Cherry R, et al: Adherence of bacteria to human foreskins. *J Urol* 140:997, 1998.
17. Blass EM, Hoffmeyer LB: Sucrose as an analgesic for newborn infants. *Pediatrics* 87:215, 1991.
18. Genini F, Johnston CC, Faucher D, et al: Topical anesthesia during circumcision in newborn infants. *JAMA* 270:850, 1993.
19. Lander J, Braoy-Fryer B, Nazarali S, et al: Comparison of ring block, dorsal penile nerve block, and topical anesthesia for neonatal circumcision: A randomized clinical trial. *JAMA* 278:2157, 1997.
20. Gee WE, Ansell JS: Neonatal circumcision: A ten-year overview with comparison of the Gomco clamp and the Plastibell device. *Pediatrics* 58:824, 1976.
21. Stock JA, Kaplan GW: Ketoconazole for prevention of postoperative penile erection. *Urology* 45:308, 1995.

Joel M.H. Teichman

Nocturnal Enuresis

How Common Is Nocturnal Enuresis?

Normal Childhood Development of Urinary Control

Nocturnal enuresis is defined as wetting the bed while sleeping in individuals who are beyond the age of expected dryness, usually around 5 years of age. Despite the fact that most children attain volitional control of micturition by age 5 years, nocturnal enuresis occurs in 20% of children aged 5 years, 7% of children aged 7 years, 5% of children aged 10 years, 3% of adolescents, and 1% of adults. In fact, an estimated 5 to 7 million children have nocturnal enuresis in the United States. Of these children, more than 60% wet the bed one or more times per week. The male to female ratio is 1.4 to 1. Nocturnal enuresis is the most common voiding problem seen in the office-based pediatric practice.

The spontaneous resolution rate is 15% per year. Because most children with nocturnal enuresis do resolve spontaneously in time, some clinicians tend to ignore nocturnal enuresis. However, nocturnal enuresis carries a significant psychosocial burden, especially for older children. Many nocturnal enuretic children will have problems with sleepover activities. They will either avoid such events, or have enuretic events during sleepovers. These children will encounter problems when asked to participate in sleepovers or at camp, or may refrain from inviting friends to play in their bedroom due to urine odor. The result may be embarrassment, poor self-esteem, social isolation, and impaired psychosocial development. Adolescent bedwetters may have problems relating to their peers. The costs of additional linen and laundry of linen and pajamas attributable to nocturnal enuresis may exceed $1000 per year per enuretic child. For these reasons, nocturnal enuresis should be addressed by clinicians when patients present with the problem.

In normal infants, bladder emptying occurs as a reflex mediated by the sacral micturition center (S2-4). In the micturition reflex, bladder filling triggers bladder stretch receptors, which triggers the micturition center to transmit efferent parasympathetic nerve impulses to the bladder, causing detrusor contractions that are coordinated with somatic efferents that inhibit the urethral sphincter. Thus, in response to bladder filling, there is a simultaneous reflex contraction of the bladder and bladder outlet relaxation, with complete evacuation of the bladder.

In infants, bladder emptying occurs often during the day and night. Between 6 and 12 months of age, the frequency of emptying decreases as the infant begins to develop supraspinal inhibition of this reflex. By 2 years of age, most children appreciate bladder fullness and can communicate the sensation. By 3 to 4 years of age, most children are able to postpone urination through cortical inhibition of the sacral micturition reflex. By 5 years of age, normal children can postpone micturition indefinitely, and micturition is "voluntarily" initiated only by the child releasing the cortical inhibition, which allows the involuntary sacral micturition reflex to proceed. In this fashion, nocturnal continence is maintained because the child does not release the cortical inhibition during sleep.

The typical sequence of bladder and bowel control is, first, daytime bladder control followed by daytime bowel control, nocturnal bowel control, and finally, nocturnal bladder control. Transient regressions or delays in toilet training are normal. Girls tend to reach these milestones sooner than boys, just as occurs with other developmental milestones.

Nocturnal urine output is also diminished in normal children and adults. There is a normal diurnal variation of arginine vasopressin (antidiuretic hormone), and vasopressin increases during sleep. The increased vasopressin causes increased urine osmolarity and decreased urine output during the night, which further aids in maintaining continence at night.

Causes of Nocturnal Enuresis

Nocturnal enuresis is multifactorial. Generally, it is caused by a delay in maturation of normal mechanisms that preserve continence during sleep. Thus, the nocturnal enuretic child tends not to reduce nocturnal urine production, fails to relax the bladder during sleep, and fails to arouse from sleep as the bladder fills. The balance between nocturnal urine production and bladder capacity is particularly important.

Urine overproduction during sleep may result from a lack of normal circadian variation in urine excretion. It has been postulated that patients do not sufficiently secrete arginine vasopressin and thus have low urinary osmolarity and increased urine volume. Failure of vasopressin secretion and high urine output of low osmolarity are seen in only some, but not all, nocturnal enuretic patients.

Bladder capacity in nocturnal enuretic children may be functionally reduced during sleep. Most nocturnal enuretic children have a normal bladder capacity while awake. Most of these children also have no daytime detrusor instability, and 70% of patients have no detrusor instability during sleep. Even in the 30% of children with nocturnal detrusor instability, daytime cystometrograms are normal. It is hypothesized that these children have a bladder contraction during sleep when their bladder reaches full capacity.

Failure of arousal from sleep may be a problem in enuretics. Parents claim that their nocturnal enuretic children sleep heavier than their non-enuretic children, although sleep studies typically show no difference from non-enuretics. Sleep arousal defects are often present, however, implying that enuretics fail to wake from sleep (as opposed to sleeping too deeply). Of note, adults with nocturnal enuresis tend to have enuretic episodes primarily during light sleep, in contrast to most children.

There is a familial predisposition to nocturnal enuresis. Children are more likely to have nocturnal enuresis if their parents had nocturnal enuresis (Table 5–1). Genetic studies show familial cohorts, citing specific abnormalities on the long arm of chromosome 13. The markers 13q13 and 13q14.2 are called ENUR1. Inheritance appears to be autosomal dominant with incomplete penetrance. Monozygotic twins are more likely than dizygotic twins to have nocturnal enuresis when one of the twins is enuretic, further demonstrating the genetic component. The fact that specific genetic factors have been identified is important to dispel notions that enuresis is behavioral.

There is no evidence that psychopathology causes nocturnal enuresis. Rather, the majority of affected patients have emotional problems secondary to the enuresis. The majority of enuretic children are psychiatrically normal. Rarely, specific psychosocial stressors may precipitate temporary secondary nocturnal enuresis. Nocturnal enuresis is not caused by excessive drinking before bed.

Table 5–1

Familial Predisposition to Nocturnal Enuresis

Parents With History of Nocturnal Enuresis	Risk of Offspring With Nocturnal Enuresis
0	15%
1	43%
2	77%

Differential Diagnosis

The differential diagnosis of nocturnal enuresis includes conditions with large urinary volumes (diabetes mellitus, diabetes insipidus, chronic renal failure, renal tubular acidosis, sickle cell disease); conditions with neurogenic bladder (spina bifida, spinal cord tumors, detrusor instability); bladder and bladder outlet conditions (cystitis, posterior urethral valves in boys, ectopic ureter in girls, interstitial cystitis); and perineal conditions that can result in urethral irritation (pinworms, vulvovaginitis).

Key History

The clinician should elicit a voiding history and voiding diary, along with information about any prior workup or therapy that has been instituted. For most children with primary nocturnal enuresis, the history will be straightforward, with no other urologic or medical problems present. The severity of enuresis is estimated by volume (large wet spots versus small drops of urine in pajamas or bed), the number of enuretic episodes per night, and the average number of enuretic nights per week. The clinician should also inquire whether the child has been previously dry at night. A history of nocturnal dryness for at least 6 months prior to enuresis defines secondary nocturnal enuresis. Secondary enuresis may indicate psychosocial stressors, but does not necessarily exclude "organic" nocturnal enuresis.

The history should focus on trying to identify or exclude specific etiologic abnormalities. A history of excessive thirst and polyuria suggests diabetes mellitus, diabetes insipidus, chronic renal failure, renal tubular acidosis, or sickle cell disease. Daytime voiding behavior is important, be-

cause children with both day and nighttime enuresis should be evaluated for true incontinence or Hinman syndrome (an acquired dyssynergic voiding pattern between the detrusor and sphincter). Obstructive voiding complaints (poor force of urinary stream, intermittency, sense of incomplete emptying, straining to void) suggest bladder outlet obstruction from either posterior urethral valves or Hinman syndrome. Urgency, frequency, and incontinence suggest detrusor instability. A history of "Vincent's curtsy," a squatting posture in girls where the heel compresses the perineum to obstruct the urethra and prevent incontinence, suggests detrusor instability. Urgency, frequency, and small voided volumes, with or without bladder pain, suggest interstitial cystitis, which can occur in children and adults. A history of urinary infections is important and warrants imaging to exclude structural abnormalities. (See Chapter 2.)

Bowel history and toileting practices should be elicited. Constipation may cause nocturnal enuresis. A neurologic history is relevant to determine if there are causes of a neuropathic bladder. Gait problems may indicate a spinal cord pathology (spina bifida), which may cause a neuropathic bladder. Overall growth rates (Friedman curves) are useful, and a failure to achieve appropriate growth may indicate chronic renal failure (a cause of polyuria).

Patients with renal tubular acidosis also tend to form stones, so a history of calculi should be elicited. Because these patients also suffer from a metabolic acidosis, they are prone to demineralize bones, and suffer from osteomalacia and growth abnormalities. A history of multiple fractures is often present.

Psychosocial history is relevant, although rarely the cause of nocturnal enuresis. Developmental milestones should be elicited. Most children reach day and night urine and bowel continence by age 5 years. Children who are slow to achieve urinary milestones tend to be slow to achieve other developmental milestones. Toilet training history (when started, if successful, ease of training) should be elicited.

Physical Examination

Overall patient appearance should be noted. Height, weight, and blood pressure are important (for general health and evidence of hypertension). The abdomen is examined for masses (giant hydronephrosis from ureteropelvic junction obstruction, vesicoureteral reflux, or bladder distension from posterior urethral valves). The back is inspected for midline abnormalities, sacral skin tuft, and asymmetry of the gluteal cleft, all of which may indicate spina bifida. A genital exam is done and the position of the urethra noted. Evidence of urinary leakage or secondary skin excoriation may be apparent. A vaginal exam is relevant for vaginal discharge, which suggests vulvovaginitis, or for an ectopic ureter, which may leak urine into the vagina. Rectal examination should elicit sphincter tone and presence of constipation. A neurologic exam is done with attention to deep tendon reflexes and perineal sensation and reflexes.

Laboratory Tests

Urinalysis (dipstick and microscopy) is indicated to look for infection (pyuria and bacteruria) and renal disease (proteinuria, casts, hematuria) and to screen for diabetes (glycosuria). Specific gravity is typically normal, although some nocturnal enuretics may have a low specific gravity. A low specific gravity may also indicate a concentration defect, suggesting renal insufficiency.

If infection is present, urine culture is indicated, and an imaging evaluation is indicated to exclude structural abnormalities. The typical imaging evaluation in children begins with renal/bladder ultrasound and voiding cystourethrogram. The voiding cystourethrogram should be delayed until after the urine is sterilized, to avoid the risk of seeding the upper tract with bacteria. Other imaging tests may be warranted depending on the results of the ultrasound and voiding cystourethrogram (see Chapter 2).

If neuropathic causes are suspected, urodynamic studies are indicated. An abnormally large bladder capacity may be seen in sensory or motor abnormalities of the bladder (spina bifida, spinal cord injury or tumor). Neurologic imaging may be warranted (MRI for spina bifida or spinal cord tumor). In spina bifida patients, the lumbosacral spine is usually abnormal on the scout film of the voiding cystourethrogram. Long-standing diabetes mellitus in adults often causes a sensory defect of the bladder, and later, a combined sensory and motor neurogenic bladder.

A 24-hour voiding log is essential. Normal bladder capacity in children is estimated by the formula: bladder capacity in ounces equals age in years + 2. Most enuretics have normal bladder capacity. Frequent, small voided volumes suggest interstitial cystitis, or detrusor instability (particularly if there is incontinence, too).

Management

General

It is important that a therapeutic relationship be established between the clinician and both patient and family. Because behavioral therapy requires cooperation, diligence, and long-term compliance, the clinician needs to communicate a realistic agenda. It is worthwhile to describe the anatomy and physiology of voiding in simple terms, and explain why enuresis occurs. Anatomic flip charts or diagrams are useful. This discussion is important both to family and child, as they will appreciate that the problem is physical, and not because the child is psychologically weak. It is therefore relevant to establish a supportive tone. Some families may already have punished, shamed, or ridiculed the enuretic child, further reinforcing poor self-esteem. A nonjudgmental request by the clinician will be useful to persuade the family to change this behavior. If the family appears to be dysfunctional or abusive, counseling or social service referral may be indicated.

The clinician should also discuss these matters with the child, using language that is age appropriate. Because these children have poor self-esteem, the clinician should communicate that nocturnal enuresis is common, affects classmates and family, and that the condition does not indicate that the child is "abnormal." Additionally, the clinician should communicate to the child that enuresis is not the child's fault.

Positive reinforcement is important to motivate the child. The clinician should establish a reward system, suggesting that the family keep a diary in which parents give the child two stars for a dry night, or one star for a night of reduced wetness. The stars can be placed into the diary, so that the child sees that progress is rewarded over time.

Behavioral Therapy

Behavioral therapy is the single most effective modality for treating enuresis. The most widely practiced form of behavioral therapy involves a bedwetting alarm. The alarm is a small device with a patch (moisture-sensing device) placed near the urethra or genitals. When the patch senses wetness, it triggers either a sound or vibratory alarm to awaken the child so that further bladder emptying can be prevented. Some authors feel the vibratory alarm is more effective than a sound alarm to arouse the child. Additionally, the patch may be examined in the morning for wet spots, which permits a rough estimate of the volume of enuresis. The family can record in the diary whether a large or small wet spot was present. Although the progression of large to small wet spots demonstrates improvement, even a small wet spot indicates continued nocturnal enuresis. The objective is to achieve a minimum of 3 consecutive weeks of complete nocturnal dryness.

The current bedwetting alarms are different than older models that were large, placed in a remote position, and used a buzzer that lead to buzzer ulcers. The current alarms are safe, inexpensive, and easy to use (Table 5–2).

The alarm uses operant conditioning to train the enuretic child to awaken upon the time of detrusor contraction. The enuretic is instructed that upon awakening, he or she should contract the pelvic floor muscles (primarily levator ani) at the time of a detrusor contraction. A sustained pelvic floor muscle contraction causes the detrusor to relax. The ultimate goal is to condition the child to arouse and awaken as their bladder fills, prior to enuresis, so as to inhibit the detrusor. The overall success rate of enuresis alarms is about 70%.

Conditioning with an alarm may be enhanced with five maneuvers. First, the clinician makes a written contract with the family that outlines what to do. Second, the clinician stresses the importance of full arousal. Third, the child remakes the bed after each wetting episode. Fourth, and most importantly, the clinician uses overconditioning. In

Table 5–2

Current Alarm Devices for Primary Nocturnal Enuresis

ALARM DEVICE	MANUFACTURER	MANUFACTURER TELEPHONE NO.	APPROXIMATE COST
Nite Train'r	Koregon Enterprises, Beaverton, OR	800-544-4240	$69
Nytone Enuretic Alarm	Nytone Medical Products, Salt Lake City, UT	801-973-4090	$54
Potty Pager	Ideas for Living, Boulder, CO	800-497-6573	$50
Sleep Dry	Star Child Labs, Aptos, CA	800-346-7283	$45
Wet-Stop	Palco Labs, Santa Cruz, CA	800-346-4488	$65

overconditioning, the child reaches a point of dryness for 3 consecutive weeks with the alarm. Then, the child is taught to drink 16 to 32 ounces of water before bed (to effect increased urine volume and increased bladder distension). The alarm is still used. Typically, enuretics will regress and have bedwetting episodes for about 1 week with the extra fluid and urine volume. Overconditioning is continued until 14 consecutive dry nights are achieved. Then the extra fluid and the alarm are stopped. Fifth, pelvic floor muscles exercises are taught (Kegel exercises). The use of these five maneuvers may increase long-term success by an additional 10%.

The alarm is not useful if the family and child are not motivated. Specifically, if the motivation is lacking such that the alarm sounds, the child wets, but does not awaken and go to the bathroom, then the conditioning exercise fails. The use of a written contract and explanation of realistic outcomes with the family may enhance family and patient motivation. Further, if the child has multiple enuretic episodes per night, the alarm would pose a risk of sleep deprivation. In this situation, the alarm may still be the best option.

Alternative use of the alarm is to arouse the child to void before enuresis occurs. This maneuver is not ideal, however, as the normal person does not need to awaken and void during the night to remain dry throughout sleep. An additional technique that has been described involves a noncontact alarm (a regular alarm clock). The alarm is set to sound and awaken the patient at a set time in sleep before enuresis; when awakened, the child goes to the bathroom to void. The initial success rate is about 70% but the relapse rate approaches 15% after cessation. This technique is simple, but again, the normal child does not need to awaken during sleep and void. Logically, the ultimate objective of behavioral therapy is not to train the child to awaken to void, but rather to suppress detrusor contraction as the bladder fills.

Other forms of behavioral therapy include hypnosis and trained awakenings. Success rates are as high as 90% but relapse rates exceed 20%.

Medical Management

DESMOPRESSIN

Desmopressin increases urine concentration and osmolarity, thereby decreasing urine output. The typical dose is to begin with 10 µg nasal spray, or a 100- to 400-µg oral dose, given at bedtime. The nasal spray is more expensive than the oral tablets. Desmopressin is effective for short-term therapy and may be indicated for patients when they go on sleepovers or for camp. It also is more effective in patients with a family history of nocturnal enuresis compared to those with a negative family history. Desmopressin is particularly effective in patients who have nocturnal enuresis with no daytime incontinence, urgency, or evidence of detrusor instability (monosymptomatic primary nocturnal enuresis).

Desmopressin has been used continuously up to 1 year in duration with good results and no evidence of increased side effects. A potential adverse effect of desmopressin is water intoxication (which if severe and left untreated may produce hyponatremia and seizures). More common and fortunately less severe side effects include nasal stuffiness and epistaxis (from the nasal spray). All forms of desmopressin may cause headaches, abdominal pain, nausea, and bad taste.

IMIPRAMINE

Tricyclic antidepressants have multiple mechanisms of action. For nocturnal enuresis, imipramine may lighten sleep (increase the ratio of non-REM to REM sleep) and make arousal easier as the bladder fills. The best studied tricyclic antidepressant for this indication is imipramine, typically started as a 25-mg oral dose 1 hour before bedtime, and increased to 50 mg after 2 weeks in children aged 7 to 12 years, and up to 75 mg in older children. The optimal duration of treatment is unknown and some authors recommend weaning children after 6 months of therapy. Weaning should involve incremental reductions of 25 mg over 3 to 4 months, with alternate night

Figure 5–1

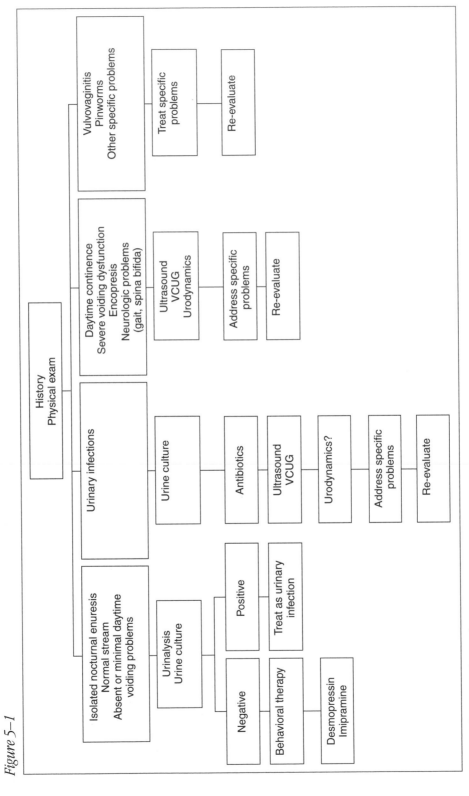

Algorithm for nocturnal enuresis.

dosing for the last week. Abrupt discontinuation, rather than weaning, may produce temporary lethargy, depression, and other withdrawal symptoms. The success rate is between 10% and 60%, and relapse is likely after discontinuation of imipramine.

Imipramine also acts as an anticholinergic drug, thus inhibiting the detrusor. Side effects include dry mouth, anxiety, sleep problems, constipation, and cardiac arrhythmias. It is unlikely that the anticholinergic effect is helpful, as anticholinergic drugs overall (oxybutynin, tolterodine, hyocyamine, probantheline) are not useful in nocturnal enuresis unless detrusor overactivity is present. Tricyclic antidepressants should also be used with caution, as fatal overdose has been reported. The clinician should instruct the parents to keep tricyclic antidepressants in a secure location, where the child cannot accidentally access the medication. If the clinician is not confident that the medication can be kept secure, or if compliance with exact dosing is an issue, tricyclic antidepressants should be avoided.

Treating Specific Abnormalities

For enuretic children with specific abnormalities detected, the underlying disorders should be addressed and enuresis reevaluated after management. Urinary infection is an unlikely cause of enuresis, but when present and treated successfully, 28% of children will become dry. Thus, the value of specific antibiotic management is clear. But the need to reassess the child is evident, because the majority of these children (with cystitis and enuresis) will still have enuresis after successful cystitis management.

Algorithm

The approach to diagnosing and managing nocturnal enuresis is shown in Fig. 5–1. In general, behavioral therapy is the mainstay of management for primary nocturnal enuresis. Drug therapy should be used in addition to behavioral therapy, and currently is considered best used for short-term therapy. Drug therapy does not cure enuresis, but may be used as a temporary measure until enuretic patients are able to wake and void on their own. Adults with nocturnal enuresis may be refractory to all options. A prolonged management approach using all available modalities may be necessary in adults.

Bibliography

Cendron M: Primary nocturnal enuresis. *Am Fam Physician* 59:1205–1213, 1999.

Issenman RM, Filmer RB, Gorski PA: A review of bowel and bladder control development in children: How gastrointestinal and urologic conditions relate to problems in toilet training. *Pediatrics* 103(suppl): 1346–1352, 1999.

Moffatt M: Nocturnal enuresis: A review of the efficacy of treatments and practice advice for clinicians. *J Dev Behav Pediatr* 18:49–56, 1997.

Norgaard JP, Djurhuus JC, Watanabe H, et al: Experience and current status of research into the pathophysiology of nocturnal enuresis. *Br J Urol* 79: 825–835, 1997.

Vandersteen DR, Husmann DA: Treatment of primary nocturnal enuresis persisting into adulthood. *J Urol* 161:90–92, 1999.

Warzak WJ: Psychosocial implications of nocturnal enuresis. *Pediatr Clin* 32(suppl):38–40, 1993.

Part

2

Common Adult Genitourinary Problems

J. Curtis Nickel

Urinary Tract Infections in Adults

Introduction

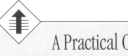

A Practical Classification System for General Practice

Many clinicians have become complacent in their attitude towards the diagnosis and treatment of urinary tract infection (UTI). We are sure of our ability to diagnose urinary tract infections, have become adept in development of new antibiotics that appear to keep us one step ahead of bacterial resistance emergence, and remain confident that we can continue to do this indefinitely.

In reality, our microbiologic diagnostic methods have not really advanced over the last half century, microbial resistance is increasing more rapidly than ever before, antimicrobial research appears to be in stagnation, and infection of the urinary tract continues to cause significant morbidity and even mortality. We have not decreased the number of individuals suffering symptoms and morbidity of such infections. We continue to spend billions of health care dollars on antimicrobial treatment, hospitalization, and other treatments. There is also a significant economic loss to society in lost work time.

Urinary tract infections continue to occupy a large proportion of the primary care clinician's practice. Urinary tract infections result in millions of office visits per year, are the leading cause of gram-negative sepsis in hospitalized patients, and catheter-associated infections are thought to significantly increase mortality rates in hospitalized patients. Thus, we should not become complacent about this very significant health care problem, and clinicians need to develop a rational and coherent management plan. Primary care clinicians must maintain an interest in urinary tract infection, must understand the mechanisms that result in such infection, and need to develop a rational, therapeutic strategy that incorporates the most up-to-date evidence-based information available to them.

Over the years a great number of systems have been proposed to allow clinicians to classify their patients with UTIs.[1,2] The only useful classification systems are those that can be used in clinical practice to rationalize and direct management strategies. Only two systems have emerged to fulfill this criterion, and only these two will be used in the discussion in this chapter.

The most familiar system is a descriptive one (Table 6–1) that categorizes infections by the specific organ system involved. Although easy to understand, it is not as clinically useful as the second system (Table 6–2), which simply divides urinary tract infections into two categories. This categorization of UTIs into uncomplicated ("simple") and complicated allows the physician to develop a rational diagnostic treatment algorithm that is useful in clinical practice. Both of these classification systems will be used in this chapter, with an emphasis placed on first deciding whether or not the patient has an uncomplicated or complicated urinary tract infection, developing a general diagnostic plan dependent on this, and finally directing a specific management and therapeutic strategy based on the final descriptive diagnostic classification (Fig. 6–1).

Table 6–1

Organ (Location)-Specific Classification of UTIs

Urethritis
Prostatitis
Cystitis
Pyelonephritis

Table 6–2

Uncomplicated/Complicated Classification of UTIs

UNCOMPLICATED ("SIMPLE") UTI
Infection of the urinary tract with no predisposing or associated factors • Cystitis in premenopausal female • Recurrent cystitis in premenopausal female • Unobstructed pyelonephritis
COMPLICATED UTI

Infection associated with an anatomic, metabolic, immunologic, neurogenic, or foreign body factor
1. Anomaly causing obstruction, stasis, or reflux
   • Prostatic hyperplasia
   • Neurogenic bladder
   • Strictures
   • Vesicoureteral reflux
   • Other congenital anomalies
2. Foreign body
   • Urinary catheter, stent, nephrostomy tube
   • Instrument manipulation (cystoscope)
3. Infected urinary stones
   • Struvite (infection-induced) calculi
   • Secondarily infected calculi
4. Immunologic or biologic disorders allowing bacterial persistence
   • Chronic bacterial prostatitis
   • Immunosuppression
   • Pregnancy
   • Diabetes

Uncomplicated Urinary Tract Infection

Simple Cystitis

Episodic bacterial cystitis in premenopausal (and usually sexually active) women is the easiest UTI to understand.[1–3] Patients with this uncomplicated UTI complain of pain on micturition, urinary frequency, urgency, suprapubic discomfort, and occasionally hematuria. Laboratory findings include at least 10 leukocytes per spun high-power field on microscopy and bacteruria of at least 10^3 colony-forming units per mL of urine.

These infections occur because of a change in the balance between the defense factors of the host and the virulence of enteric bacteria. Host defenses include competitive inhibition by favorable bacteria (lactobacilli) within the vagina and the distal urethra (effectively competitively inhibiting the colonization by potential uropathogenic bacteria from the gut), immunologic and chemical antimicrobial factors within the urine, the mucosa of the bladder and urethra, and the mechanical, repetitive washing/evacuation action of the bladder by the very act of voiding itself. When there is some subtle defect or alteration in these host defenses or an increase in virulence of particular bacteria, colonization of the vagina and distal urethra by uropathogenic bacteria occurs and subsequently the scenario is set for the establishment of bacterial cystitis. Sexual intercourse, some types of reversible contraception (antispermicide cream, diaphragm), and ineffective voiding routine can all contribute to the propensity for development of such infections in susceptible individuals.

The presentation of simple cystitis is characteristic and well recognized by both primary care clinicians and their patients, and the treatment is simple. Pyuria is established by either microscopy or dipstick (leukocyte esterase or nitrites), and in the case of a first episode, a midstream urine culture is indicated. The most likely organism is *Escherichia coli* followed by *Staphylococcus saprophyticus*, but other bacteria can also be involved in simple cystitis. The patient is started on a short course of a first-line antibiotic (Table 6–4).

It appears from a review of the literature that 3 days of treatment is superior to single-dose therapy, and in the particular case of simple cystitis, longer therapy may offer no further advantages.

Figure 6–1

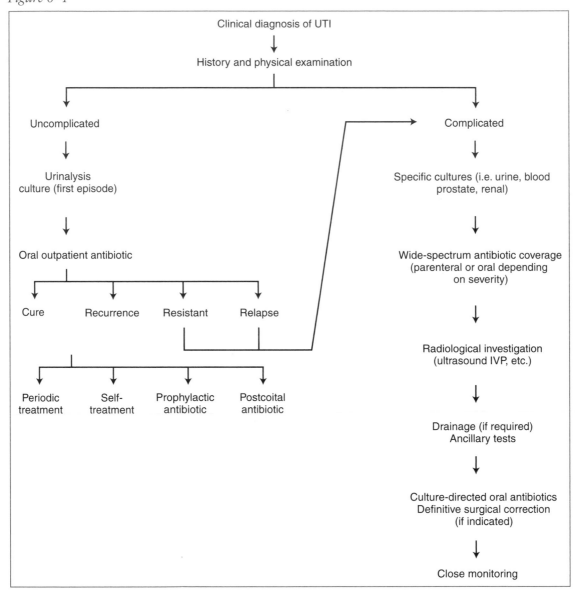

Clinical management of UTI.

The antibiotics of choice for simple cystitis include the fluoroquinolones, trimethroprim-sulfamethoxazole (or trimethroprim alone), or nitrofurantoin. The dose, adverse effects, and potential drug interactions should be familiar to all clinicians (Table 6–4).

Recurrent Simple Cystitis

Many susceptible, sexually active, premenopausal women develop constellations of recurrent infections. These can occur at a rate of 1 or 2 per year or even 1 or 2 per month. A treatment goal for

Table 6–3

Treatment Options for Recurrent Cystitis in Females

1. Episodic physician directed antimicrobial therapy
2. Self-treatment directed antimicrobial therapy
3. Long-term low-dose prophylactic antimicrobial therapy
4. Postcoital antimicrobial therapy

these patients is not only amelioration of symptoms but prevention of further infections, and reducing morbidity when infections do occur. Although debatable, there appears to be little benefit in repeating investigations such as urinalysis and culture in patients with recurrent simple cystitis. Patients who have suffered one or two episodes of simple cystitis will be able to distinguish and self-diagnose another subsequent episode. If treatment fails after 48 hours, however, the patient should be instructed to seek medical attention. At that time, the physician should consider a either resistant organism or a more complicated infection.

Table 6–3 outlines the various treatment options available to the physician for patients with recurrent simple cystitis. The patients need not and should not have to wait until the next available appointment to see their physician for antibiotic prescription for each individual episode of cystitis. This will increase the morbidity, time loss at work, and costs associated with recurrent infections.

The most effective therapeutic plan for the prevention of recurrent cystitis is low-dose antimicrobial prophylaxis. Any of the front-line medications can be taken at one quarter of the regular daily dose, usually in the evening for a protracted period of time (6 to 12 weeks). This in itself will significantly reduce the rate of recurrent urinary tract infections and in many cases breaks the cycle of recurrent infections. If a patient continues to have infections after cessation of this low-dose prophylaxis, then a prolonged course of antimicrobial prophylaxis with alternate-day therapy may be considered. Alternatively, in sexually active young women, postcoital antibiotic dosing (one dose of a front-line antibiotic taken after intercourse) has been suggested to reduce the rate of recurrent urinary tract infections.

Table 6–4

Antimicrobial Regimes for Uncomplicated UTIs

ANTIBIOTIC	DOSE	DURATION
Cystitis		
Trimethoprim (TMP)	200 mg	q 12 h × 3 days
Trimethoprim/sulfamethoxazole (TMP/SMX)	160/800 mg	q 12 h × 3 days
Norfloxacin	400 mg	q 12 h × 3 days
Ciprofloxacin	250 mg	q 12 h × 3 days
Ofloxacin	200 mg	q 12 h × 3 days
Nitrofurantoin	100 mg	q 6 h × 3 days
Macrocrystalline nitrofurantoin	100 mg	q 12 h × 3 days
Pyelonephritis (Oral Therapy[a])		
TMP/SMX	160/800 mg	q 12 h × 14 days
TMP	200 mg	q 12 h × 14 days
Norfloxacin	400 mg	q 12 h × 14 days
Ciprofloxacin	500 mg	q 12 h × 14 days
Ofloxacin	300 mg	q 12 h × 14 days

[a] Following initial parenteral dose of antibiotics (gentamicin/ampicillin).

In reasonably intelligent, motivated patients, a self-treatment program can be helpful. In this case, a supply of antibiotics with appropriate instructions is issued to the patient. When she develops symptoms of simple cystitis, she will take a 3-day course of the front-line antibiotic prescribed. If she is not improving by 48 hours, she will contact her physician, for an evaluation that should include urine culture and a prescription of a different antibiotic. The patient should keep a diary of the number of times she requires self-treatment, and this can be reviewed with her physician at periodic health care visits. It has been the experience of most clinicians who have used the self-treatment program that patients do not take antibiotics indiscriminately but judiciously, and treat themselves only when convinced that cystitis has developed and will not resolve spontaneously.

Acute Nonobstructive Pyelonephritis

Acute, uncomplicated, nonobstructive pyelonephritis is a clinical syndrome characterized by fever, chills, flank pain, and a positive urine culture (greater than 10^3 CFU/mL) with associated pyuria. This syndrome occurs almost exclusively in the same patient population that develops simple, uncomplicated cystitis—premenopausal women.

The great majority of episodes result from E. coli, with other organisms such as S. saprophyticus, Klebsiella pneumoniae, and Proteus mirabilis making up less than a quarter of these episodes. Most E. coli isolated from patients with acute, uncomplicated pyelonephritis have a phenotypic expression of P-fimbriae, although this interesting finding currently plays no role in the primary care clinician's treatment algorithm.

It can usually be expected that women with no anatomic or functional problems (see "Acute Complicated Pyelonephritis" later in the chapter) who are otherwise healthy will respond promptly to antibiotic therapy, and there is almost no long-term morbidity. If possible, patients diagnosed with acute, uncomplicated

pyelonephritis can be managed as outpatients (Table 6–5). An initial single parenteral dose of IV or IM antibiotic (ampicillin plus gentamicin or equivalent cephalosporin antibiotic) is helpful, and then the patient is discharged home on oral therapy (Table 6–5). Follow-up, including repeat cultures and an abdominal ultrasound to rule out structural abnormalities, can be arranged once the patient has clinically improved, but the rate of underlying congenital urinary abnormalities is quite low (Fig. 6–2).

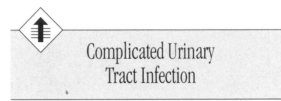

Complicated Urinary Tract Infection

Complicated UTIs are associated with predisposing factors that decrease antibacterial defense mechanisms of the urinary tract.[1-3] These structural or functional abnormalities include indwelling catheters, anatomic abnormalities of the urinary tract causing stasis or obstruction, urolithiasis, malignancy, abnormal (neurogenic) bladder function, foreign bodies, and immunologic problems (Table 6–2). These infections are characterized by systemic symptoms (fever, sepsis), persistence, progression, and relapse.

The approach to complicated UTIs is entirely different from that of an uncomplicated infection. The patient must be thoroughly assessed with urine and blood cultures, assessment of renal function, hospitalization (in many cases), wide-spectrum intravenous antibiotic therapy, hemodynamic support (if associated with sepsis), rapid evaluation of the genitourinary tract with radiologic investigation and in many cases endoscopy, and early initiation of urinary drainage procedures. Definitive therapy may require close monitoring of urine cultures, suppressive antibiotic therapy, prophylactic antibiotic therapy, and/or surgery (Fig. 6–1).

Although E. coli still causes a significant number of complicated infections, the majority are caused by other bacteria including Enterococcus faecalis,

Figure 6–2

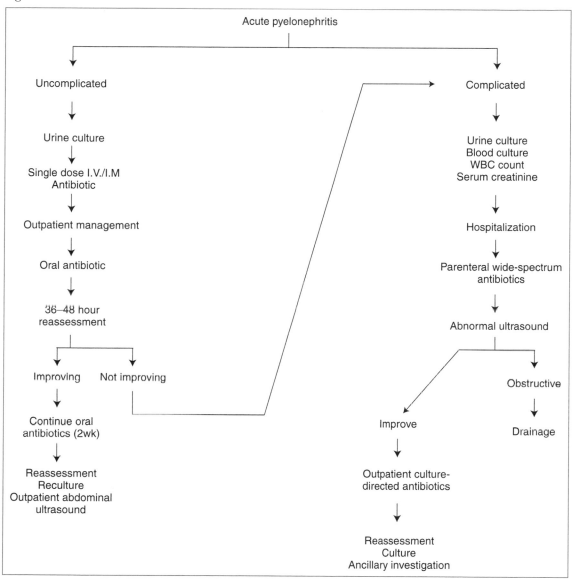

Treatment algorithm for acute pyelonephritis.

Pseudomonas, Proteus, Serratia, Klebsiella, and *Enterobacter.* Combination therapy with several antibiotics is usually required to cure complicated UTI associated with sepsis. Combination therapy with a beta-lactamase inhibitor and beta-lactam, aminoglycoside and beta-lactam, and macrolides and fluoroquinolones are very effective in treating complicated UTIs (Table 6–6).

The patient should be continued on parenteral drugs until the fever has abated and the clinical danger has passed. The patient should then be treated with culture-specific oral drugs. To illus-

Table 6–5

Important Considerations in Outpatient Antibiotic Use[a]

ANTIMICROBIAL	COMMENTS	ADVERSE EFFECTS	DRUG INTERACTIONS
Fluoroquinolones (norfloxacin, ciprofloxacin, ofloxacin)	• Safe • Wide-spectrum activity for gram-negative (and some gram-positive) bacteria • High tissue penetration	• GI symptoms • CNS symptoms • Photosensitivity	• Theophylline • Caffeine • Warfarin • Antacids
Nitrofurantoin (and macro-crystalline nitrofurantoin)	• High urinary concentration • Acts against *E. coli, S. saprophyticus*, and enterococci • Not in vaginal secretions (decrease yeast vaginitis)	• GI symptoms • Skin rashes • Peripheral polyneuropathy (rare) • Pulmonary hypersensitivity reaction (rare) • Hepatitis (rare)	• Magnesium salts
Aminopenicillins (ampicillin, amoxicillin)	• Long experience • Increasing bacterial resistance	• Yeast vaginitis • Hypersensitivity reactions (rash, anaphylaxis) • GI symptoms	• Allopurinol • Birth control pills
Penicillin plus beta-lactamase inhibitor (amoxicillin plus clavulinic acid and ampicillin plus sulbactam)	Useful against most beta-lactamase-producing strains of *E. coli, S. aureus, S. epidermidis, Klebsiella, Proteus*	Same as with aminopenicillins	Same as with amino-penicillins
Trimethoprim/sulfamethoxazole	Synergistic bacteriocidal activity against most gram-positive and gram-negative uropathogens	• Anaphylaxis • Hematological effects • Rash • Folate deficiency • Stevens–Johnson syndrome (rare)	• Warfarins • Sulfylureas • Phenytoin
Trimethoprim	Like TMP/SMX but perhaps less toxic	Similar to TMP/SMX	Similar to TMP/SMX
Cephalosporins (cephalexin)	Active against most gram-positive and many gram-negative uropathogens	• Hypersensitivity • Penicillin allergy • Drug fever	• Alcohol • Warfarin • Heparin • Vitamin K

[a] The practicing physician must be aware not only of the advantages of oral antibiotic use for the therapy of UTIs but of adverse effects and potential drug interactions associated with each drug.

Table 6–6

Antimicrobial Regimes for Complicated UTIs

Single Agent
- Beta-lactams
  Penicillins (piperacillin)
  Cephalosporins (ceftazidime)
  Carbapenems (imipenem)
  Monobactems (aztreonam)
- Fluoroquinolones (ciprofloxacin, ofloxacin)

Combination Therapy
- Beta-lactamase inhibitors and beta-lactam (clavulinic acid and amoxicillin)
- Aminoglycosides and beta-lactam (gentamicin and ampicillin)
- Aminoglycoside and cephalosporin (gentamicin and ceftazidime)

trate this approach, a number of complicated UTIs are described next, along with a rational management plan.

Acute Complicated Pyelonephritis

Acute pyelonephritis associated with obstruction, renal abnormalities, reflux, or stones, and all pyelonephritis in children, is recognized as a complicated UTI.[1,2] In these patients, attention must be paid to the integrity of the kidney and the development of bacteremia and sepsis. Patients with severe systemic symptoms, high fever, and nausea and vomiting should be hospitalized and parenteral therapy administered until fever has resolved. Therapy in this case would be gentamicin (usually with ampicillin to cover *Enterobacter*), trimethoprim/sulfamethoxazole, ceftriaxone, ciprofloxacin, or ofloxacin.

If symptoms do not resolve rapidly (and even when they do), further evaluation should be done, including abdominal ultrasonography, plain x-ray of the abdomen, and perhaps an intravenous pyelogram. In some patients, CT of the kidney is necessary to determine the extent of the disease and to rule out the presence of perinephric or renal abscess in patients who are not responding. With infections complicated with obstruction, stones, and so forth, the obstruction must be relieved; otherwise a pyonephrosis (pus building up under pressure in an obstructed collecting system) can develop. This can cause serious renal damage and sepsis. In this case a percutaneous nephrostomy would be the treatment of choice. Occasionally gas can be associated with pyelonephritis. Close monitoring is all that is necessary if the gas is within the collecting system. However, if gas develops within the renal parenchyma (emphysematous pyelonephritis), the advice and help of a urologic specialist is indicated for consideration of surgery (nephrectomy) or percutaneous drainage.

Catheter-Associated UTI

Catheters are routinely used in primary care settings to facilitate drainage of the urinary tract in incontinent patients who have lower urinary tract obstruction, or to allow urinary output determinations in ill patients.[4–6] Catheter associated sepsis is still the leading cause of gram-negative sepsis leading to mortality in our hospitals today. However, because all catheters become colonized with bacteria, indiscriminate antibiotic therapy of asymptomatic bacteruria associated with catheters will just lead to the emergence of resistant bacterial strains.

Therefore, the best advice for the management of infections associated with catheters is to remove the catheter as soon as possible, or perhaps switch to intermittent catheterization. If a catheter has to remain in place, even for a short period of time, strict adherence to a closed urinary drainage system is mandatory to reduce the emergence of bacterial colonization in subsequent infection. Antibiotic prophylaxis in patients at risk who are to undergo short-term catheterization (less than

3 days) may be indicated. If the patient does become symptomatic, wide-spectrum antibiotic therapy will help suppress the symptoms; but unless the catheter is removed, the infection will return. For patients with long-term catheterization, it may be appropriate to remove the catheter and then replace it after several hours of appropriate antibiotic therapy.

Urinary Stones

Struvite (or infection) stones are a serious threat to the integrity of the urinary tract.[7] They can occur in the bladder associated with stagnant urine or in a damaged kidney. They are caused by urinary tract infection with a urease-splitting bacteria (usually *Proteus mirabilis*), which results in precipitation of magnesium-ammonium-phosphate crystals and a subsequent emergence of a soft crystalline and matrix stone that can take the structural shape of the renal pelvis (hence its name, staghorn calculus). Calcium oxalate and other types of stones that are not formed from infection can become secondarily infected and lead to similar problems within the urinary tract. Infections associated with stones cannot be cured with antibiotic therapy alone and the stone must be removed (either endoscopically, percutaneously, or with extracorporal shock-wave lithotripsy or open surgery). Antibiotics should be prescribed during and for sometime after the stone is removed. If any stone remains, it is most likely that the infection will recur.

Pregnancy

It is now generally acknowledged that a pregnant woman who develops simple cystitis or even asymptomatic bacteriuria has a higher likelihood of suffering from acute pyelonephritis of pregnancy.[2] Pyelonephritis in pregnancy predisposes to both maternal and fetal morbidity. Short courses (even a single dose or 48-hour short course) are useful in these patients as long as repeat culture shows no evidence of bacteriuria. However, these women need to have repeated monitored cultures at each clinical visit.

If patients have recurrent episodes, low-dose prophylaxis medication, such as nitrofurantoin at night, could be indicated. Women with recurrent cystitis have been successfully treated using nightly prophylaxis and postcoital antibiotics as described in the "Recurrent Simple Cystitis" section earlier in the chapter.

Hospitalization is generally recommended for "simple" acute pyelonephritis in pregnant patients because of the small percentage who develop acute respiratory distress syndrome after initiation of antibacterial therapy. However, new research suggests that some patients may be managed as outpatients in selected cases. Drugs suggested for therapy during acute pyelonephritis in pregnancy include gentamicin (with or without ampicillin), aztreonam, a cephalosporin, or trimethoprim/sulfamethoxazole (except in the last trimester). Fluoroquinolones should be avoided in pregnant women because of teratogenicity, as should trimethoprim and/or sulfamethoxazole in the third trimester.

Urinary Tract Infection in the Elderly

Urinary tract infection is the most frequent bacterial infection in the elderly.[8,9] Its optimal management is essential to clinicians providing primary care to older populations of patients. Institutionalized elderly have an even higher incidence of urinary tract infections, related not only to long-term indwelling catheterization but also to impaired immune defense, impaired bladder function, and other factors. Bacteriuria can exist in anywhere from 5% to 30% of older patients (compared to a prevalence of less than 5% in young women). Although *E. coli* is still the single most frequent organism isolated, there is an increased prevalence of gram-positive organisms as well as those bacteria more commonly associated with complicated UTIs. Mixed infections also frequently occur in the elderly; however, potential difficulties in obtaining an adequate urine sample for culture must always be considered by the primary care physician.

Symptomatic urinary tract infection in the elderly usually presents with clinical symptoms similar to those in younger patients. They should be treated in a similar way: classification as complicated or uncomplicated and treatment directed based on that diagnosis. However, because of poor bladder emptying associated with aging, most infections are complicated. In patients with complicated UTI secondary to obstructive uropathy (high residual urine), stones, tumors, or strictures, long-term prophylactic or suppressive therapy may be required to prevent symptomatic recurrences.

Many studies have attempted to determine the real morbidity and mortality resulting from asymptomatic bacteriuria. Although some studies suggest that asymptomatic bacteriuria in the elderly is associated with decreased survival in both men and women, other studies have failed to confirm this association. Given the relatively limited morbidity identified with asymptomatic bacteriuria in the elderly, it would seem appropriate that antimicrobials not be used to treat asymptomatic bacteria. In fact, it may be counterproductive in that most bacteriuria usually recurs and in many cases with a more resistant organism if treatment has previously been given. Others have suggested if asymptomatic bacteriuria occurs with pyuria, treatment is indicated; however, based on various outcome studies, this recommendation for treatment of asymptomatic bacteriuria is also not currently justified.

Prostatitis

ACUTE BACTERIAL PROSTATITIS

Prostatitis is usually thought of as a complicated UTI.[10, 11] Acute bacterial prostatitis is a significant infection of the prostate gland associated with generalized symptoms of impending or real sepsis. The patient presents with suprapubic and perineal pain, difficult painful urination, fever, and other signs of systemic infection. Following a clinical diagnosis based on history and physical examination alone, culture of the urine and blood is all that is necessary at the initial step before proceeding with therapy. If the patient has an obstructed bladder outlet (as is usual), insertion of a Foley catheter will provide relief. Sometimes a urethral catheter is too painful and difficult to insert or will have to be removed because of discomfort. In that case a suprapubic cystotomy would be indicated.

Wide-spectrum intravenous antibiotics should be continued until the patient is afebrile. This usually means an admission to hospital. If the patient's fever is not responding in 36 to 48 hours, ultrasonography—preferably a transrectal ultrasound approach—or alternatively a CAT scan is indicated to rule out prostatic abscess that would require surgical drainage. Otherwise the patients usually improve within 36 to 48 hours and can be switched to culture- and sensitivity-directed oral antibiotic therapy. Oral antibiotic therapy should be continued for at least 4 weeks. The best therapy is a fluoroquinolone, trimethoprim/sulfamethoxazole, or trimethoprim alone.

CHRONIC PROSTATITIS

Patients with a chronic prostatitis syndrome present with a long history (at least 3 months) of genital, urinary, and perineal pain associated with variable obstructive and irritative voiding symptoms. A major sexual symptom is pain on ejaculation. In these patients, categorization of the infection based on culture and microscopy can be very important in deciding appropriate long-term treatment. Although urologists tend to use the more elaborate four-glass culture of the lower urinary tract, it is difficult or even impossible for most clinicians to do this. Instead, the pre- and postmassage test (PPMT) is advocated. In this test, a urine specimen is taken just before and just after a vigorous prostate massage. The urine specimens before and after prostate massage (labeled pre-M and post-M) are subjected to culture (routine culture and sensitivity as for any other urine specimen) and microscopy of the centrifuged specimen. Patients with uropathogenic bacteruria and inflammatory cells in the post-M specimen compared to the pre-M specimen are diagnosed with chronic bacterial prostatitis. This is quite rare and will only account for about 5% of patients. Incidentally, the findings on prostate massage are not definitive for either chronic prostatitis or specifically for one type of prostatitis or another (Fig. 6–3).

Each patient should be treated with definitive antibiotic therapy for as long as 6 to 12 weeks. The antibiotics that have demonstrated the best prostate drug levels and efficacy include all the available fluoroquinolones and trimethoprim-sulfamethoxazole (or trimethoprim alone). Suppressive prophylactic antibiotics may be indicated for patients with relapsing or recurrent bacterial prostatitis.

The majority of patients show no excessive uropathogenic bacteruria in the post-M specimen. Those with excessive leukocytes (greater than 5 white blood cells per high-power field) in the post-M specimen can be categorized as chronic nonbacterial prostatitis. Because it is unclear whether some of these patients' symptoms maybe due to unculturable or cryptic infections, a 6-week trial of antibiotics is indicated. Again, as in chronic bacterial prostatitis, the fluoroquinolones or trimethroprim/sulfamethoxazole is appropriate. Because of the possibility of *Chlamydia* or *Ureaplasma* causing the symptoms, a trial of tetracycline (Vibramycin) or erythromycin may also be helpful. Alpha-blockade for patients with obstructive symptoms can be helpful. In those with boggy, tender prostate glands, repetitive prostate massage (done 2 or 3 times a week for 6 weeks) combined with antibiotics is also beneficial. If this is not helpful, urologic consultation is required.

PROSTATODYNIA

Patients who have no evidence of pathogenic bacteruria or inflammatory infiltrate (leukocytosis) in the post-M specimen are diagnosed with prostatodynia. Because this may not be due to prostate pathology at all, it may be more appropriate to call this pelvic floor myalgia or chronic pelvic/perineal pain syndrome. Due to of the vagaries of diagnosis, at least one short course (4 weeks) of antibiotics is indicated. If this is of no benefit, antibiotics should not be used again. Therapy that is helpful includes alpha-blockers (terazosin), analgesics (and/or anti-inflammatories), and muscle relaxants (diazepam) either sequentially, or better, concurrently. If this fails to provide any benefit to the patient, urologic consultation may be helpful. Some of these patients may have interstitial cystitis (see Chapter 9). Unfortunately, however, the urologist will likely also find no pathology and will have few other options to offer this particular patient. Individual psychotherapy and supportive therapies as well as other alternative medical approaches may be of benefit to the patient with pelvic floor myalgia. In the end, he needs to be treated like any other chronic pain syndrome patient.

Summary

Primary care clinicians are and should be the first contact for patients presenting with UTIs, whether uncomplicated or complicated. Clinicians need to periodically review the etiologic and diagnostic considerations and be sure that they understand the constantly evolving principles of microbial therapy. More importantly, the committed primary care physician must develop a personal evidence-based diagnostic approach and a rational therapeutic plan for patient care in the field of infectious disease of the urinary tract.

Figure 6–3

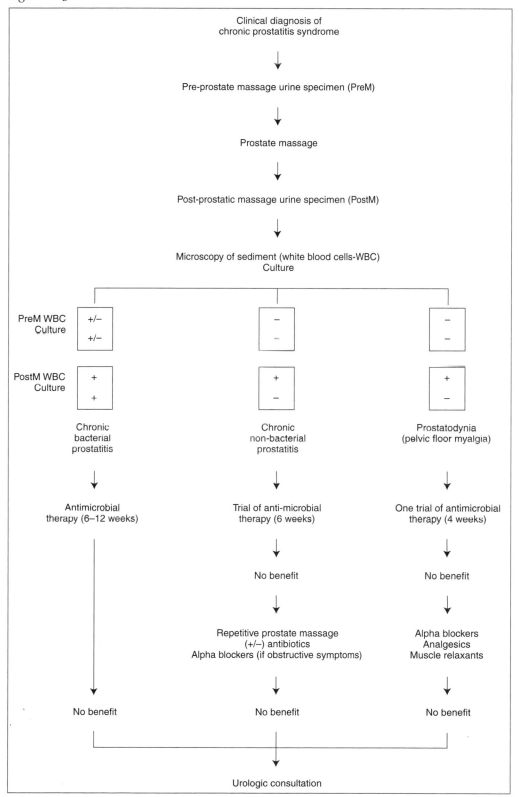

Clinical diagnostic algorithm for chronic prostatitis syndromes.

References

1. Nickel JC: Special consideration in the management of complicated urinary tract infections. In Harrison LH (ed): *Management of Urinary Tract Infections. International Congress and Symposium Series.* New York, Royal Society of Medicine Services, 1990, pp 89–99.

2. Nickel JC: A practical approach to urinary tract infections. *Can J Diagnosis* 10:64, 1993.

3. Nickel JC: The battle of the bladder: The pathogenesis of uncomplicated cystitis. *Int Urogynecol J* 1:218, 1990.

4. Nickel JC, Feero P, Costerton JW, Wilson E: Incidence and significance of bacteriuria in postoperative, short-term urinary catheterization. *Can J Surg* 32:131, 1989.

5. Nickel JC: Catheter-associated urinary tract infections: A new perspective on an old problem. *Can J Infect Cont* 6:38, 1991.

6. Nickel JC: Catheter-associated urinary tract infections. In Mandell GL, Sobel JD (eds): *Atlas of Infectious Diseases. Urinary Tract Infections and Infections of the Female Pelvis.* Philadelphia, Current Medicine, 1997.

7. McLean RJC, Stickler DJ, Nickel JC: Biofilm mediated calculus formation in the urinary tract. *Cells Materials* 6:165, 1996.

8. Nickel JC, Pidutti R: A rational approach to urinary tract infections in older patients. *Geriatrics* 47:49, 1992.

9. Nickel JC: Severe urinary tract infection in elderly men and women: A rational approach to diagnosis and treatment. In Sinclair A, Woodhouse K (eds): *Acute Medical Illness in the Elderly.* London, Chapman & Hall, 1995, pp 213–234.

10. Nickel JC: A practical approach to the management of prostatitis. *Techniques Urol* 1:162,1995.

11. Nickel JC: Prostatitis: Myths and realities. *Urology* 51:362, 1998.

For More Detailed Reading

Kunin CM (ed): *Detection, Prevention and Management of Urinary Tract Infection.* Baltimore, Williams & Wilkins, 1997.

Mulholland SG (ed): *Antibiotic Therapy in Urology.* Philadelphia, Lippincott-Raven, 1996.

Bergan T (ed): *Urinary Tract Infections.* Basel, Karger, 1997.

Dalhoff A: *Pharmacokinetics of Selected Antibacterial Agents.* Basel, Karger, 1998.

Stephen Lynch

Chapter 7

Urethritis

How Common Is Urethral Discharge?

Discharge in Males and Females

Urethral discharge is largely caused by sexually transmitted diseases (STDs). The two most common pathogens causing urethral discharge are gonorrhea and chlamydia.

In 1995, there were nearly 400,000 cases of gonorrhea reported to the United States Centers for Disease Control and Prevention (CDC), although the Institute of Medicine estimates that as many as 800,000 cases of gonorrhea occur annually. The cost of gonorrhea exceeds $1 billion annually.

The CDC estimates that there are over 4 million cases of chlamydia annually at an annual cost in excess of $2 billion. Thus, urethral discharge (and urethritis and vaginitis) may be presumed to affect over 4 million people annually at a significant cost to health care resources. Because STDs tend to be underreported, the actual number of people affected and costs may be significantly higher.

This chapter develops the differential diagnoses of a segment of sexually transmitted diseases: urethritis and urethral discharge. Sexually transmitted diseases that manifest primarily as genital ulcerations or as cutaneous lesions are covered in Chapter 15.

Regardless of the presenting symptom, there are several important precepts when treating any STD. First, the patient or partner, although infected with a communicable disease, may not be symptomatic. Second, the patient may have contracted not one but multiple sexually transmitted pathogens. Third, contingent upon the varied sexual practices of the inoculated patient and the type of pathogen encountered, the infection may involve multiple sites. Fourth, the patient's sexual consorts should be examined and treated. Fifth, patient education about safe sexual practice should be provided.

Males who present to primary care clinics complaining of a urethral discharge should be considered to have an STD until proven otherwise. On the other hand, female patients will rarely describe a urethral discharge as their initial complaint. Instead, female patients are more likely to describe a vaginal discharge, but not all vaginal discharges are sexually acquired.

Nonsexually acquired vaginal discharges include monilial vaginitis, bacterial vaginosis, or a physiologic discharge. The primary care clinician must be able to discriminate these nonsexually acquired diseases from the sexually acquired mucopurulent cervicitis associated with gonococcal and chlamydial infections.

Defining Urethritis and Urethral Discharge

Men with urethritis may be symptomatic or asymptomatic. Symptoms of urethritis include a purulent or mucoid discharge, urethral tingling, itching, or dysuria. The diagnosis of urethritis is established by finding at least one of the following: (1) a frankly purulent urethral discharge; (2) if the discharge is scant and mucoid, the finding of at least five polymorphonuclear (PMN) leucocytes per oil-immersion field (1000X); or (3) for men with urethral dysuria but who have no discharge, examination of a centrifuged sample of the first 5 to 10 mL of urine may establish the diagnosis of urethritis. The presence of 15 or more PMNs per high-power field (400X) in this initially voided urine sample indicates urethritis. This finding must be supported by the lack of significant PMNs in a midstream urine sample obtained at the same time. PMNs in a midstream sample indicate a bladder infection. If these criteria of urethritis are present, then the primary care clinician may begin empiric antimicrobial therapy to treat both *Neisseria gonorrhoeae* and *Chlamydia trachomatis.*

Key History

All male patients presenting with a urethral discharge and all female patients presenting with a mucopurulent cervicitis should be asked in a nonjudgmental fashion about (1) the number of sexual contacts in the last 2 months (more than one partner increases the risk of having acquired an STD), (2) gender preferences (because this information may provide a clue regarding sexual practices), and (3) preferences of sexual practice (vaginal, oral, anorectal-receptive). A history of intravenous drug use, or of sex relations with intravenous drug users, places patients at risk for hepatitis B, hepatitis C, and human immunodeficiency virus (HIV). The use of condoms should be ascertained.

Physical Examination

The physical examination should include inspection of the skin in the genital region and also of the soles, palms, trunk, and perineum. Disseminated gonococcal infections may present with a skin rash predominantly on the extremities. The inguinal and femoral areas should be inspected for adenopathy, and if there has been oropharyngeal exposure, then cervical adenopathy should be addressed as well. Gonorrhea and other STDs may involve regional lymph nodes.

The female genital examination should include inspection of the external genitalia, a speculum

examination, a bimanual examination, and inspection of the anus and perineum (which may all be infected by gonorrhea). The male genital examination should include an inspection of the external genitalia including the entire glans penis and prepuce by complete retraction of the foreskin. Urethritis from chlamydia or gonorrhea may coexist with other cutaneous STDs such as syphilis or HPV. The scrotum should be inspected with particular attention directed to the epididymis. Both gonococcus and chlamydia commonly cause epididymitis in men less than 35 years of age. For both men and women, if there is a history of receptive anal intercourse and the patient has rectal complaints, anoscopy should be performed. If there is a history of oropharyngeal exposure, inspection of the oral cavity is indicated.

Laboratory Evaluation

For any patient presenting with an STD, screening laboratory studies should be done. A syphilis serology should be done in all patients who have not had one done in the last 3 months. HIV testing and follow-up counseling of HIV results should be offered to patients in at-risk groups.

All men should have (1) a urethral Gram's stain; (2) an assessment of the presence of chlamydia via antigen detection test or culture of the urethra, or alternatively via microbial nucleic acid probes of the urine or of the urethral discharge; and (3) an assessment of *N. gonorrhoeae* that can be accomplished through either nucleic acid probes or through cultures. If there is a history of anal or oral contacts, these areas should be cultured for *N. gonorrhoeae.* Men should also have serologic testing for syphilis and HIV testing and counseling.

All women should have (1) an endocervical specimen for Gram's stain; (2) a vaginal secretion specimen for a potassium hydroxide study and for a wet mount for microscopic examination; and (3) cultures, antigen detection tests, or nucleic acid probes should be sent from the endocervix and the anus for both chlamydia and gonorrhea. If the patient has had a hysterectomy, then the urethra should be substituted as the source for the endocervical specimen. Oral cultures are indicated if there is a history of oral sex. Women should also have serologic testing for syphilis and receive HIV testing and counseling.

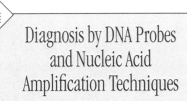

Diagnosis by DNA Probes and Nucleic Acid Amplification Techniques

New tests to diagnose *C. trachomatis* and *N. gonorrhoeae* include *nonamplified* DNA probe hybridization techniques and *amplified* nucleic acid techniques (Table 7–1). Nucleic acid amplification methods offer improved specificity over traditional assays and in the future may circumvent the need for cultures in legal cases. The problem with molecular amplification techniques involves the potential for cross-contamination within the laboratory if specimens, reagents, and equipment are not stringently handled. Nonamplified hybridization methods have a specificity of 97% and a sensitivity of 95%.[1–4] The nucleic acid amplification methods have even greater sensitivity and are sensitive enough to detect pathogens in the first-voided urine. Nonamplified tests may not be sufficiently sensitive to detect infection when using urine samples and should not be used on urine samples.

The ability to use first voided urine samples avoids the intrusiveness of obtaining intraurethral specimens and may increase compliance in the screening of asymptomatic male sexual contacts. This screening may lead to a reduction in the reservoir of the asymptomatic male carriers.

In females, the endocervix is the primary site of infection. The urethra may be uninvolved in up to 30% of females who have chlamydial infections. Recent studies, nonetheless, have shown detecting *C. trachomatis* by screening the urine of asymptomatic women to be sensitive.

Noninvasive DNA methods of screening asymptomatic partners may reduce the reservoir of asymptomatic male and female carriers. Presently the American Academy of Family Practice and the Centers for Disease Control advocate annual screening of sexually active, asymptomatic females (described later). Informed that diagnosis no longer requires the placement of a swab in the penile urethra, asymptomatic males may be more likely to agree to evaluation. Another advantage of DNA techniques is the speed of diagnosis. Results are available within 8 hours.[1–4]

Classification of Male Urethritis

Urethritis is usually classified as either gonococcal or nongonococcal. In the United States, non-

Table 7–1

Diagnosis by DNA Probes and Nucleic Acid Amplification Techniques

TEST	MECHANISM	MANUFACTURER
PACE 2C	Nonamplified DNA hybridization	GenProbe
LCR	Ligase chain reaction nucleic acid amplification	Abbott
PCR	Polymerase chain reaction nucleic acid amplification	Roche Molecular Systems
TMA	Transcription-mediated nucleic acid amplification	GenProbe

gonococcal urethritis is two times more common than gonococcal urethritis. The etiologic agent causing gonococcal urethritis is *N. gonorrhoeae.* The etiologic agents causing nongonococcal urethritis (NGU) in order of prevalence are *C. trachomatis, Ureaplasma urealyticum, Trichomonas vaginalis,* perhaps a new agent, *Mycoplasma genitalum,* and rarely, herpes simplex virus. The uncertainty of diagnosis may complicate nongonococcal urethritis management. Not all of the agents causing NGU are known, and those known are not easily cultured.

Distinction between gonococcal and nongonococcal urethritis cannot be reliably made on clinical grounds. However, in general, the symptoms of a gonococcal urethritis are more pronounced than that of NGU. Patients with gonococcal urethritis are more likely to complain of dysuria and are more likely to have a copious purulent discharge. Additionally, those with gonococcal urethritis are more likely to have a shorter duration of symptoms. The incubation period for gonococcal urethritis is 2 to 6 days, and due to the more pronounced symptoms, the affected patient seeks care sooner than those with NGU do. The usual incubation period for chlamydia is 7 to 35 days, and because of the paucity of symptoms in some individuals infected with chlamydia, presentation may be delayed beyond 1 month from the time of sexual contact.[5]

In men, a urethral discharge or urethritis is the most common manifestation of a sexually transmitted disease (STD). For the male patient with the presenting complaint of a urethral discharge, the most common diagnosis is an STD. A diagnosis of a mucopurulent urethral discharge is an STD until proven otherwise. One condition that should be differentiated from a mucopurulent discharge is terminal dribbling of urine postmicturition. This condition, sometimes associated with urethral strictures or urethral diverticula, is easily differentiated from a sexually transmitted urethritis. In terminal dribbling, the leakage is consistent with urine and not mucopurulent. Furthermore, the leakage occurs postvoiding and is not persistent between voids.

Urethral discharges are rarely associated with nonsexually transmitted genitourinary disease processes. The common nonsexually acquired processes such as prostatitis and bacterial cystitis almost never have urethral discharge as a predominant complaint. In contrast, epididymitis may be a presenting complaint of a sexually transmitted disease, even in the patient who denies having had a urethral discharge.

Gonococcal Urethritis

Gonococcal urethritis is the most frequently reported infectious disease in the United States. It is acquired almost exclusively by sexual contact, often from partners who are asymptomatic. Men exposed to females harboring gonorrhea have a 20% chance of acquiring gonorrhea with a single sexual contact.[6] Florid symptoms of urethritis develop in 85% of men within 14 days; 15% will have mild to no symptoms. Coinfection with *C. trachomatis* occurs in 15% to 25% of males infected with gonorrhea. Therapy should be directed at both pathogens.

In contrast, women who encounter men with the infection have a 50% rate of transmission from a single contact.[7] Less than 20% will have florid symptoms of a purulent cervical discharge. Nonspecific symptoms will be present in 70%, and may contribute to an untreated reservoir of disease.

Typically the infected male develops a purulent discharge within 5 days of inoculation. Dysuria is usually present. If the symptoms are ignored or left untreated, men may develop complications of *N. gonorrhoeae* infections such as epididymitis, urethral stricture disease, and disseminated gonococcal infections. Macular skin lesions and a multiarticular tenosynovitis characterize disseminated gonococcal infections. The "arthritic" inflammation does not involve the joint, but is confined to the tendon sheaths. Less frequently, men may have only a scant discharge and minimal dysuria. When symptoms are minor, infection may go unnoticed. These individuals may account for an unmeasured reservoir of male disease carriers.

Women account for a larger proportion of asymptomatic carriers than men. Up to one half of infected women are asymptomatic. Untreated women may develop Bartholin's or Skene's gland abscesses, rectal infections, and pelvic inflammatory disease (PID) including salpingitis and tubo-ovarian abscesses. PID is associated with tubal scarring, leading to complications of infertility and tubal ectopic pregnancies. Pharyngeal infections are possible in individuals who practice oral–genital sexual contact. Disseminated gonococcal infections may complicate untreated infections. These complications of untreated gonococcal urethritis should be stressed to patients so that hopefully they will be inclined to report their sexual contacts. Additionally, to lure identification and treatment of consorts, clinicians should stress that testing of asymptomatic individuals does not always involve urethral swabbing. Fortunately with today's DNA amplification techniques, it appears that even testing of the first voided urine may be adequate to identify those infected. By examining the urine, one can avoid the uncomfortable urethral instrumentation. Asymptomatic partners may be more willing to undergo urine testing than urethral swabbing.

Screening Women at High Risk for Gonorrhea

Because gonococcal infections are often asymptomatic in women and because asymptomatic infections can lead to tubal scarring, infertility, and ectopic pregnancies, the Centers for Disease Control (CDC) advocates screening of women at high risk. The prevalence of *C. trachomatis* cervical infections in sexually active female adolescents varies from 8% to 15%.[8] The routine screening of this young population will reduce the reservoir of

asymptomatic carriers as well as reduce the complications associated with chlamydial salpingitis.[9] The CDC guidelines state that screening should be extended to sexually active asymptomatic females younger than 20 years of age, and older than 20 years with risk factors for STD infections defined as new or multiple sexual partners in the last 3 months or inconsistent use of barrier contraceptives. Similarly the U.S. Preventive Services Task Force Guidelines state that women 14 to 20 years of age should be tested for *C. trachomatis* whenever they present for health care (at least once a year), regardless of whether their sexual behavior places them at risk. Older women should be tested if they have more than one sexual partner, if they have begun a new sexual relationship since the last test, or if they have been diagnosed with another STD. The American Academy of Family Practice also recommends screening of asymptomatic sexually active females.

The ability to detect both gonorrhea and chlamydia in women using voided *urine* assays subjected to nucleic acid amplification techniques is sensitive and specific. Presently, urine-based nucleic acid amplification testing is not advocated for the screening of asymptomatic men. Nonetheless, the estimated prevalence of chlamydia in asymptomatic, sexually active men may be as high as 11%.[10] In clinical practices where the prevalence of STDs is low, the sensitivity of urine testing via nucleic acid amplification techniques is poor.

Presumptive Laboratory Diagnosis

In settings where clinicians have ready access to Gram stains (emergency rooms, hospital-based clinics), presumptive diagnosis of *N. gonorrhoeae* urethritis can be made if the clinician sees gram-negative intracellular diplococci in the microscopic examination of the urethral discharge. For male subjects, this finding of intracellular diplococci carries a sensitivity and specificity of >95%. If the gram-negative diplococci are only extracellular, or if their morphology is atypical, only 20% of cultures will be positive. If there are no diplococci seen, but there are more than 4 polymorphonuclear cells per oil immersion field, then the presumptive diagnosis is nongonococcal urethritis (NGU) and the patient should be treated empirically.

For female patients, the examination of the cervical or urethral specimens for intracellular diplococci is less sensitive than examination of the male urethral discharge. Only half of symptomatic women infected with *N. gonorrhoeae* will have a positive Gram stain showing intracellular diplococci. Despite a sensitivity of only 50%, the specificity remains similar to that seen in males, nearly 95%.[11] This specificity is due to the presence of commensal vaginal flora that are morphologically similar to *N. gonorrhoeae*. With a sensitivity of only 30% to 60%, one should rely more heavily on culture or DNA probes for establishing the diagnosis.

The diagnosis of rectal infection and pharyngitis based on Gram's stain is imprecise. In women who have mucopurulent cervicitis due to gonococcus, approximately 40% will have a rectal infection as well. Typically, these infections are asymptomatic and they may occur due to proximity, not necessarily due to anal sexual penetration.[12] In the case of pharyngeal infection, Gram's stain is imprecise because other *Neisseria* species are known to be commensal oral flora.[13]

Specimen Collection for Culturing

N. gonorrhoeae should be plated onto selective culture media such as modified Thayer–Martin and placed in a CO_2-enriched atmosphere, either via a CO_2-generating tablet, a candle jar, or a CO_2 incubator. Cultures should be taken from all sites of known sexual contact depending upon the individual's sexual practice habits (urethra, cervix, rectum, pharynx).

DNA Amplification Probes

Commercially available DNA amplification probes allow for testing of *N. gonorrhoeae* and *C. trachomatis* simultaneously (Table 7–1). The sensitivity and specificity of these probes are good provided that the laboratory uses standardized techniques to avoid intralaboratory cross-contamination with other specimens. Results can be available within 8 hours of specimen submission. For rectal and pharyngeal sources, the sensitivity of these DNA techniques may be questionable. Culture documentation, in lieu of or in addition to DNA amplification testing, is advocated in cases of medical-legal importance.

Surveillance for Development of Antimicrobial Resistance

Although DNA amplification probes are reliable and yield results more quickly than traditional culturing and enzyme techniques, they do pose a problem in that they do not identify antimicrobial resistance. Penicillinase-producing *N. gonorrhoeae* were first reported in the mid-1970s. This is a plasmid-mediated resistance, but there are also chromosomal mutations that have caused antimicrobial resistance. Chromosomal-mediated resistance is thought to be responsible for strains that are resistant to spectinomycin and are likely responsible for the emerging cases of fluoroquinolone resistance. The CDC monitors the development of antimicrobial resistance through the culture reporting of gonorrhea from 26 sites across the United States. This project is called the Gonococcal Isolate Surveillance Project. Culturing is mandatory for those individuals with persistent symptoms after a course of antimicrobial therapy. Although reexposure is the most likely cause for treatment failure, one must rule out emergence of a resistant strain.

Management of Gonococcus

Table 7–2 shows the recommended antibiotic regimens for gonococcal infections of the urethra, cervix, and rectum. Table 7–3 shows the recommended antibiotic regimes for gonococcal pharyngitis.

Table 7–2

Recommended Treatment from the 1998 CDC Guidelines for Uncomplicated Gonococcal Infections of the Cervix, Urethra, and Rectum[a]

Cefixime 400 mg orally in a single dose, (curing 97.1% via oral dosing) OR Ceftriaxone 125 mg IM in a single dose, (curing 99.1% via IM dosing) OR Ciprofloxacin 500 mg orally in a single dose OR Ofloxacin 400 mg orally in a single dose, PLUS azithromycin 1 g orally in a single dose OR Doxycycline 100 mg orally twice a day for 7 days Alternative regimen for treatment of patients who cannot tolerate cephalosporins and quinolones: Spectinomycin 2 g IM in a single dose

[a] Other clinical considerations: Fluoroquinolones are contraindicated in pregnancy, in nursing mothers, and in children less than 17 years of age. Fluoroquinolones will not cure syphilis, whereas ceftriaxone, a 7-day regimen of doxycycline, or erythromycin, will.

FOLLOW-UP AND TEST OF CURE

Patients who have uncomplicated gonorrhea and who are treated with any of the recommended regimens need not return for a test of

Table 7–3

Recommended Treatment from the 1998 CDC Guidelines for Gonococcal Infection of the Pharynx[a]

Ceftriaxone 125 mg IM in a single dose OR Ciprofloxacin 500 mg orally in a single dose OR Ofloxacin 400 mg orally in a single dose, PLUS azithromycin 1 g orally in a single dose OR Doxycycline 100 mg orally twice a day for 7 days

[a] Gonococcal infections of the pharynx are more difficult to eradicate than infections at urogenital and anorectal sites.

cure unless symptoms persist.[14] Patients with persistent symptoms after treatment should be evaluated by culture for *N. gonorrhoeae*, and antimicrobial susceptibility testing should be performed on any gonococci isolated. Infections identified after treatment usually result from reinfection rather than treatment failure.

MANAGEMENT OF SEXUAL PARTNERS

Clinicians face a dilemma with the sexual partners of patients with STDs such as gonorrhea, chlamydia, or syphilis. Should partners be evaluated and treated only if proven to be infected? If this strategy were employed, then clinicians would have to examine these patients, obtain appropriate confirmatory tests, and follow up with test results and contact the partner with these results to initiate treatment. Or should partners be treated empirically on the basis of having been a sexual contact of someone with an STD alone? This strategy risks potential overtreatment with antibiotics. However, this strategy is more easily implemented and avoids potential reinfection by partners who are carriers, avoids further transmission of the STD to other sexual partners, and obviates the need for the clinician to examine and follow up with the partner. Thus, empiric treatment of the partner is warranted.

Chlamydia Trachomatis

Microbiology

C. trachomatis is an important pathogen in men with urethritis. *C. trachomatis* accounts for 30% to 40% of the cases of NGU.[16] It is isolated in 30% to 40% of symptomatic men compared to 0% to 3% of asymptomatic men.[18] *C. trachomatis* is an obligate intracellular parasite. The parasite has a propensity to infect only squamocolumnar and columnar epithelia. This organism causes a urethritis or an epididymitis in men and a cervicitis or an ascending genital tract infection in women. It has not been incriminated as a cause of vulvo-vaginitis in women, nor is it a cause of cystitis in men or women. When establishing the diagnosis via a Gram's stain or culture, it is important that the urethral swab specimen contain epithelial cells. Examination or culturing of the discharge alone will not suffice. The swab specimen collection must be vigorous enough to contain the host epithelial cells, not just the PMNs found in the urethral discharge. Adequate swabbing of the cervical os or a sample from within the endocervical canal must be obtained in women.

Clinical Manifestations

The serotypes causing the sexually transmitted *C. trachomatis* urethritis are serovars D through K. The serovars A, B, Ba, and C are associated with endemic trachoma (blindness), while serovars L1, L2, and L3 are associated with lymphogranuloma venereum. In addition to urethritis, serovars D through K have also been associated with epididymitis, Reiter's syndrome, proctitis, cervicitis, endometritis, salpingitis, tubal scarring, and ectopic pregnancies. Some studies indicate that *C. trachomatis* is a more common cause of PID than *N. gonorrhoeae*, and that *C. trachomatis* infection is more likely to result in tubal scarring than *N. gonorrhoeae* infection.

It is not always easy for the clinician to distinguish between gonorrhea and chlamydia clinically. Some general differences may help to distinguish between pathogens. Generally, chlamydia is a more indolent illness than gonococcal urethritis. The typical male patient with chlamydia has had symptoms for 3 to 4 weeks before seeking medical attention, whereas the patient with gonococcal urethritis typically gives a history of 3 or 4 days of urethral discharge.[15] The patient with chlamydia may have mild or no dysuria and only a scant discharge that is mucoid but not purulent. Both dysuria and urethral discharge are present in only 38% of patients with chlamydia,

whereas 78% of patients harboring *N. gonorrhoeae* have these two symptoms.

Management Recommendations for Chlamydia and Other Nongonococcal Urethritis

Diagnosis

All patients presenting with a urethritis should be tested for chlamydia and gonococcus. Commercial availability of DNA amplification probes allows for the simultaneous detection of *C. trachomatis* and *N. gonorrhoeae* with one urethral swab. The presumptive diagnosis of chlamydia is based on the exclusion of intracellular diplococci on Gram's stain of the urethral discharge and the confirmation that the patient indeed has a urethritis (PMNs on Gram's stain or first voided urine, as discussed earlier). Note that these presumptive diagnostic criteria make gonorrhea unlikely, and chlamydia likely, but do not confirm chlamydia over other NGU causes.

Antibiotic Regimens

Table 7–4 shows current recommended antibiotic regimens for chlamydia and other non-gonococcal urethritis.

Ureaplasma Urealyticum

Ureaplasma urealyticum is not always pathogenic in men with NGU from whom it is isolated. It is a common commensal organism of the genital tracts

Table 7–4

Treatment Recommendations for Nongonococcal Urethritis from the 1998 CDC Guidelines for STDs

Azithromycin 1 g orally in a single dose

OR

Doxycycline 100 mg orally twice a day for 7 days

The safety and efficacy of azithromycin in persons less than 15 have not been established. Pregnant women should be treated with erythromycin base, 500 mg orally four times a day for 14 days.

Alternative Regimens

Erythromycin base 500 mg orally four times a day for 7 days

OR

Erythromycin ethylsuccinate 800 mg orally four times a day for 7 days

OR

Ofloxacin 300 mg twice a day for 7 days

If only erythromycin can be used and a patient cannot tolerate high-dose erythromycin schedules, one of the following regimens can be used:

Erythromycin base 250 mg orally four times a day for 14 days

OR

Erythromycin ethylsuccinate 400 mg orally four times a day for 14 days

of asymptomatic sexually active women and men who have no evidence of urethritis. *U. urealyticum* is believed to account for another 15% to 25% of NGU cases.[17] Rates of genital colonization are related to sexual activity, and those with multiple sexual partners are more likely to be colonized.[19] Further evidence that *U. urealyticum* represents a sexually acquired pathogen is validated by showing a better clinical response of symptomatic men to treatment for NGU when the antibiotic regimen chosen has activity against *U. urealyticum* than when one chooses a regimen specific for chlamydia. Outside of research settings, there are no easily available methods for culturing *U. urealyticum*. Men with urethritis due to ureaplasma are usually effectively treated with the tetracyclines commonly prescribed for chlamydia urethritis (Table 7–4). However, 10% of ureaplasma may be resistant to tetracycline, and here treatment with erythromycin or azithromycin is recommended.[20]

Mycoplasma Genitalium

The role of *Mycoplasma genitalium* in causing urethritis is controversial.[21] Since the advent of polymerase chain reaction technology, the evidence that *M. genitalium* is a true urethral pathogen has increased. In 103 men with symptoms of urethritis, *M. genitalium* was detected by PCR in 24.[22] It accounts for urethritis in less than 5% of male urethritis. Commercially available diagnostic tests to identify these organisms are not available. Treatment is similar to that for chlamydia (Table 7–4).

Trichomonas Vaginalis

Trichomonas vaginalis is a flagellated protozoan transmitted by sexual contact. It accounts for less than 5% of male urethritis. However, this pathogen is responsible for up to 25% of clinically evident vaginitis syndromes seen in women's health clinics.

The protozoan may be recovered in greater than 30% of male consorts. Infected males are commonly asymptomatic, and they may be able to clear the pathogen spontaneously.[23] There have been rare cases where the transmission of *Trichomonas* was attributed to close physical but not sexual contact. Nonetheless, most experts consider this to be a sexually transmitted disease.

The symptoms of ***Trichomonas*** in males are commonly limited to a slight meatal itch. In females, the symptoms generally include a profuse, malodorous vaginal discharge and dysuria. In 90% of cases, the urethra and the vagina are infected. Because the organism displays a propensity to infect squamous epithelium, the cervix (composed of columnar epithelium) is usually spared. The presence of a concomitant cervical infection should direct the clinician to consider additional STDs. As many as 50% of women infected with *T. vaginalis* have gonorrhea.

During physical examination of the female genitalia, the clinician usually encounters a thin, profuse grayish vaginal discharge that may be frothy. Punctate hemorrhages, or "strawberry cervix," are the classic description, but present in less than 10% of cases.

Wet Prep Diagnosis

T. vaginalis is a unicellular, motile pear-shaped protozoan with four flagella, a posterior axostyle, and an undulating surface membrane. It is only slightly smaller than squamous epithelial cells and moves in a twitching motion. Microscopic visualization is accomplished by wet mount inspection of an unstained specimen from the vaginal discharge, urethral exudate, or first morning voided specimen in men. The specificity and sensitivity of this test are 100% and 75%, respectively. Establishing the diagnosis is based on the wet prep, not on culture. Metronidazole is the treatment of choice. Cure rates using 250 mg orally three times a day for 7 days are slightly superior to a single oral dose of 2 g, 95% versus 85%, respectively.[24] Currently, the Centers for Disease Control recommend a 2-g single dose.

Treatment of Recurrent or Persistent Symptoms of Urethritis

The most common reason for recurrent or persistent symptoms is reinfection. Other explanations may be (1) poor patient compliance if a multidose regimen was initially chosen; (2) infection with an atypical pathogen such as *T. vaginalis, M. genitalium,* or *U. urealyticum;* or (3) emotional repentance or guilt. Because of the remorsefulness associated with contracting an STD outside the marriage, some patients develop persistent symptomatology despite lack of clinical evidence that urethral inflammation persists. Symptoms alone,

without evidence of a urethritis or a positive culture, are not a basis for retreatment.

If one believes poor patient compliance or reexposure to an untreated partner is likely, then retreatment with the initial regimen is recommended. Otherwise, one should treat persistent urethritis as if it were due to an atypical pathogen (*T. vaginalis, M. genitalium,* or *U. urealyticum*). The treatment of atypical pathogens includes metronidazole for the treatment of *T. vaginalis* combined with the addition of erythromycin for the treatment of doxycycline-resistant *Ureaplasma.*

The recommended antibiotic regimens for atypical pathogens are shown in Table 7–5.

Algorithms

Figs. 7–1 and 7–2 show the algorithms for urethral and vaginal discharges, respectively. Fig. 7–3 shows the algorithm for persistent urethritis after treatment.

Other Manifestations and Complications of Urethritis

Reiter's Syndrome

Less than 5% of men with NGU develop Reiter's syndrome. Reiter's syndrome is a symptom triad

Table 7–5

Treatment of Atypical Pathogens

Metronidazole 2 g orally in a single dose, PLUS erythromycin base 500 mg orally four times a day for 7 days
OR
Erythromycin ethylsuccinate 800 mg orally four times a day for 7 days

Figure 7–1

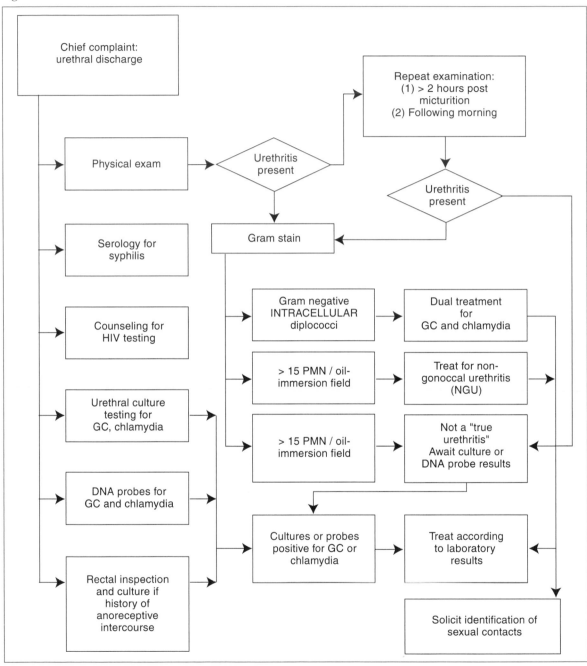

Algorithm for urethral discharge. (GC = gonorrhea)

Figure 7–2

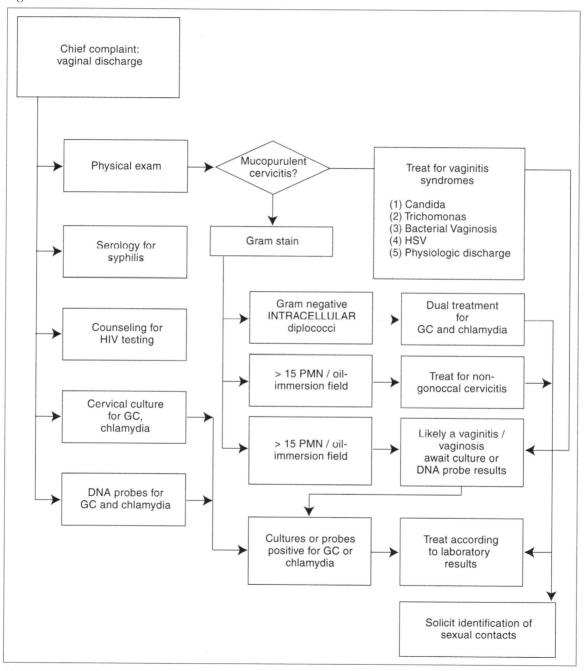

Algorithm for vaginal discharge. (GC = gonorrhea; HSV = herpes simplex virus)

Figure 7–3

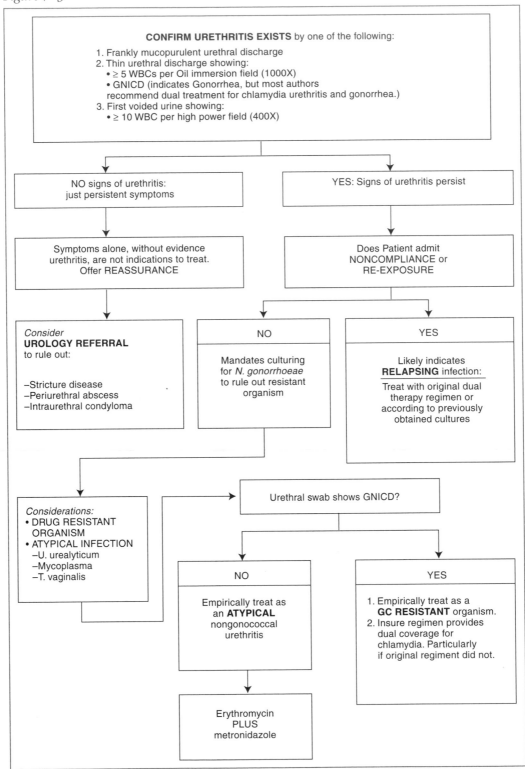

Algorithm for persistent urethritis after treatment. (GNICD = gram negative intracellular diplococci;
GC = gonorrhea)

of arthritis, conjunctivitis, and urethritis. Other associated findings include two cutaneous lesions: balanitis circinata and keratoderma blenorrhagica. Balanitis circinata is a scalloped psoriaform plaque of the glans penis. Keratoderma blenorrhagica is a similar psoriasis-like lesion located on the palms and soles of the feet. Typically the syndrome develops 3 to 6 weeks after a chlamydial infection.[27] The syndrome may represent an idiosyncratic immune response to a chlamydial infection, and appears to be associated with HLA-B27 seropositivity.[28] For most affected individuals, the syndrome resolves spontaneously in 4 to 6 months. Arthritis tends to be the most persistent feature of the syndrome. Reiter's syndrome may also follow *Shigella* dysentery.[29]

Persistent Urethritis

The most common etiology of persistent urethral discharge after dual treatment for *N. gonorrhoeae* and *C. trachomatis* is reinoculation from an untreated individual. Other etiologies to consider are (1) emergence of a resistant strain of gonococcus, (2) infection with an atypical pathogen, or (3) development of one of two persistent urethritis syndromes. The emergence of a resistant strain is diagnosed by culturing the discharge. An atypical pathogen is not easy to diagnose, but simply treated empirically with erythromycin and metronidazole as described earlier. Two other persistent urethral syndromes are described next. Persistent urethral syndromes generally fall into one of two classes: chronic urethritis and noninfectious urethrodynia. The etiology of both of these entities is not clearly understood.

Chronic urethritis is defined as a persistent urethral discharge, associated with inflammatory cells (polymorphonuclear leukocytes or PMNs), but negative for either *N. gonorrhoeae* or *C. trachomatis* infection. Usually there is a clear antecedent acute urethritis episode before the symptoms became chronic. Typically these patients have been treated for *N. gonorrhoeae* and *C. trachomatis*, as well as for atypical pathogens such as

T. vaginalis and *U. urealyticum*, and they have faithfully avoided reinoculation. Yet they still have signs and symptoms of urethritis. Symptoms may improve on antibiotics, only to relapse at completion of therapy. The etiology of the relapsing nature of this syndrome may be explained in part by our incomplete knowledge of all pathogens responsible for nongonococcal urethritis. Simply, we have not yet identified the causative agent.[30] Patients with signs of a persistent urethral discharge should be evaluated by a urologist. These patients may have developed urethral stricture disease, intraurethral condyloma, or periurethral abscesses.[31]

Noninfectious urethrodynia can be differentiated from chronic urethritis by two findings. First, patients with noninfectious urethrodynia have persistent urethral discomfort or "burning," but essentially no urethral discharge. Although their original urethral discharge may have been documented to be a true sexually acquired infection, their recurring symptoms are not supported by physical findings. Second, patients with noninfectious urethrodynia do not improve with antibiotic treatment. Often these patients will frequently "strip" or "milk" their urethra in search for a discharge. The search, if repeated often enough, will result in a reactive urethritis associated with a scant discharge.[32] These patients should be instructed not to strip the urethra. Often these patients feel guilty about undisclosed sexual events with someone other than their established sexual companion. The treatment for these patients is reassurance that they do not harbor a venereal infection. Antibiotics are not indicated.

Epididymitis

In sexually active males less than 35 years of age, epididymitis is frequently associated with an STD. Although *N. gonorrhoeae* may cause epididymitis, the most common pathogen in this age group is *C. trachomatis*.[33] Patients with a sexually transmitted epididymitis may not complain of a urethral discharge. The absence of a urethral discharge should not dissuade the practitioner from treating the epididymitis.[34]

For men over the age of 35, most cases of epididymitis are related to urinary tract infections with coliform bacteria. This age distinction is not particularly important when deciding on the appropriate antibiotic therapy. Epididymitis, regardless of the cause, is best treated for 10 to 14 days with a fluoroquinolone. Fluoroquinolones treat all common etiologies: *C. trachomatis, N. gonorrhoeae*, and coliforms. The age distinction is important for other reasons, however. If the epididymitis represents an STD, sexual contacts should be interviewed and treated. Additionally, cystourethroscopy or other anatomic evaluations of the lower urinary tract are not indicated in males with a single bout of an uncomplicated "venereal" epididymitis. However, in the older male with prostatic enlargement, epididymitis is more likely a consequence of a coliform cystitis. In these individuals a urologic investigation for correctable anatomic abnormalities should be pursued.

Urethral Stricture

Similar to fallopian tube obstruction seen as a complication of sexually transmitted diseases in females, urethral strictures may be seen as a complication of STDs in males. Urethral strictures are associated with both gonorrhea and nongonorrheal urethritis. Prompt antibiotic treatment and eradication of pathogens lessens the likelihood of stricture formation. Strictures do not develop acutely, but typically become symptomatic more than 15 years after the episode of urethritis.[35]

Controversies

The ideal antibiotic regimens are not known. One controversial issue is whether longer antibiotic regimens (with high cure rates but lower patient compliance) are preferable to shorter antibiotic regimens (with lower cure rates but higher patient compliance). For example, for nongonococcal urethritis (Table 7–4), clinicians should consider the following factors when choosing a 1-g single-dose azithromycin versus a 14-day doxycycline as the initial regimen for treatment of NGU. The clinical cure rate for chlamydial infection with doxycycline is 90%, whereas the cure rate with single-dose azithromycin is 83%. The clinical cure rate for *U. urealyticum* is 45% for doxycycline and 47% for azithromycin.[25] The cost comparison for the two regimens was $24 for azithromycin versus $2 for doxycycline.[26] Although neither agent is absolutely effective, particularly with respect to ureaplasma infections, using a single-dose regimen will maximize compliance. Thus, despite being more expensive and less effective compared to doxycycline, azithromycin may be considered the treatment of choice for patients whose compliance seems poor.

Pitfalls to Avoid

Several pitfalls should be avoided. First, it is important to consider multiple pathogens in each patient with urethritis. Thus, the clinician should always test for gonorrhea and chlamydia. Likewise, syphilis and HIV testing are indicated, as these infections are commonly seen in patients with urethritis.

Second, do not ignore the sexual partner. It is relevant to educate the patient to seek treatment for his or her partner. Reporting to the appropriate agency may facilitate partner contact and treatment. Failure to treat the partner exposes the patient to reinfection and leaves untreated a reservoir for propagating STDs.

Third, make sure patients are followed after treatment to ensure eradication of pathogens. Fourth, educate patients to engage in safe sex (condom use) to minimize the risk of subsequent infection.

Emerging Trends

Antibiotic resistance has been rising over time. Antibiotic resistance to gonorrhea has been particularly problematic in Southeast Asia and likely will be increasingly problematic in the United States. It is possible that other pathogenic organisms that cause urethritis, such as chlamydia, will develop antibiotic resistance. This problem underscores the need to prevent STDs. Routine condom use diminishes the risk of transmitting gonorrhea or chlamydia during intercourse.

Note: The author is a full-time federal employee. This work is in the public domain. The views expressed are those of the author, and are not to be construed as official or as reflecting those of the Department of Defense, the Army Medical Department or the U.S. Air Force.

References

1. Stary A, Kopp W, Zahel B, et al: Comparison of DNA-probe test and culture for the detection of *Neisseria gonorrhoeae* in genital samples. *STD* 20:243–247, 1993.
2. Hale YM, Melton ME, Lewis JS, Willis DE: Evaluation of the PACE 2 *Neisseria gonorrhoeae* assay by three public health laboratories. *J Clin Microbiol* 31: 451–453, 1993.
3. Limberger RJ, Biega R, Evancoe A, et al: Evaluation of culture and the Gen-Probe PACE 2 assay for detection of *Neisseria gonorrhoeae* and *Chlamydia trachomatis* in endocervical specimens transported to a state health laboratory. *J Clin Microbiol* 30: 1162–1166, 1992.
4. Iwen PC, Walker RA, Warren KL, et al: Evaluation of nucleic acid-based test (PACE 2C) for simultaneous detection of *Chlamydia trachomatis* and *Neisseria gonorrhoeae* in endocervical specimens. *J Clin Microbiol* 33:2587–2591, 1995.
5. Jacobs NF, Kraus SJ: Gonococcal and nongonococcal urethritis in men: Clinical and laboratory differentiation. *Ann Intern Med* 82:7, 1975.
6. Hooper RR, et al. Cohort study of venereal disease: I. The risk of gonorrhea transmission from infected women to men. *Am J Epidemiol* 108:136, 1978.
7. Thin RNT, Williams IA, Nicol CS: Direct and delayed methods of immunofluorescent diagnosis of gonorrhea in women. *Br J Vener Dis* 47: 27, 1970.
8. Biro FM, Reising SF, Doughman JA, et al: A comparison of diagnostic methods in adolescent girls with and without symptoms of *Chlamydia* urogenital infection. *Pediatrics* 79:76–83, 1987.
9. Hillis S, Nakashima A, Amsterdam L, et al: The impact of a comprehensive chlamydia prevention program in Wisconsin. *Fam Plann Perspect* 27:108–111, 1995.
10. Shafer MA, Schachter J, Moncada J, et al: Evaluation of urine-based screening strategies to detect *Chlamydia trachomatis* among sexually active asymptomatic young males. *JAMA* 270:2065–2070, 1993.
11. Holmes KK: Lower genital tract infections in women: Cystitis, urethritis, vulvovaginitis, and cervicitis. In Holmes KK, et al (eds): *Sexually Transmitted Diseases*. New York, McGraw-Hill, 1990, pp 527–545.
12. Klein EJ, et al. Anorectal gonococcal infections. *Ann Intern Med* 86:340, 1977.
13. Hook EW, Holmes KK: Gonococcal infections. *Ann Intern Med* 102:229, 1985.
14. Williams JM, Brillman JC: Sexually transmitted diseases. In Brillman JC, Quenzer RW (eds): *Infectious Disease in Emergency Medicine*, ed 2. Philadelphia, Lippincott-Raven, 1998, pp 667–702.
15. Jacobs NF, Kraus SJ: Gonococcal and nongonococcal urethritis in men: Clinical and laboratory differentiation. *Ann Intern Med* 82:7, 1975.
16. Centers for Disease Control and Prevention: Recommendations for the prevention and management of *Chlamydia trachomatis* infections. *MMWR* 42(suppl RR-12):1–39, 1993.
17. Bowie WR: Urethritis in males. In Holmes KK, Mardh PA, Sparling PF, Wiesner PJ (eds): *Sexually Transmitted Diseases*, ed 2. New York, McGraw-Hill, 1990, pp 627–639.
18. Schmid GP, Fontanarosa PB: Evolving strategies for the management of nongonococcal urethritis syndromes. *JAMA* 274:577, 1995.
19. McCormack WM, Lee YH, Zinner SH: Sexual experience and urethral colonization with genital mycoplasmas. *Ann Intern Med* 78:696, 1973.

20. Stimson JB, Hale J, Bowie WR, et al: Tetracycline resistant *Ureaplasma urealyticum*: A cause for persistent non-gonococcal urethritis. *Ann Intern Med* 94:192, 1981.

21. McCormack WM, Lee YH, Zinner SH: Sexual experience and urethral colonization with genital mycoplasmas: A study in normal men. *Ann Intern Med* 78:696–698, 1973.

22. Horner PJ, Gilroy CB, Thomas BJ, et al: Association of *Mycoplasma genitalium* with acute nongonococcal urethritis. *Lancet* 342:582–585, 1993.

23. Rein MF: Current therapy of vulvovaginitis. *Sex Transm Dis* 8:316, 1981.

24. Rein MF, Muller M: Trichomonas vaginalis. In Holmes KK, Mardh PA, Sparling PF, et al (eds): *Sexually Transmitted Diseases*. New York, McGraw-Hill, 1984, p 525.

25. Stamm WE, Hicks CB, Martin DH, et al: Azithromycin for empirical treatment of the nongonococcal urethritis syndrome in men: A randomized double-blind study. *JAMA.* 274:545–549, 1995.

26. Erbelding EJ, Quinn TC: Urethritis treatment. In: *Dermatology Clinics: Sexually Transmitted Diseases* 16:735–738, 1998.

27. Martin DH, Pollock S, Kuo CC, et al: Chlamydial trachomatis infections in men with Reiter's syndrome. *Ann Intern Med* 100:207–213, 1984.

28. Kahn M, Kahn M: Diagnostic value of HLA-B27 testing in ankylosing spondylitis and Reiter's syndrome. *Ann Intern Med* 96:70–74, 1982.

29. Ford DK: Reiter's syndrome: Current concepts of etiology and pathogenesis. In Hobson D, Holmes KK (eds): *Nongonococcal Urethritis and Related Infections*. Washington, DC, American Society for Microbiology, 1977.

30. Bowie WR: Urethritis in males. In Holmes KK, Mardh PA, Sparling PF, et al (eds): *Sexually Transmitted Diseases*. New York, McGraw-Hill, 1984, pp 638–650.

31. Krieger JN, Hooton TM, Brust PJ, et al: Evaluation of chronic urethritis. *Arch Intern Med* 148:703–707, 1988.

32. Rein MF: Urethritis. In Mandell GL, Douglas RG, Bennett JE (eds): *Principles and Practice of Infectious Diseases*. New York, Wiley, 1984, pp 720–729.

33. Berger RE, Alexander ER, Monda GD, et al: *Chlamydia trachomatis* as a cause of "idiopathic" epididymitis. *N Engl J Med* 298:301, 1978.

34. Berger RE, Alexander ER, Harnisch JP, et al: Etiology, manifestations and therapy of acute epididymitis: Prospective study of 50 cases. *J Urol* 114:121, 1979.

35. Kibukamusoke JW: Gonorrhoea and urethral stricture. *Br J Vener Dis* 41:135, 1965.

R. Duane Cespedes
Edward Tieng

Chapter 8

Urinary Incontinence

How Common Is Urinary Incontinence?

Urinary incontinence has been estimated to affect approximately 13 million people in the United States with an annual cost of more than 16 billion dollars. The prevalence of incontinence is higher in females and the elderly, but incontinence should not be considered normal in females nor considered a normal feature of aging.

The overall prevalence of incontinence in adults 15 to 64 years old ranges from 1.5% to 5% in men and 10% to 30% in women. In a series of randomly selected women 30 to 59 years old, 26% reported episodic urinary incontinence, with 14% perceiving urinary incontinence as a social or hygienic problem. Community-dwelling patients older than 60 years of age have a 15% to 35% prevalence of incontinence, with females twice as likely to be incontinent. The highest prevalence of incontinence is found in institutionalized patients, with 53% of patients experiencing problematic urinary incontinence. In fact, urinary incontinence is one of the major reasons for institutionalization of the elderly.

Incontinence not only affects the patient physically but psychologically as well. Patients with urinary incontinence oftentimes alter their behavior to compensate for this problem. In an attempt to prevent any incontinence accidents, many patients become very knowledgeable of all the toilet facilities around them, always carrying a supply of absorbent products and even a change of clothing, and may use perfumes in an attempt to cover up a perceived uriniferous odor. In addition, one report noted that 40% of women with incontinence avoid sexual activity. The overall result of incontinence in these patients is a reduction of social activities and a degradation of quality of life.

The cost of incontinence to society is substantial. It has been estimated that incontinence costs $11.2 billion annually in the community and $5.2 billion in institutionalized care. For comparison, the annual cost of management of urinary incontinence in these patients is more than the combined annual cost of coronary artery bypass surgery and renal dialysis.

Although the majority of urinary incontinence evaluations are performed by a urologist or urogynecologist, knowledgeable primary care providers can perform the initial evaluation and implement nonsurgical treatments with referral of more complicated patients or those who fail initial interventions. This chapter will discuss the diagnosis and treatment of all categories of urinary incontinence. For primary care providers who desire an in-depth discussion of incontinence and helpful diagnostic algorithms, the Department of Health and Human Services has recently updated the Clinical Practice Guidelines for urinary incontinence.

Definition of Incontinence and Classifications

Urinary incontinence is defined as the involuntary loss of urine that causes a social or hygienic problem. There are many etiologies for urinary incontinence, with multiple possible treatment options depending on the type of incontinence and the underlying disease process. The most commonly used classification of urinary incontinence is based upon symptomatology. This classification includes transient incontinence, stress incontinence, urge incontinence, mixed incontinence, continuous incontinence, overflow incontinence, and nocturnal enuresis (Table 8–1). In addition, the severity or grade of incontinence within each category can also be quantified (Table 8–2).

Transient Incontinence

A number of medical conditions and medications have been identified that may cause or ex-

Table 8–1

Classification of Different Types of Urinary Incontinence

> **Transient:** Leakage due to potentially reversible cause; most common in the elderly
>
> **Stress:** Leakage occurs with increased abdominal pressure
>
> **Urge:** Leakage occurs due to uninhibited bladder contraction
>
> **Mixed:** Leakage due to both urge and stress incontinence
>
> **Continuous:** Continuous leakage both day and night; may be due to a fistula
>
> **Overflow:** Leakage due to a failure of the bladder to empty
>
> **Nocturnal enuresis:** Leakage that occurs at night; usually refers to condition prevalent in young children

Table 8–3

Potential Causes for Incontinence in the Elderly (DIAPPERS)

> **D**elirium
>
> **I**nfection
>
> **A**trophic vaginitis
>
> **P**harmacologic
>
> **P**sychological
>
> **E**ndocrine
>
> **R**estricted mobility
>
> **S**tool impaction

acerbate urinary incontinence. In many cases, the incontinence can be cured or greatly improved by identifying and treating these factors, and therefore this type of incontinence has been categorized as "transient" or reversible. Transient incontinence is much more common in the elderly, where functional limitations in addition to concurrent diseases and medications are much more frequent.

A useful mnemonic for remembering these potentially reversible causes is "DIAPPERS" (Table 8–3). When elderly patients complain of incontinence that appears to have presented rather acutely, these possible reversible causes should be entertained before proceeding on to more advanced diagnostic studies or treatments. Incontinence in the elderly is covered in greater detail in Chapter 10.

Table 8–2

Grading System for Stress Urinary Incontinence

> **Grade I:** Patient loses urine only with sudden severe increases of abdominal pressure, but never at rest or in the supine position
>
> **Grade II:** Incontinence with minimal to moderate degrees of physical stress such as walking, changing to a standing position, but not while supine.
>
> **Grade III:** Severe incontinence without significant relationship to physical activity or position

Stress Incontinence

Stress urinary incontinence (SUI) is defined as urinary leakage secondary to an increase in abdominal pressure in the absence of a bladder contraction or an overdistended bladder. One cause of SUI commonly seen in females is due to a loss of urethral support, which allows excessive mobility of the urethral sphincter and has been called urethral hypermobility. Activities such as coughing, laughing, sneezing, exercise, or sudden changes in position, which raise intra-abdominal pressure, can cause rotational descent of the urethral sphincter into a position where it does not function normally. There are multiple possible reasons for urethral hypermobility to develop, but the most common reasons include multiparity, intrinsic tissue weakness, and advancing age. The urinary sphincter itself is usually normal in these patients, and treatments that immobilize the bladder neck in the normal retropubic position will usually cure the incontinence. It is important to note that the loss of support that allows the urethra to become hypermobile oftentimes affects other areas of the vagina, and concurrent cystocele, rectocele, or uterine prolapse may be found on physical examination.

Stress incontinence may also be due to a poorly functioning urinary sphincter, called intrinsic sphincter deficiency (ISD). In these patients, the sphincter is intrinsically "weak" and cannot resist the increased intra-abdominal pressure that occurs with coughing or even mild physical activity. These patients, who are often elderly or may have had prior incontinence procedures, usually have more severe urinary leakage than patients with stress incontinence due to urethral hypermobility.

On physical exam, the urethra usually has minimal mobility; however, urethral mobility and intrinsic functional strength each exist as a continuum, with a variable degree of either abnormality present in a given patient. The contribution of each component in causing the incontinence can be quantified on physical exam and using an abdominal leak point pressure (ALPP), which will be described later. The distinction between these two types of stress incontinence (urethral hypermobility versus ISD) is important because the treatment options are different. An older classification of female stress incontinence, which is still sometimes used, categorizes patients radiographically into "types" as seen in Table 8–4.

Stress incontinence is rare in men, but may occur in congenital abnormalities such as myelomeningocele, after certain neurologic injuries, or after surgical procedures (e.g., radical prosta-

Table 8–4
Classification of Stress Urinary Incontinence

> **Type 0:** Typical history of stress incontinence, but no demonstrable leakage on physical or urodynamic examination. This failure to demonstrate incontinence is likely secondary to momentary voluntary contraction of the external urethral sphincter during the examination or undiagnosed urge incontinence.
>
> **Type I:** Bladder neck is closed at rest, and with increased intra-abdominal pressure there is minimal descent of the bladder neck, no cystocele is present, and urinary incontinence occurs.
>
> **Type II:** The bladder neck is closed at rest; however, with increased intra-abdominal pressure, there is a downward rotation of the urethra associated with a cystocele and urinary incontinence.
>
> **Type III:** The bladder neck and proximal urethra are open at rest without detrusor contraction, and incontinence occurs with minimal effort and minimal urethral rotation. (Previously called a "pipestem" urethra, now called intrinsic sphincter deficiency, or ISD.)

tectomy). In almost all cases the leakage is secondary to intrinsic sphincter deficiency requiring treatment somewhat different than females with this condition.

Urge Incontinence

Urinary urgency is a sudden and severe desire to void. The most severe form of urgency, in which the patient is unable to make it to the bathroom before leakage occurs, is called urge incontinence. Urge incontinence results from an involuntary bladder contraction that the patient is unable to adequately suppress, with resulting incontinence.

Urgency and urge incontinence are common in the elderly, and oftentimes have no identifiable etiology. This type of urge incontinence is called idiopathic detrusor instability, and has recently been referred to as overactive bladder.

If the involuntary detrusor contractions are due to neurologic conditions such as multiple sclerosis, a cerebrovascular accident, or Parkinson's disease, this is called detrusor hyperreflexia. These patients usually have complex reasons for their leakage and should be referred for evaluation and treatment by a urologist.

Some elderly men with bladder outlet obstruction due to prostatic enlargement (benign prostatic hyperplasia) may also complain of urgency or urge incontinence. In this situation, the treatment must be directed towards resolution of the obstruction, as treatment with medications for urge incontinence may lead to painful urinary retention. Again, referral to a urologist for evaluation and treatment is appropriate.

In some cases urge incontinence can be precipitated by reversible causes (as noted under "Transient Incontinence" earlier in the chapter), such as urinary tract infection, medications, fecal impaction, or even bladder cancer. Additionally, many patients with stress incontinence have concomitant urgency or even urge incontinence. This combination of incontinence is called mixed incontinence.

Mixed Incontinence

Mixed incontinence is defined as a mixture of both stress and urge incontinence. One study found that mixed incontinence is the most common type of incontinence in females, accounting for 55% of incontinent women over 60 years of age, followed by pure stress incontinence at 27%, and pure urge incontinence at 9%.

In most cases, one type of leakage is more significant than the other. As noted, many patients with stress incontinence also complain of urgency or even concomitant urge incontinence. This can oftentimes be demonstrated on urodynamics where stress incontinence, precipitated by a cough, is followed by an involuntary bladder contraction. This phenomenon is called stress-induced urge incontinence. The pathophysiology of why this occurs has not been completely elucidated, but it is thought to occur when the proximal urethra partially opens, stimulating a reflex bladder contraction. In most cases, this type of urgency is cured or improved with successful treatment of the stress incontinence.

Continuous Incontinence

Continuous leakage may occur due to an overdistended bladder (called overflow incontinence, described in the next section), severe sphincter weakness, or a bypassing of the normal urinary tract, called extraurethral incontinence. These patients leak both day and night and in some cases have little or no desire to void. Common etiologies for this type of incontinence include urinary fistulas such as vesicovaginal fistulas or in congenital anomalies in which the ureter(s) end at sites other than the bladder.

Overflow Incontinence

Overflow incontinence is due to a failure of the bladder to empty, causing an increase in bladder volume until bladder pressure overcomes sphincter pressure, resulting in continuous day and nighttime leakage. In the acute setting, the patient will usually complain of severe pain, but if the retention develops very slowly, the patient may have no pain at all. These patients can usually be identified because they will leak while sleeping in bed with little or no desire to void. This condition most commonly occurs in men, associated with urinary obstruction secondary to prostatic hyperplasia and less commonly from urethral stricture disease. Diabetic neuropathy, neurologic lesions, or procedures that either decrease bladder sensation or impair the bladder's ability to contract can also cause overflow incontinence. Overflow incontinence is rare in women but may occur after initiating anticholinergic medications, after incontinence procedures in which the urethra is obstructed, or from urethral obstruction from severe pelvic prolapse.

Nocturnal Enuresis

Nocturnal enuresis refers to incontinence that occurs during sleep. This condition is prevalent in young children, with spontaneous resolution in almost all children by age 18. Nocturnal enuresis in adults is rare and usually indicates a significant abnormality in the bladder or urinary sphincter. In some cases, injudicious use of sleeping aids can lead to nocturnal enuresis in patients with urgency, because the bladder begins to empty before the patient has time to awaken.

Evaluation of the Patient with Incontinence

History

The basic evaluation of urinary incontinence begins with a detailed history focusing on the specific symptoms of incontinence and its characteristics, along with a focused medical, neurologic, and genitourinary history. Certain risk factors for incontinence should be assessed, and the precise nature of the incontinence should be described. It is important to remember that although an accurate history is helpful in guiding the physician's diagnostic evaluation, therapeutic decisions can rarely be based on history alone. It should be noted that the following suggested historical and evaluative methods described are similar to the Clinical Practice Guidelines published in 1996 with some modifications based on personal experience.

KEY QUESTIONS

The history should begin with an evaluation of the characteristics of the urinary incontinence and its duration. An incontinence questionnaire completed by the patient prior to the office visit can facilitate the incontinence history (Table 8–5). Specifically, the history should focus on differentiating stress from urge incontinence. For example, determine if the incontinence is associated with cough, sneezing, laughing, or activity (stress incontinence), or with a sudden desire to urinate and the inability to reach a bathroom in time (urge incontinence). Determine if the symptoms were associated with any special circumstances or precipitating causes (e.g., hematuria, painful urination, acute illness, childbirth, new medication), whether the symptoms have progressed or have stayed constant, and whether the onset was acute or gradual. If the incontinence is continuous both day and night, then overflow incontinence, a urinary fistula (vesicovaginal or ureterovaginal), or an ectopic ureter should be considered. All patients with hematuria or continuous incontinence need an evaluation to determine the cause.

Voiding patterns and degree of leakage should also be assessed during the history. Is there a history of frequent small voids? Some patients have an intrinsically small bladder or have a sensory ur-

Table 8–5

Incontinence History Questionnaire

1. Do you ever leak urine or lose control of urination?   Yes   No

2. If you leak urine, do you know when it happens or do you just find yourself wet?
    Know when it happens   Find myself wet

3. How often do you wet yourself or your pads when you cough or sneeze?
    Never   Few times/year   Few times/month   Few times/week   Daily

4. How often do you wet yourself or your pads when you engage in physical activity (running, jumping, aerobics, or lifting)?
    Never   Few times/year   Few times/month   Few times/week   Daily

5. How often do you wear pads or other forms of protection because of the wetting?
    Never   Few times/year   Few times/month   Few times/week   Daily

6. If leakage is daily, on average, how many pads do you use a day?_____

7. On average, how wet are they when you change them?
    Dry   Moist   Damp   Wet   Soaked

8. How often do you lose control of urination and wet yourself or your pads because you feel a strong urge and can't stop it?
    Never   Few times/year   Few times/month   Few times/week   Daily

9. On a scale of 0 to 10 (*0* is not at all, *10* is intolerable), how badly does the urinary leakage bother you?_____

gency problem such as interstitial cystitis, which is treated differently. What is the longest time between voids? How many pads are worn? What type of pads (thin day pads versus thick absorbent pads)? Are they completely soaked or lightly damp? Patients who soak through their pads usually have urge incontinence.

Obstructive or bladder weakness symptoms should also be assessed with questions such as: Is there a need to strain to void? Do you feel like you empty your bladder completely? How is the force of your urinary stream? How many times are you getting up at night to go to the bathroom? Patients who drink a large amount of fluid will often complain of nocturia. Do you have any leaking at night while in bed? Do you leak at night because you are unable to get up to the bathroom in time or do you wake up already wet? Leakage in bed can be a sign of a severe underlying disorder such as a poorly compliant bladder. Are you aware that you are leaking? Patients who are unaware that they are leaking usually have stress incontinence.

VOIDING LOG

A simple method of determining a patient's voiding habits and degree of urinary leakage is to obtain a voiding log (Table 8–6). The voiding log should include at least 2 or 3 days, and should represent the patient's typical urinary habits. Documentation of voided volumes, frequency, nocturia, incontinent episodes, and number of pads used and degree of pad wetness over a 24- to 72-hour period is helpful in diagnosing the degree and type of incontinence. Patients with urge incontinence will often complain that the leakage "soaks through my pants and runs down my leg," because in contrast to the small volumes leaked with stress incontinence, in urge incontinence, a large portion of the bladder may be emptied before the patient can terminate the bladder contraction.

Large volume or frequent voids may be indicative of an undiagnosed medical problem such as diabetes or heart failure. Dysuria and hematuria may indicate an urinary infection. Any history of hematuria, gross or microscopic, with a negative urine culture requires further evaluation of the upper and lower urinary tracts to rule out a malignancy. Occasionally, incontinence and frequency are related to the excess production of urine. Inquiries should be made about the type and amount of fluid intake and any history of diuretic use. Excessive caffeine intake can exacerbate urge incontinence by producing a diuresis. Diuretics should be taken in the morning to reduce the severity of nocturia.

BOWEL PATTERNS

In addition to urinary complaints, bowel movements should also be assessed, especially in the elderly. Any history of fecal incontinence, constipation, or fecal impaction should be evaluated.

UNDERLYING MEDICAL PROBLEMS

The patient's past medical history may also give insight into the etiology of the urinary incontinence. Medical problems such as poorly controlled diabetes may cause a diuresis resulting in frequency and urgency. In addition, long-term diabetes can cause neurologic damage leading to an inability to empty the bladder. A neurologic history such as multiple sclerosis, a herniated intervertebral disk, and spinal cord trauma may also cause urinary incontinence. Inquiries should be made about changes in vision, muscle weakness, tremors, numbness or tingling, or history of paralysis. Parkinson's disease, multiple sclerosis, and prior strokes are frequently associated with bladder overactivity and urge incontinence. It is also important to obtain an obstetric history to include a history of vaginal tears or trauma to the perineal region. In addition, a history of acute urinary retention would indicate that overflow incontinence may be a factor.

Prior surgical procedures are also important to know. Prior attempts to treat incontinence may have caused urethral obstruction, which may cause urgency, urge incontinence, or incomplete voiding. Patients with obstruction may complain of pelvic pain due to the high intravesical pressure

Table 8–6

Voiding Diary

Name: _____   Date: _____

TIME OF URINATION	VOIDED VOLUME (ML)	URGE INCONTINENCE? (YES OR NO)	STRESS INCONTINENCE? (YES OR NO)	PAD CHANGED? (YES OR NO)
TOTALS				

Incontinence is any undesired leakage of urine.

Stress incontinence is leakage with coughing, sneezing, or activity.

Urge incontinence is leakage due to inability to make it to the bathroom before urination starts.

generated, whereas patients with large postvoid residuals will often have frequent urinary tract infections. Radical pelvic procedures such as radical hysterectomy or abdominoperineal resection of the rectum can cause neurologic injury to the bladder, leading to a variety of complex voiding abnormalities or incontinence. In addition, any history of radiation therapy may cause tissue damage to the bladder or sphincter, leading to irritative voiding symptoms or stress incontinence. In some cases, severe bladder fibrosis occurs, yielding a small, poorly compliant bladder. All of these abnormalities will require urodynamics for evaluation.

Certain medications may also cause or worsen urinary incontinence and are thought to be perhaps the most common cause of reversible incontinence in primary care practice. Tricyclic antidepressants, sympathomimetics, anticholinergic agents, and some over-the-counter cold medications (including antihistamines and sympathomimetics such as over-the-counter decongestants) may precipitate bladder outlet obstruction or impair detrusor contractions, causing urinary retention and overflow incontinence, especially in males. Sympatholytic agents such as alpha-adrenergic blockers, diazepam, alpha-methyldopa, and phenothiazines may cause or exacerbate stress urinary incontinence by lowering smooth or skeletal urethral muscle tone.

Due to their frailty and diminished physiologic reserve secondary to increased age, the elderly are prone to transient urinary incontinence from various factors. These factors are summarized using the mnemonic "DIAPPERS" (Table 8–3). Many of these problems may be easily corrected with simple medical management without the need for more invasive treatments.

Physical Examination

A general physical exam should start with observation of a patient's gait while ambulating into the office. An abnormal gait may suggest a neurologic abnormality. In cases where neurologic disease is suspected, a neurologic screening exam should be performed. Examination of the lower extremity functions (innervated by the lower thoracic, lumbar, and sacral nerves) may provide indirect evidence regarding urinary function. Reflex contraction of the pelvic musculature in response to the anal sphincter and bulbocavernosus reflexes provides evidence of the integrity of the S2–4 sacral reflexes. However, it is important to note that these reflexes are not present in all patients. A neurologic consultation should be obtained in any patient with abnormal neurologic findings.

ABDOMINAL EXAM

The abdominal exam should consist of a general overview of the abdomen, identifying any prior surgical scars and observing for any evidence of a distended bladder. A postvoid residual utilizing either office ultrasound or catheterization should be obtained immediately after the patient voids. Normally, urine residuals should be less than 50 mL. In males, great care should be taken in obtaining a catheterized postvoid residual so as not to injure the urethra or prostate. In females, the

catheter used to perform the postvoid residual can also be used to fill the bladder, which is required for evaluating incontinence and pelvic prolapse.

PELVIC EXAM

The pelvic examination in females should start with an assessment of the estrogen status of the genitalia. Hypoestrogenic atrophy of the vaginal mucosa, especially in the postmenopausal female, may indicate similar atrophic changes in the urethra, which may contribute to urinary leakage. A recent Pap smear should be documented. The female patient should then be examined with a moderately full bladder in the supine lithotomy position to check for prolapse and incontinence.

Q-TIP TEST

The degree of urethral hypermobility can be assessed using the "Q-tip test." It is performed by inserting a well lubricated cotton-tipped swab gently into the urethra past the level of the bladder neck, which is the area of greatest resistance. The resting angle is measured from the horizontal and the patient is then asked to strain. The degree of deflection of the Q-tip is measured, and hypermobility is defined as greater than a 30-degree change.

STRESS MANEUVERS

The swab is then removed and the patient is asked to slowly strain to increase intraabdominal pressure and demonstrate leakage. Occasionally, no leakage will be demonstrated due to voluntary contraction of the external sphincter. The patient may then perform a half sit-up followed by three spontaneous coughs to try to demonstrate leakage. If a large cystocele is present, the urethra may be obstructed, preventing incontinence; therefore prior to straining or coughing, the cystocele should be reduced using a vaginal pack. If no urinary incontinence is demonstrable in the supine position, the evaluation should be repeated in the standing position, the usual position for urinary loss in most patients. If no leakage is noted after these maneuvers, stress incontinence is unlikely and urge incontinence is the probable reason for the incontinence.

If urinary incontinence is demonstrated, a Bonney–Marshall test may be performed to determine whether a urethral suspension procedure may improve urinary leakage. This is performed by elevating the anterior vaginal sulci adjacent to either side of the urethra while the patient is straining and determining whether the incontinence is eliminated. Care must be taken not to directly compress the urethra while performing this test.

Lastly, an assessment of the urethra and vaginal prolapse should be documented. A "bulge" in the area of the urethra may indicate a urethral diverticulum, whereas prolapse of the anterior wall indicates a cystocele (Fig. 8–1) and prolapse of the posterior wall indicates a rectocele (Fig. 8–2).

EXAMINATION IN MEN

In males, the majority of cases of urinary incontinence are due to postsurgical changes such as prostatectomy for obstruction or cancer or ab-

Figure 8–1

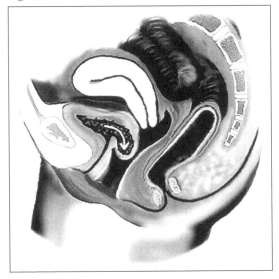

When the anterior vaginal wall becomes weak and no longer provides adequate support for the bladder, a cystocele, as depicted here, may develop.

Figure 8–2

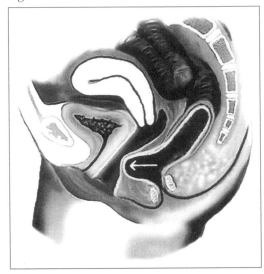

When the posterior vaginal wall becomes weak and no longer provides adequate support for the rectum, a rectocele, as depicted here, may develop.

dominoperineal resection for rectal carcinoma. The examination is more simplified compared to the female examination because males rarely demonstrate urethral hypermobility. With a full bladder, the male patient is placed in the standing position and instructed to strain forcefully. Any demonstrable leakage is likely due to intrinsic sphincter deficiency. However, it is important to remember that these patients may also have concomitant urge incontinence that may contribute to urinary leakage. A careful history may be able to differentiate between the two. Males with no prior history of pelvic surgery or neurologic trauma who complain of leakage almost always have urge incontinence which may be secondary to obstruction due to benign prostatic hyperplasia (BPH). Additionally, severely obstructed patients may have overflow incontinence.

Diagnostic Studies

Once the physical examination is complete, certain tests may be used to confirm the diagnosis and cause of the urinary incontinence. Initial tests should include urinalysis and urine culture to rule out urinary tract infections. In addition, the presence of any hematuria in the absence of an infection requires further evaluation to rule out malignancy. Urinary cytology should be obtained for patients with unexplained urinary urgency, especially with a history of tobacco use, to rule out the possibility of transitional cell carcinoma of the bladder. Female patients presenting with severe pelvic prolapse can have ureteral obstruction, and a BUN and creatinine as well as a renal ultrasound should be obtained to evaluate for upper tract obstruction.

Uroflowmetry

Uroflowmetry is measurement of the urine flow rate. Although this test is usefully performed using specialized equipment, it can be crudely assessed using a stopwatch. With a relatively full bladder, patients are instructed to void into a device that measures the amount of urine output over time. Uroflowmetry is helpful in male patients with symptoms of bladder obstruction because standardized nomograms allow classification of the flow rate into obstructed or nonobstructed categories (Fig. 8–3). Unfortunately, no useful nomograms exist for female patients and uroflowmetry cannot be used to diagnose the type of incontinence in women. Additionally, uroflowmetry is unable to accurately distinguish between obstruction and a weak bladder contraction in males or females without simultaneously measuring detrusor pressure.

Urodynamics

Urodynamic evaluation can be helpful in determining the precise etiology of the urinary incontinence. Urodynamic studies can determine the capacity, sensation, and overall function of the bladder with great precision. Additionally, sphincter function, mobility, and degree of anterior vaginal wall prolapse can be assessed. These studies range from relatively simple urodynamic studies to sophisticated multichannel fluoroscopic studies that may include pressure/flow studies and videorecording.

Figure 8–3

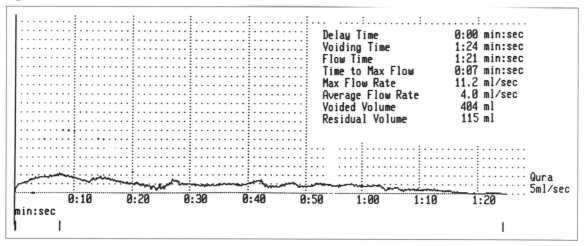

Delay Time	0:00 min:sec
Voiding Time	1:24 min:sec
Flow Time	1:21 min:sec
Time to Max Flow	0:07 min:sec
Max Flow Rate	11.2 ml/sec
Average Flow Rate	4.0 ml/sec
Voided Volume	404 ml
Residual Volume	115 ml

This is the flow rate study from a man with symptomatic prostatic obstruction. The maximum flowrate of 11.2 mL/second is well below normal, and the residual urine volume is excessive. Note the undulating flow rate tracing, which indicates that the patient is straining to void.

Simple urodynamic studies may give an overview of the patient's symptoms. This may be performed easily in the office during the pelvic examination. Under sterile conditions, a catheter is inserted into the bladder to determine the postvoid residual. Once the bladder is completely emptied, a 60-mL catheter (bayonnette) tipped syringe is connected to the end of the catheter and the bladder is slowly filled under gravity in a retrograde fashion with saline or water at room temperature. As the water level in the syringe falls, its meniscus represents the intravesical pressure. The syringe is refilled anytime the level reaches the tip of the syringe. The first sensation (when something is felt within the bladder), first desire to void, strong desire to void, and total bladder capacity are evaluated while the bladder is slowly filled. The volumes at these points are recorded. Detrusor instability is seen with the patient experiencing a sudden urge to void with rapid efflux of fluid back into the syringe or even around the catheter. However, a rise in intravesical pressure may also be due to an increase in intra-abdominal pressure or poor bladder wall compliance. Once the bladder capacity is obtained, the volume is then reduced to approximately 200 to 300 mL and examination is performed to determine the presence of stress urinary incontinence and any other pelvic abnormalities such as prolapse (as previously described).

Sophisticated multichannel urodynamic studies that measure precise bladder and urethral pressures should be considered when gross urodynamic studies are inconclusive, urinary leakage cannot be demonstrated clinically, a history of postsurgical incontinence is present, a history of neurologic disease (including cerebrovascular accident, multiple sclerosis, spinal cord trauma, Parkinson's disease, or myelodysplasia) exists, or there is any history of prior incontinence operations (Fig. 8–4). The main advantage of these urodynamic studies is the ability to record and display multiple parameters simultaneously, thus minimizing the likelihood of misinterpretation of findings. Due to the cost of the equipment and complexity of performing the evaluation, these studies are usually performed by a urologist or urogynecologist.

The testing performed during multichannel urodynamics can be divided into individual functional tests. For example, a cystometrogram is a test of detrusor function. Using a pressure-transducing catheter in either the bladder, rectum, or both, bladder sensation, capacity, compliance, and magnitude of voluntary and involuntary detrusor contractions are measured. Usually, the bladder is filled at a rate of 50 to 100 mL per minute with saline or radio-opaque contrast if fluoroscopy is used. Similar to simple urodynamics, sensation is measured at specific pressures along with observing for the presence of abnormal detrusor contractions.

Whereas the cystometrogram is a test of bladder function, the abdominal leak point pressure (ALPP) is a test of sphincteric function. This test is usually performed in the patient who complains of stress incontinence or has incontinence of unknown etiology. Basically, the ALPP is the lowest pressure at which urinary leakage occurs during an increase in intra-abdominal pressure (Fig. 8–5). To perform this test, the bladder is filled to approximately half full (200 mL is standard) and the patient is instructed to strain until leakage occurs. If no leakage occurs or the patient cannot generate pressures greater than 100 cm H_2O, then vigorous coughing can be used. An ALPP below 60 cm H_2O is indicative of intrinsic sphincter deficiency (ISD), pressures between 60 and 100 cm H_2O indicate combined ISD and urethral hypermobility, and pressures greater than 100 cm H_2O are associated with pure urethral hypermobility (Fig. 8–6). This data can be helpful in deciding which method of treatment should be undertaken.

Of note, significant pelvic prolapse can falsely elevate the ALPP; therefore, prolapse should be reduced prior to measuring the ALPP. If radioopaque contrast is used as the filling agent, fluoroscopy may be used to obtain a radiographic view of the lower urinary tract during bladder filling, leakage, and voiding.

In cases where a patient has a voiding abnormality such as urgency, urge incontinence, straining to void, or incomplete bladder emptying and it is not clear whether the cause is bladder outlet obstruction or a "weak" bladder, a pressure-flow

Figure 8–4

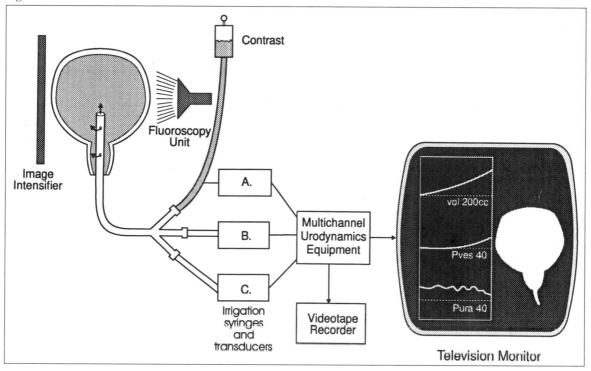

The typical videourodynamics equipment used in a urodynamics laboratory. (Reprinted by permission from McGuire EJ, Cespedes RD, et al: Videourodynamic studies. *Urol Clin North Am* 23:309, 1996.)

Figure 8–5

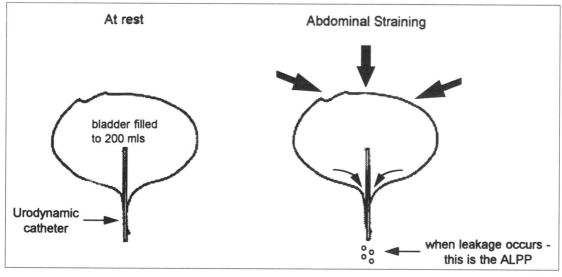

With the bladder filled to 200 mL, the patient is asked to strain until leakage occurs. The bladder pressure at the time of leakage is the abdominal leak point pressure (ALPP).

Figure 8–6

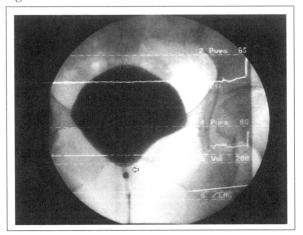

This is a fluorourodynamic photograph at the time of leakage while the patient is straining. The patient was found to have an ALPP of 65 cm H_2O, consistent with intrinsic sphincter deficiency. The arrow is at the level of the incompetent bladder neck and proximal urethra. The patient underwent a pubovaginal sling procedure with excellent results.

Figure 8–7

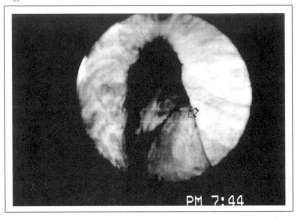

This is a cystoscopic view of an obstructing prostate with the prominent median lobe at the arrow.

study can be performed. This test allows for the simultaneous measurement of bladder pressure and urine flow rate by placing pressure-transducing catheters in the bladder and rectum (to subtract intra-abdominal pressure, which may be elevated if the patient strains) and then having the patient void into a machine to measure the flow rate. This test is most commonly performed on older males to rule out prostatic obstruction and occasionally in females after an incontinence procedure to rule out iatrogenic obstruction.

Cystourethroscopy

Cystourethroscopy utilizing a cystoscope allows for direct visualization of the urethra and bladder. This study is a useful adjunctive test in that it may identify other potential causes of urinary incontinence such as a tumor, fistula, urethral diverticulum, urethral strictures, obstructing prostate, foreign bodies, and stones (Fig. 8–7). Additionally, abnormalities of the bladder such as inflammation

and bladder wall thickening can be evaluated. The sphincter can also be visually inspected for mobility and coaptation characteristics.

Additional Studies

Urethral pressure profilometry (UPP) allows for the static measurement of urethral pressure, which has been used to categorize the type of incontinence. Unfortunately, a significant overlap of UPP values in continent and incontinent females limits the predictive value of the UPP. Additionally, technical problems such as variability with the orientation of the catheter, variation with speed of withdrawal of the catheter, and differences with bladder filling may all effect the urethral pressure. Although this test was previously used quite frequently, it has been basically supplanted by the ALPP, which has been found to be more accurate.

Electromyography (EMG) studies have most commonly been used to measure the electrical activity of the external urethral sphincter in patients with neurologic abnormalities involving the spinal cord. Basically, a normal voiding reflex requires two processes to happen: The sphincter must first open and the bladder must subsequently generate sufficient pressure. An EMG can be used to ensure that the sphincter is functioning normally during voiding. EMG recordings may be performed using either surface electrodes or needle electrodes placed in the perineal area. Surface electrodes are more comfortable for the patient but are not as accurate as the needle electrodes. During a normal EMG, as the bladder fills, the EMG waves become stronger, whereas when voiding is initiated, the EMG waves disappear.

A pelvic MRI may occasionally be of use in female patients when a urethral diverticulum is suspected but cannot be identified on cystoscopy or other radiologic studies. In general, this test is ordered by the urologist only after the preliminary studies are nondiagnostic. Patients with a urethral diverticulum typically present with the 3 "D's": *dysuria, postvoid dribbling, and dyspareunia.* In addition, some women present with urgency and or urge incontinence secondary to urethral irritation or recurrent UTIs that cannot be eradicated despite appropriate antibiotic treatment. The majority of urethral diverticula are thought to be acquired secondary to an infection of the periurethral glands.

An intravenous pyelogram (IVP), renal ultrasound, or a CT scan are often used by urologists to identify potential reasons for hematuria; however, these tests are rarely indicated in the incontinent patient without hematuria. The decision to perform these tests is usually made after referral to a specialist.

Treatment Options for Incontinence

Nonsurgical Treatment Options

BEHAVIORAL THERAPY

Depending on the type of incontinence, there are a number of possible treatment options. The 1992 Department of Health and Human Services guidelines recommended that "surgery, except in very specific cases, should be considered only after behavioral and pharmacological interventions have been tried." Although few patients will be cured with conservative therapy, almost all patients with incontinence may benefit from some form of conservative therapy. Many patients with mild to moderate stress or urge incontinence may be satisfied with the improvement and not desire further treatment. The most common nonsurgical treatment options include pelvic muscle exercises, biofeedback, bladder retraining, vaginal cones, and electrical stimulation.

PELVIC MUSCLE EXERCISES   Pelvic muscle exercises (PME) are believed to strengthen the musculature responsible for urethral resistance and reflex contraction of the pelvic floor, thereby improving incontinence during episodes of increased abdominal pressure and unstable bladder contractions. Popularized by Kegel in the 1940s and 1950s, patients were taught to isolate the pubococcygeus muscles and contract them vigorously without simultaneously contracting the abdominal and gluteal muscles. The goal is to promote increased resting muscular tone (improves stress incontinence) and the ability to terminate undesired reflex bladder activity (improves urge incontinence). Some studies have found that Kegel exercises are effective in reducing urinary incontinence in men following prostate surgery.

For the pelvic floor exercises to be of benefit, they must be performed correctly. This is best done by assisting the patient in isolating the correct pelvic muscles to contract. Written or verbal instructions may be insufficient to teach the patient how to properly perform these exercises. During the initial pelvic examination, while the patient is in the lithotomy position, the perineum is gently retracted posteriorly and the patient is instructed to tighten the pelvic muscles. The examiner should assess the patient's ability to isolate the pelvic muscles while keeping the abdomen, thighs, and buttocks at rest. Patients may be instructed to contract the levator muscles as if to hold in a tampon. Interruption of the urinary stream may also determine if the exercise is being done properly, but may occasionally lead to dysfunctional voiding if the exercises are routinely performed during voiding.

Once the patient is able to successfully isolate and contract these muscles, they are instructed to perform 10 pelvic floor contractions for 10 to 20 seconds at least 3 or more times daily. Patients should be informed that it may take up to 6 to 12 weeks before there is any noticeable improvement in stress incontinence; however, the degree of improvement may increase for up to 6 months. One study has shown that among elderly females, Kegel exercises have a 16% cure rate with 54% rate of improvement of urinary incontinence (both urge and stress incontinence). Others have reported improvement rates as high as 84% in highly selected and well-motivated patients. For patients who are unable to isolate or contract their pelvic muscles, biofeedback and/or electrical stimulation help with learning these exercises.

BIOFEEDBACK   Biofeedback uses electromyographic or pressure readings to provide visual or auditory feedback to the patient regarding the status of the pelvic floor musculature (Fig. 8–8). The perineometer consists of a vaginal chamber attached to a manometer, which measures perineal muscle contractions and provides visual feedback for the patient. In addition, surface electromyelography is used to identify which muscles are contracting, enabling the patient to determine whether the abdominal, gluteal, or thigh muscles are being used to compensate for weakness in the pelvic floor. The goal of biofeedback is assist the patient in objectively measuring improvement in the ability to isolate and subsequently strengthen the correct pelvic floor muscles.

BEHAVIORAL MODIFICATION/BLADDER RETRAINING   The basic concept of behavioral modification or "bladder retraining" is to combine multiple conservative treatment modalities to help the patient increase the time interval between voiding and to improve continence under conditions of physical activity

and urinary urgency. Patients undergo reeducation in the use of the pelvic floor muscles (as noted earlier) in maintaining continence during increases in abdominal pressure and to inhibit the bladder when an undesired detrusor contraction is initiated. This regimen helps to reestablish the cortical inhibition of reflex bladder activity that is abnormal in many patients with detrusor instability. The adjunctive use of biofeedback techniques improves the effectiveness of these exercises. Additionally, fluid and dietary modifications along with timed voiding regimens are also used.

Traditionally employed to treat urge incontinence and urgency, patients with stress incontinence secondary to urethral hypermobility and other mild forms of incontinence may benefit from behavioral modification. Patients are instructed to void on a set schedule during the day, regardless of whether there is an urge to urinate. Initially, patients are instructed to void at 1-hour intervals, gradually increasing the interval between voiding until there is approximately 3 to 4 hours between voids. All other desires to void are inhibited using pelvic floor contractions, or with the use of relaxation or distraction techniques, even if it initially results in some incontinence. Relaxation and distraction techniques include deep breathing and slowly counting to 100. The eventual goal is to gain voluntary control over all bladder contractions. As many female patients drink large volumes of fluid, they are encouraged to drink smaller volumes, keeping up with thirst, but preferably at least nothing 2 to 3 hours before sleeping at night. Although short-term improvement rates range as high as 80%, rarely are these patients "cured" of their urinary incontinence using behavioral modification alone.

VAGINAL CONES   Another form of biofeedback is the use of weighted vaginal cones. These progressively weighted cones are individually placed into the vagina, starting with the lightest cone, and are retained while in the upright position and while walking. The usual regimen is to retain the cone for at least 15 minutes each session, with at least one and preferably three or more sessions

Figure 8–8

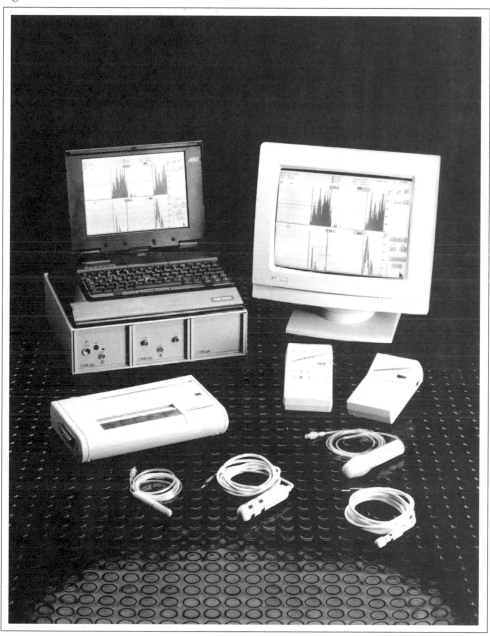

An example of the biofeedback and pelvic floor stimulation equipment available for behavioral therapy. (Courtesy of Incare Medical Products, Libertyville, IL.)

per day. Tactile biofeedback occurs when the patient senses that the cone is falling out and contracts the isolated pelvic floor musculature to retain the cone. The weight is gradually increased as tolerated by the patient, in essence progressively strengthening the pelvic musculature. This technique appears to be more effective in younger women as some older patients may be either reluctant in using intravaginal techniques or may have such severe pelvic floor weakness that they are unable to retain even the lightest cone.

ELECTRICAL STIMULATION   Electrical stimulation (ES) of the pudendal region has been shown in selected cases to improve both stress and urge incontinence, depending on the stimulation techniques. In detrusor instability, a lower frequency is generally used to increase the inhibitory impulses to the bladder. On the other hand, striated muscles are better stimulated at higher frequencies. The electrode, oftentimes placed in a vaginal probe, is ideally placed close to the pudendal nerves, allowing for effective excitation of primarily the levator ani muscles. Home electrical stimulation devices are available (Fig. 8–8) that combine biofeedback and ES, and are generally well received by patients. However, this technique is relatively contraindicated in pregnancy, those patients with a history of cardiac arrhythmias or pacemakers, and those patients with poor sensory perception in the perineal/vaginal region. The majority of patients who respond to electrical stimulation therapy will experience improvements within 6 weeks. Some studies have shown an improvement rate as high as 87%.

Sacral nerve stimulation has been used in severe refractory urge incontinence; however, the placement of this device requires specialized surgical equipment and knowledge.

Pharmacologic Therapy

Pharmacotherapy is available for both stress and urge incontinence. Used in conjunction with behavioral therapy, especially with urge incontinence, these medications may be very effective.

The pharmacotherapy is directed in relaxing the detrusor with urge incontinence, or augmenting intrinsic urethral tone in patients with stress urinary incontinence. Depending on the type of incontinence, medications may be used to selectively relax the bladder, relax the bladder *and* tighten the sphincter, or increase bladder outlet resistance (Table 8–7).

ANTICHOLINERGICS   The medications used to relax the bladder typically have anticholinergic effects, which decrease the nervous system's impulses to the bladder. These medications are usually used to treat urgency and urge incontinence. Unfortunately, the majority of these medications lack uroselectivity, and thus have many side effects associated with the anticholinergic properties: dry mouth, constipation, blurred vision, decreased sweating, and glaucoma exacerbation. Commonly used medications in this class include oxybutynin (Ditropan and Ditropan XL), hyoscyamine (Levbid), propantheline bromide (Pro-Banthine), and tolterodine (Detrol). Tolterodine represents a new class of anticholinergics with a decreased affinity for the salivary gland, thereby decreasing the severity of dry mouth. Ditropan XL uses standard oxybutynin but delivers the drug such that once a day dosing is possible and the severity of dry mouth may be decreased. All of these medications increase the capacity of the bladder, thereby increasing the time between voids. As unstable bladder contractions usually occur near bladder capacity, the number of urge incontinence episodes should decrease. Unfortunately, none of these drugs increase the "warning time," which is the time between the sensation that undesired voiding is starting and subsequent urinary leakage. Additionally, none of these medications will totally eliminate undesired detrusor contractions.

Anticholinergic medications should be avoided in males with possible prostatic obstruction due to the risk of acute urinary retention. Additionally, these medications should be avoided in patients who work or play outside in hot weather, in patients with severe cardiovascular disease, in patients with Alzheimer's disease, and in patients

Table 8–7

Pharmacologic Therapy for Urge and Stress Incontinence

INDICATION	MEDICATION	MECHANICS	DOSAGE	SIDE EFFECTS	CONTRAINDICATION
DETRUSOR INSTABILITY	Oxybutynin (Ditropan, Ditropan XL)	Anticholinergic, musculotropic	5 mg bid-tid (XL: 5–20 mg/day)	Dry mouth, decreased sweating, blurred vision, constipation	Glaucoma, cardiovascular disease, BPH
	Hyoscyamine (Levbid)	Anticholinergic	0.375 mg bid-tid	Same as above	Same as above
	Propantheline bromide (Pro-Banthine)	Anticholinergic, muscarinic	15–30 mg Q 4–6h	Same as above	Same as above
	Tolterodine (Detrol)	Selective anticholinergic (bladder)	1–2 mg bid	Same as above, dry mouth less severe	Same as above
	Imipramine (Tofranil)	Anticholinergic (central and peripheral), muscarinic, mild alpha-adrenergic	10–50 mg bid	Same as above, hypertension, orthostatic hypotension, arrhythmias, impotence	Same as above, MAO inhibitors (cause central nervous system toxicity)
	Flavoxate HCl (Urispas)	Mild anticholinergic, antispasmodic	100–200 mg tid-qid	Mild anticholinergic properties	Glaucoma, cardiovascular disease, BPH
STRESS INCONTINENCE	Ephedrine	Alpha-adrenergic	25–50 mg qid	Hypertension, anxiety, tremors, insomnia, arrhythmias, palpitations	Hypertension, hyperthyroidism, BPH, elderly
	Pseudoephedrine	Alpha-adrenergic	30–60 mg qid	Same as above	Same as above
	Phenylpropanol-amine (Entex LA)	Alpha-adrenergic	25–75 mg bid	Same as above	Same as above
	Estrogen	Vaginal trophicity, enhances alpha-adrenergic response	Vaginal cream biw-tiw × 6–12 weeks	? Increased risk of endometrial and breast cancer	History of breast cancer

with narrow-angle glaucoma, who may develop a precipitous rise in intraocular pressure.

Tricyclic antidepressants are advantageous in treating mixed incontinence due to their alpha-adrenergic and anticholinergic properties. Bladder outlet resistance is increased due to alpha-adrenergic stimulation, while detrusor relaxation occurs due to anticholinergic properties. Imipramine (Tofranil) is the most commonly used tricyclic antidepressant for treating urinary incontinence. Side effects of these medications include hypertension, orthostatic hypotension (especially in older patients), and those associated with the anticholinergic properties. In addition, tricyclic antidepressants may cause arrhythmias in higher doses and should be kept away from small children.

SYMPATHOMIMETICS Sympathomimetics stimulate the alpha-adrenergic receptors in the internal sphincter, thereby increasing smooth muscle tone with some improvement of mild stress incontinence in selected patients. Unfortunately, few studies have shown significant improvement of these agents in the treatment of stress urinary incontinence. Some commonly used medications in this category include Sudafed, which contains pseudoephedrine; and Entex and Dexatrim, both of which contain phenylpropanolamine as the active ingredient. Potential side effects of these medications include nausea, anxiety, insomnia, dry mouth, and hypertension. Sympathomimetic agents should be used cautiously in patients with hypertension, hyperthyroidism, arrhythmias, or coronary artery disease.

ESTROGEN In postmenopausal women, estrogen replacement therapy may increase urethral resistance as well as enhance the sensory threshold for involuntary detrusor contractions. In addition, estrogenization may also enhance the alpha-adrenergic contractile response of the urethral smooth muscle and may improve the results of concurrently used sympathomimetic agents. It has been reported that up to 70% of women with mild stress incontinence may have some improvement with estrogen therapy. Estrogen is usually given as an oral supplement or as a vaginal cream if the side effects of oral administration preclude its use. Patients with an intact uterus will also need concurrent progesterone therapy. Contraindications to estrogen use include a history of endometrial cancer and in most cases of breast cancer.

Surgical Treatment Options

There are many surgical options for urinary incontinence depending on the etiology of the incontinence. Patients with stress incontinence should be aware that although surgery offers a better chance for a long-term cure, there are more potential complications than non-surgical approaches. In addition, the success rate of surgery to treat urinary incontinence decreases with the increasing number of attempts for correction. Women of child-bearing age should be counseled that an operation may be damaged or undone by subsequent pregnancy, labor, and delivery.

PERIURETHRAL BULKING

For older patients with intrinsic sphincter deficiency (ISD) and minimal urethral mobility, a minimally invasive option includes periurethral injections of bulking agents. Historically, many agents have been used, but most were abandoned due to either safety reasons of lack of efficacy. Currently, glutaraldehyde cross-linked (GAX) bovine collagen (Contigen, CR Bard, Covington, GA) is the only FDA-approved bulking agent. Because of a 2% to 5% risk of a hypersensitivity reaction, a subdermal skin test is performed at least 30 days prior to the first injection. The procedure can be performed in an outpatient clinic setting with local anesthetic utilizing an endoscope especially made for transurethral injection. The prepackaged collagen is injected submucosally into the bladder neck region (proximal urethra) until the urethral lumen is closed. It is not uncommon for female patients to require 2 or even 3 injections (for a total of 10 mL) due to the absorbable content of the collagen. Injections are normally spaced at least 4 to 6 weeks apart to allow tissue healing. The most common complication is temporary urinary retention, occurring in 4% to 12% of patients, with resolution usually occurring within 48 hours. Cure rates are reported as high as 70% in selected patients, but periodic reinjections will be required every 1 to 3 years to remain dry.

Males with ISD secondary to a prostatectomy or certain neurologic diseases can also be treated with collagen injection (Fig. 8–9). Males may require 4 or 5 injections and up to 30 mL of colla-

Figure 8–9

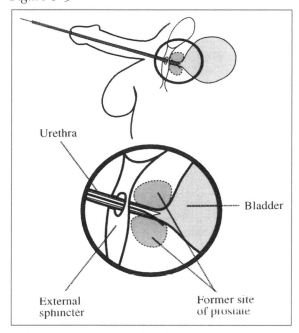

In the postprostatectomy male, collagen is injected into the bladder neck area utilizing specialized endoscopic equipment.

gen to obtain continence. Significant improvement is obtained in approximately 60% of patients, and they also require periodic reinjections to remain dry.

BLADDER SUSPENSION SURGERY

For patients with urethral hypermobility as the cause of their stress urinary incontinence, the commonly performed treatment options include various retropubic urethropexies, needle suspension procedures, and pubovaginal slings. Although surgical techniques vary, the basic reason why all of these procedures work is that they provide support for the urethra and bladder neck so that when intra-abdominal pressure causes the urethra to move downward, the urethral lumen is compressed and remains closed.

The Marshall, Marchetti, and Krantz (MMK) retropubic suspension procedure was first de-scribed in 1949 for the treatment of stress urinary incontinence. A low suprapubic (Pfannenstiel) incision is made and the retropubic space is developed. The superior wall of the vagina near the lateral edge of the urethra is sutured to the pubic periosteum, thereby fixating the bladder neck. Although the MMK has a reported cure rate of 70% to 90%, a relatively high incidence of urethral obstruction as well as osteitis pubis (an inflammation of the pubic periosteum) has been reported.

Burch described another method for retropubic suspension of the urethra in 1961. The Burch procedure differed from the MMK by suturing the lateral vaginal fascia to Cooper's ligament, creating a hammock-like support for the urethra using the vaginal wall (Fig. 8–10). Due to the lateral placement of these sutures, the Burch retropubic suspension has a much lower incidence of urethral obstruction. The average cure rate for this procedure is similar to the MMK procedure at approximately 80% overall.

The first needle suspension urethropexy was performed by Pereyra in 1959. This procedure requires a vaginal incision for exposure to the paravaginal space. A nonabsorbable suture is placed

Figure 8–10

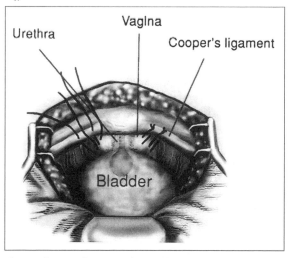

The Burch procedure is performed by suspending the lateral vaginal wall to Cooper's ligament. The suspended vaginal wall provides support for the hypermobile urethra.

bilaterally in a helical fashion through the strong paraurethral tissues. A special needle passer is introduced through a small suprapubic incision and passed down to the paravaginal space using fingertip guidance. The sutures are then pulled up into the suprapubic incision and secured over the rectus fascia. The urethra is thereby supported by a "hammock" of vaginal tissue. Short-term success rates as high as 94% have been reported; however, many variations of this procedure have been utilized, and the long-term cure rates appear to be inferior to either retropubic suspensions or sling procedures. The beneficial aspect of this procedure is that postoperative morbidity is generally less than most other procedures for urethral hypermobility.

Suburethral or pubovaginal slings were first described as early as 1907 by Giordano who utilized gracilis muscle to encircle the urethra. Since then, many other materials have been used to support the urethra including autologous fascia, synthetic grafts, and most recently, cadaveric fascia. Again, many different techniques have been described, but most involve opening the paravaginal space at the level of the bladder neck transvaginally. A low abdominal (Pfannenstiel) incision is then made to the level of the rectus fascia. If autologous fascia is used, a 1.5 by 10 cm sling is harvested from the rectus fascia and the defect closed. If cadaveric fascia or synthetic material is used, a needle passer is introduced just above the pubic symphysis and passed to the vaginal incision similar to a needle suspension. The sutures that have been previously sewn into the ends of the sling are then passed from the vaginal incision to the suprapubic incision. The fascial sling is then secured to the periurethral tissue and tied over the rectus fascia (Fig. 8–11). The sling is tied just tight enough to support the urethra; otherwise, urethral obstruction can occur. Cure rates have been reported between 80% and 95% for stress incontinence due to either urethral hypermobility or ISD. Note that in mixed incontinence, urgency and urge incontinence are improved in approximately 60% of patients.

The only acceptable long-term surgical treatment for stress incontinence in females due to ISD

Figure 8–11

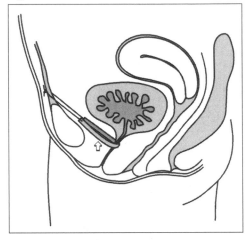

The pubovaginal sling (at the arrow) provides both support and mild urethral compression, making it the ideal choice for long-term treatment of intrinsic sphincter deficiency.

is one of the sling procedures. Although the exact incidence is not known, patients with ISD who undergo one of the other surgical procedures suffer a high failure rate. This high failure rate is one of the reasons why preoperative urodynamics is performed: to document the reason for incontinence and then pick the procedure that will most effectively treat the incontinence. More recently with the increased availability of cadaveric fascia, many urologists have simply performed pubovaginal slings on all patients, because this procedure effectively treats all types of stress incontinence and the surgical morbidity is decreased without the need to harvest fascia from the patient.

Complications of all of these procedures include bladder laceration, long-term urinary retention, and possibly a worsening of urinary urgency. Patients should be willing to perform intermittent self-catheterizations during the initial postoperative period until normal voiding is reestablished.

Males with ISD have traditionally been one of the hardest groups to treat effectively. Although collagen injection works for many patients and is minimally invasive, some patients do not respond to therapy or desire to be dry as soon as possible and don't like the prospect of repeated injections. For these patients, an artificial urinary sphincter (AUS, American Medical Systems, Minnetonka, MN) may be the answer (Fig. 8–12). This device has three main components: the cuff that encircles the bulbar urethra, the reservoir that holds the fluid, and the pump assembly that is compressed by the patient to move fluid from the cuff to the reservoir when voiding is desired. The pump assembly also has a special valve inside that slowly allows the fluid to return to the cuff

over a few minutes with subsequent restoration of continence. The AUS provides social continence in up to 85% of patients; however, patient selection is important and up to 35% of patients will need surgical revision to maintain continence. In addition, the assembly can become infected at anytime in the future and usually requires removal of all components.

Future Trends

Incontinence, like impotence, has historically been a problem that few patients talked about and few doctors asked their patients about. With the increasing awareness of this widespread problem and continuing research, advancements in the diagnosis and treatment of incontinence are occurring at a fast pace. New medications, affecting novel neural pathways, are being developed for urge incontinence. New bulking agents are being developed that are easily injected and are not degraded by the body, decreasing the number of injections needed to obtain continence and abolishing the need for reinjections. Machines that cause pelvic floor contractions through electromagnetic induction will allow treatment without even removing one's clothes. New techniques such as the use of bone anchors for sling procedures and bladder neck suspensions may decrease operative time and morbidity. Unfortunately, as evolutionary as many of these advancements are, much research and study will be necessary before we can make incontinence a disease of the past.

Figure 8–12

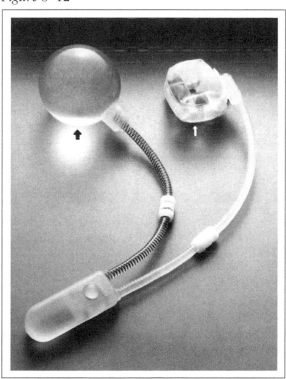

The artificial urinary sphincter has three components: the pump assembly, which transfers fluid between the reservoir (*black arrow*) and the urethral cuff (*white arrow*). The cuff is normally filled, thus maintaining continence. When voiding is desired, the patient squeezes the pump, transferring fluid from the cuff to the reservoir. A special valve in the pump assembly allows the fluid to slowly (3 to 5 minutes) return to the cuff.

Note: The authors are full-time federal employees. This work is in the public domain. The views expressed are those of the authors, and are not to be construed as official or as reflecting those of the Department of Defense, the Army Medical Department or the U.S. Air Force.

Bibliography

Cespedes RD, Cross CA, McGuire EJ: Urinary incontinence: Putting minimally invasive therapies to best use in urinary incontinence. *Contemp Urol* 8:37–44, 1966.

Couillard, Webster GD: Detrusor instability. *Urol Clin North Am* 22:593–612, 1995.

Cross CA, Cespedes RD, McGuire EJ: Individualizing the approach to the unstable bladder. *Contemp Urol* 8:60–73, 1996.

Diokno AC: Epidemiology and psychosocial aspects of incontinence. *Urol Clin North Am* 22:481, 1995.

Fantl JA, Newman DK, Collings J, et al: *Urinary Incontinence in Adults: Acute and Chronic Management. Clinical Practice Guideline*, no. 2, 1996 update. AHCPR pub. no. 96-0682. Rockville, MD, Agency for Health Care Policy and Research, Public Health Service, U.S. Dept. of Health and Human Services, 1996.

Griebling TL, Kreder KJ: *Female Urinary Incontinence. New Management Techniques and Technologies.* Mediguide to Urology 11(3),1998.

Haab F, Zimmern PE, Leach GE: *Diagnosis and Treatment of Intrinsic Sphincter Dysfunction in Females.* AUA Update Lesson 35 Vol. 15, 1996.

Heritz DM, Blaivas JG: Evaluation of urinary tract dysfunction. In Raz S (ed): *Female Urology*, ed 2. Philadelphia, Saunders, 1996, p 89.

Iselin CE, Webster GD: Office management of female urinary incontinence. *Urol Clin North Am* 24:625, 1998.

O'Donnell PD: The pathophysiology of incontinence in the elderly. *Adv Urol* 4, 1991.

Payne CK: *Conservative Therapy for Female Urinary Incontinence.* AUA Update Lesson 34 Vol. 15, 1996.

Rovner ES, Wein AJ: *Pharmacologic Treatment of Non-BPH Induced Voiding Dysfunction, Facilitation of Urine Storage* (part I). AUA Update Lesson 33 Vol. 17, 1998.

Rovner ES, Wein AJ: *Pharmacologic Treatment of Non-BPH Induced Voiding Dysfunction, Facilitation of Urine Storage* (part II). AUA Update Lesson 25 Vol. 17, 1998.

Urinary Incontinence Guideline Panel: *Urinary - Incontinence in Adults: Clinical Practice Guideline.* AHCPR pub. no. 92-0038. Rockville, MD, Agency for Health Care Policy and Research, Public Health Service, U.S. Dept. of Health and Human Services, 1992.

Wein AJ: Principles of pharmacologic therapy: Practical drug treatment of voiding dysfunction in the female. In Raz S (ed): *Female Urology*, ed 2. Philadelphia, Saunders, 1996, p 283.

Chapter 9

Interstitial Cystitis

How Common Is Interstitial Cystitis?

This chapter addresses interstitial cystitis (IC), a disorder that is both more common and more complex than it was originally believed to be. Often confused with other disorders such as recurrent urinary tract infection (UTI), benign prostatic hyperplasia (BPH), or prostatitis, IC affects surprisingly large numbers of both women and men.

IC is a clinical syndrome of frequency, urgency, and/or pelvic pain in the absence of any other definable pathology, such as urinary infection, carcinoma, or cystitis induced by radiation or medication. Traditionally, patients received the diagnosis of IC only if their symptoms were severe and persistent, and perhaps only if destructive changes in bladder tissue were detectable on cystoscopy or biopsy. The patient with mild or intermittent symptoms was likely to receive the diagnosis of recurrent UTI or "urethral syndrome" (which basically is IC) in women, or prostatitis or BPH in men. In reality, however, many such patients probably have an early form of IC. In fact, clinicians should rule out IC in anyone carrying a diagnosis of recurrent bacterial cystitis.

Because the diagnostic criteria published in 1987 by the National Institutes of Health (NIH) describe only advanced disease, most reports of the prevalence of IC are low, probably identifying no more than 5% of the individuals who are afflicted. Recent estimates are that IC actually affects between 0.6 and 2.5 million women in the United States, or as many as 3% to 5% of women. The disease also affects a significant number of men.

nonspecific and intermittent. Until the symptoms become more continuous, IC may be confused with other urologic or gynecologic disorders.

In women who consult urologists for their symptoms, IC is often initially diagnosed as or mistaken for recurrent bladder infections (a rare problem) or "the urethral syndrome." Women who experience pain as the primary symptom of their IC often present to the gynecologist, who may interpret their discomfort as pelvic pain and attribute it to endometriosis or various types of vaginitis or vulvodynia. In men, the disease is often confused with prostatitis or with problems associated with bladder outlet obstruction due to prostate enlargement. It is to be emphasized that whenever the aforementioned diagnoses are considered, IC should be considered as a possible alternate diagnosis.

The patient with negative urine cultures in the presence of the signs and symptoms of UTI may receive a diagnosis of "the urethral syndrome" or urgency-frequency syndrome (UFS). In a large study of 1000 successive patients presenting to outpatient centers in England for a clinical trial, for example, 50% of the patients with signs and symptoms of urinary tract infection (urgency/frequency) had negative cultures. In reporting their results, the authors concluded that these patients had "the urethral syndrome." In fact, urethral syndrome is most likely a mild early-phase form of IC, when the symptoms are intermittent.

IC is a gradually progressive disease process. Its symptoms tend to be intermittent in the beginning and more persistent as the disease advances. The clinician may see significant variance in the presentation of IC, depending on the severity of the patient's symptoms at the time of examination, as well as the length of time the disease process has been present.

Principal Diagnoses

Pathophysiology

Urinary urgency/frequency and/or pelvic pain may be caused by a number of disorders. In the early phases of the IC, patients' complaints are often

The etiology of IC, a subject of considerable debate in the current scientific literature, may involve a number of different factors. Lymphatic, infectious, neurologic, psychologic, autoimmune, and vasculitic causes have been proposed. The symptoms of urinary frequency and urgency or pain are the bladder's only response to noxious stimuli. In any given patient, any one or a combination of several mechanisms may culminate in a bladder insult that ultimately results in these symptoms. Some recent developments in the understanding of what produces IC are discussed later, under "Controversies."

Risk Factors

In examining the reported risk factors for IC, the published data may not reflect an accurate picture because the traditional diagnostic criteria for IC exclude all but end-stage disease. The traditional diagnostic criteria are based on an NIH research definition of IC, intended to facilitate multicenter clinical trials. These NIH criteria exclude 60% of patients thought to have IC. Nonetheless, the median age of diagnosis of IC is about 42 years; at the time of presentation to the urologist, the average patient has had symptoms for 3 to 4 years, a delay that is probably attributable to the fact that early IC is often initially mistaken for other disorders. The female to male ratio of cases of IC is reported as approximately 9 to 1, but this ratio does not take into account the numbers of men whose IC has been misdiagnosed as BPH or prostatitis.

The NIH criteria for the diagnosis of IC exclude individuals under the age of 18 years purely on an arbitrary basis, due to problems relating to conducting research on children. There have been a number of reports of IC in children, however. In children, a female to male ratio of 2 to 3 is reported.

Why Is Interstitial Cystitis Important?

As the syndrome of IC progresses from its generally mild early stages to the more advanced stages, an individual's symptoms increase while bladder function deteriorates. Pain is a late symptom that becomes an increasingly prominent factor, and with time the symptoms of urgency and frequency become persistent and more severe.

The individual who has had IC for 10 to 20 years may have significant secondary changes to the bladder; for example, an altered epithelium, adhesion molecules, basement membrane changes, muscle loss, and/or nerve up-regulation in peripheral nerves and centrally in the spinal column. In advanced IC, the bladder may be severely damaged; a cystoscopic evaluation may show a Hunner's ulcer (a velvety red bladder ulcer that may be mistaken for carcinoma in situ) or the presence of glomerulations (or submucosal petechial hemorrhages).

Patients with IC present with physical discomforts and with significant disruptions of their personal and occupational lives. Particularly as the disease reaches more advanced stages, the symptoms of IC place significant limits on an individual's daily activities. The disease can take a psychological as well as a physical toll. Depression can result from the chronic pain and loss of sleep that go along with advancing IC.

If the clinician uses a broad definition of IC and recognizes that the disease is significantly underdiagnosed, help can be offered to many patients with milder forms of the disease. The majority of patients with early-stage IC will respond readily to therapy and, it is hoped, their advancement to more severe end-stage disease can be prevented.

Typical Presentation

IC is a clinical syndrome with as yet no distinct pathologic tissue or serum changes to indicate its presence. It tends to develop gradually, and it may unfold over decades of a patient's life. Its symptoms vary depending on whether a patient has an early-phase, milder version of the syndrome, or a later, more advanced stage as is seen in older patients.

IC can be described in terms of its development over time. A time line (Fig. 9–1) is helpful to conceptualize this development. The severity of a patient's symptoms, and therefore the diagnosis likely to be applied, depend on the patient's location on the time line. Younger patients tend to have mild, intermittent urgency/frequency, and typically are diagnosed with recurrent bladder infections. After persistent symptoms and repeated negative cultures, they are next diagnosed with urethral syndrome. As the disease progresses further, the patient's symptoms become continuous and more severe, perhaps meeting the original NIH criteria for IC. The disease continues to destroy the bladder as the patient grows older, and eventually a diagnosis of "classic" IC is made. Overall, there is a progressive increase in symptomatology and decrease in bladder function as the patient ages and the disease takes its toll.

In some individuals, pelvic pain may be the principal component of the syndrome, with very little urgency or frequency. It is perhaps this patient population that would most likely present to the gynecologist (as chronic pelvic pain) or primary care clinician rather than to the urologist.

Key History

In evaluating a patient with urgency/frequency and/or pelvic pain, the first objective is to rule out other gynecologic or urologic disorders that can produce these symptoms. Once other disorders have been excluded, it is important to distinguish early IC from more advanced phases of the disease.

The principal symptoms of IC are the presence of abnormal sensory urgency and/or pain. Sensory urgency causes patients to report urinary frequency. Most patients with urgency and frequency will have associated bladder pain, although some patients experience pelvic pain and no urgency. One study of over 200 patients showed that approximately 15% of patients presenting with IC had little or no bladder pain, while 85% of patients presented with significant pain.

Location of Pain

It is important to determine whether a patient's pain is of bladder origin. The patient should be asked whether the pain, despite being constantly present, worsens if the bladder is not emptied. Similarly, the clinician should ask the patient if

Figure 9–1

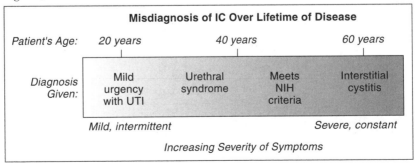

IC is a disease in a continuum. The traditional view of IC as a syndrome of fixed severity has resulted in misdiagnosis of the various phases of IC over the lifetime of the disease.

the pain improves, but does not disappear, with voiding or if it is induced by the act of voiding, but there are some patients whose pain is not affected by bladder volume or voiding. The bladder pain of IC is experienced suprapubically, in the perineum or the vulva, vaginally, in the low back, or even medial in the thighs. One third of patients experience dysuria. Men may experience pain in the scrotum or testes.

Nocturia and Frequency

The occurrence of nocturia in IC is variable. In general, 90% of patients will complain of voiding at least 1 to 2 times per night, but many patients have no nocturia. Because nocturia increases with the severity and duration of the disease, little or no nocturia will be present in the early phases. The average patient with clinically active IC voids approximately 16 times a day, with an average voided volume of 75 mL (in contrast to normal subjects who void an average of 6.5 times a day with an average voided volume of 270 mL). Thus, most patients report they void frequently, void small volumes, and may report not emptying the bladder completely because they void shortly thereafter again. A minimum for diagnostic purposes is considered to be 8 voids per day.

Overall, IC should be suspected if the patient voids more than 8 times in 24 hours and/or has associated pain in the bladder or urethra. Table 9–1 summarizes clinical data on IC reported by the author.

Dyspareunia

Between 85% and 90% of individuals with IC are female. Of those who are sexually active, the majority (75%) will complain that sexual intercourse exacerbates the symptoms. The increase in symptoms may be felt during sexual activity, immediately after, or within 24 to 48 hours. In addition, most women who are still menstruating will complain of a flare of symptoms several days to a

Table 9–1

Urinary Symptoms Reported in 225 Patients Including Frequency Distributions for Symptom Severity

Nocturia		
Mean	4.7	
90% cut-off level	1.5	(1–2 voidings)
Range	0–13	
1–2	41	18%
2–4	90	40%
4.5–8	63	28%
Daytime Frequency		
Mean	16.0	
90% cut-off level	7	
Range	5.5–40	
Urgency		
Mild	8	3.5%
Moderate	63	28%
Moderate–severe	35	15.5%
Severe	119	53%
Pain		
None	41	18%
Mild	16	7%
Moderate	82	36%

week before the onset of the menstrual cycle. Note that any woman presenting with dyspareunia and a perimenstrual flare of symptoms should first be considered to have IC or pain of bladder origin; then, after IC is excluded, she should be considered to have a gynecologic problem such as endometriosis.

Duration

Determining the duration of symptoms (Table 9–2) helps to distinguish patients with full-blown IC from those with the milder form of the disease. The diagnosis of IC is more likely if the individual has had the presence of continuous symptoms for at least 6 months. Clinically, to separate early IC from later forms of the disease is worthwhile

Table 9–2

Bladder Changes Associated With Duration of IC

	AVERAGE AT 1 YR[a]	AVERAGE AT >7 YRS[b]
Number of patients	34	42
Voidings	15.2	17.3
Voided volume (mL)	128	105
Anesthetic capacity (mL)	711	518

[a] Patients with 1 year of symptoms.
[b] Patients with >7 years of symptoms.

because early IC may need little or no therapy, and the prognosis for the patient is good.

It is important to recognize that although many individuals with IC do not meet traditional diagnostic criteria, they suffer from the disease and will benefit from therapy. Regardless of the frequency or severity of symptoms, the abnormal urgency and/or pain were sufficient to drive the patient to seek medical care.

Physical Examination

Pelvic Examination

One particular finding on physical examination helps confirm the diagnosis of IC. On pelvic examination, over 95% of patients will complain of a tender bladder base. In women, this discomfort is easily demonstrated by palpation of the anterior vaginal wall.

Ancillary Tests

Analysis of Catheterized Urine Specimen

Because the low voided volumes make midstream collection difficult to obtain, urine analysis and culture on voided specimens is not useful in patients with IC, recurrent UTI, or urethral syndrome. In these women, one sees only vaginal secretions unless a catheterized specimen is obtained. A catheterized specimen examined under the microscope should show no bacteria, and most specimens will show no red or white blood cells.

The patient presenting with gross or microscopic hematuria requires a full urologic workup to exclude the possibility of malignancy (intravenous pyelogram, cystoscopy, ± urine cytology). In addition, any male over the age of 40 should undergo at least an initial screening, consisting of urine cytology and an office cystoscopy, to rule out malignancy.

Voiding Log

A voiding log is one of the most useful and inexpensive methods to screen possible IC patients. It is particularly valuable in women whose pelvic pain is considered to have a gynecologic origin. An accurate assessment of number of daily voids and average voided volume can be determined from a 2-day voiding log, in which each voiding is measured and recorded by the patient at home. From such data, it is known that the average patient with IC voids 16 times per day. In 97% of patients, voided volume averages less than 100 mL (average, 73 mL). This compares to normal subjects who void an average of 6.5 times per day with a mean volume of 270 mL. Anyone voiding 8 or more times per day with an average volume of less than 100 mL is probably abnormal.

The voiding profile is helpful in establishing the diagnosis of IC, and may be used subsequently to create a therapeutic plan and to determine progress in therapy. The clinician should obtain one voiding log initially and one at each subsequent visit. As might be anticipated, patients with a longer disease history have a smaller functional bladder capacity, as reflected in the average voided volume and number of daily voids (Table 9–3).

Table 9–3

Voiding Profiles of 145 Patients With IC and 48 Normal Controls

VOIDING PROFILES OF 145 PATIENTS WITH IC			
	NUMBER OF VOIDINGS[a]	VOIDED VOLUME (mL)	NOCTURIA
Average	16.4	73	4.7
90% confidence limit[b]	9	100	
Range	6–39	26–235	
VOIDING PROFILES OF 48 NORMAL CONTROLS			
	NUMBER OF VOIDINGS[a]		VOIDED VOLUME (mL)
Average	6.5		270
90% confidence limit[b]	7[b]		150[c]
Range	3–13		100–600

[a] Per day.
[b] 90% of subjects had at least this level.
[c] 90% of patients above this level

The clinician may be surprised to find that many patients have abnormal voiding logs but minimal complaints of urgency/frequency. This is because the increase in urgency may be so gradual that the patient accepts it as normal; in the author's experience, patients complain more of the pain of IC than of the urgency/frequency. The voiding log is valuable in uncovering the presence of any "silent" urgency/frequency that may signal the presence of IC.

less than 125 cc and with water less than 150 mL. In 75 patients with water cystometrograms reported by Parsons, the average bladder capacity was 220 mL, with over 90% of patients having a functional volume of less than 350 mL. Except for a small (<5%) subgroup of IC patients who develop a bladder myopathy, bladder capacity will be reduced. If the cystometric portion of the CMG is normal, the patient probably has no or mild IC.

Urodynamics

A cystometrogram (CMG) can be of substantial help in establishing or ruling out the diagnosis of IC. A normal CMG essentially excludes IC. Recently published data by the NIH Interstitial Cystitis Data Base (ICDB) Study Group demonstrate that the urodynamics can be substituted for cystoscopy in diagnosis.

Because all patients complain of significant urinary urgency, this can usually be documented with cystometry. If gas is employed, the patient will have a sensation of significant urgency at

Potassium Test

The Parsons potassium test, a simple test devised by the author, is based upon the hypothesis that the bladder's ability to maintain an impermeable epithelium is impaired in individuals with IC (see "Controversies" later in the chapter). The test involves placing a 40-mL solution of 0.4 molar potassium chloride into the patient's bladder with a small (8–12 Fr) catheter. In an individual without IC, the normal impermeability of the epithelium prevents the cation from penetrating the bladder surface, and the solution provokes no symptoms of urgency or pain. In an individual with IC, the leaky epithelium allows the potassium to diffuse across the transitional cells and depolarize sensory nerves in the bladder, causing urgency or pain (Table 9–4). The test is depicted in Fig. 9–2.

Cystoscopy

Cystoscopic evaluation of the bladder is not necessary in the evaluation of a patient with symptoms of IC unless cancer is suspected. In fact, examination under local anesthesia for the purpose of diagnosing IC should be discouraged, because it offers little help in diagnosis and causes the patient severe discomfort. To rule out carcinoma in high-risk individuals (those over 40 and those with hematuria), however, cystoscopy under local anesthesia is warranted.

Table 9–4

Use of Parsons Potassium Test as a Guide to Therapy

Potassium-positive patients respond best[a] to:

- Dilation
- DMSO
- Heparin
- Pentosanpolysulfate
- Polycitra

Potassium-negative patients respond best to:

- Antidepressants
- Possibly pentosanpolysulfate

[a] Add hydroxyzine if allergies are present.

Traditionally, the diagnosis of IC via cystoscopy depended on one of two findings, a Hunner's ulcer or the presence of glomerulations or pe-

Figure 9–2

Postassium test procedure

Solution 1 = 40 mL sterile water
Solution 2 = 40 mL potassium solution (16 mEq KCl)
For potassium solution, bring 20 mEq KCl ampule up to 50 mL with water

1. Ask patient to rate baseline pain and urgency using the scales at right.
2. Place small catheter in patient's bladder.
3. Slowly, over 1–2 minutes, instill solution 1 into the bladder.
4. Ask patient to rate current pain and urgency after 5 minutes.
5. Remove solution 1 from the bladder.
6. Slowly, over 1–2 minutes, instill solution 2 into the bladder.
7. Ask patient to rate current pain and urgency after 5 minutes.
8. Remove solution 2 from the bladder and wash once with 40 ml water.
9. Ask patient to compare the two solutions using the two questions at right.

Grading scales for symptoms

Pain

None	Mild		Moderate		Severe
0	1	2	3	4	5

Urgency

None	Mild		Moderate		Severe
0	1	2	3	4	5

Questions

1. Which solution is worse?
   ____ Solution 1
   ____ Solution 2
   ____ Neither

2. Is the difference between the solutions:
   ____ None
   ____ Mild
   ____ Moderate
   ____ Severe

Instructions for performing the potassium test.

techial hemorrhages. Because not all patients with IC show these bladder changes, their absence on cystoscopy does not exclude the diagnosis of IC.

In IC, cystoscopy is primarily important as a therapeutic maneuver by performing cystoscopic hydrodistension under anesthesia, and then only in patients with severe symptoms. For patients with milder symptoms, it is best to omit cystoscopy and proceed with other therapies. If cystoscopy is to be performed for therapy, it should be done under anesthesia.

Algorithm

The diagnostic algorithm for IC (Fig. 9–3) shows that patients should be referred for a urologic evaluation immediately if they present with gross or microscopic hematuria. Males over age 40, with or without hematuria, should also be referred to the urologist for a basic screening to rule out malignancy.

Analysis and culture of a catheterized urine specimen will identify those patients with bacterial UTI. A history and physical examination are useful, but not definitive, if the urine analysis and culture are negative. If both a bacterial UTI and a high risk for malignancy are ruled out, and a history reveals 8 or more voids per day with pain on bladder filling or emptying, the diagnosis of IC may be considered. The finding of pain at the bladder base on physical examination supports the diagnosis of IC. Once IC is suspected, the primary care clinician may initiate treatment, or refer the patient to the urologist for further IC workup.

Treatment

In recent years, we have developed very good strategies for the management of IC. Most impor-

tant in these strategies is that it takes multimodality therapy to help patients with more advanced disease. Generally, patients with milder/early-phase disease require less intervention. If patients are having repetitive symptoms, it is best to place them on chronic therapy to manage the disease process.

The strategies for managing IC are so successful that it is very important not to withhold the diagnosis of IC for earlier-phase patients, such as those with "urethral syndrome" (which is IC), and to suspect that many patients with "recurrent bladder infections" have IC, as do many patients with pelvic pain who are being followed for gynecologic problems such as endometriosis. Table 9–5 summarizes the drug treatments of IC.

Principles of Therapy

The first principle in helping the IC patient is understanding what many consider the chief defect underlying the disease. That defect is thought to be the loss of the permeability regulatory mechanism of the bladder epithelium, which results in the leaking of urinary solutes (primarily potassium) into the bladder wall, triggering symptoms and causing bladder destruction (see "Controversies" later in the chapter). Thus, the first step in treating IC is correcting this problem. It has been known for approximately 20 years that heparinoids will restore the bladder surface mucus, which is the primary mechanism regulating the permeability of the epithelium. The heparinoids that have been used successfully in this regard are intravesical heparin and oral pentosanpolysulfate (Elmiron). These drugs that correct the primary problem, the defective epithelium, are the mainstays of multimodality therapy for IC (Table 9–6).

The second concept is that of neural up-regulation. Many patients with IC have a marked increase in the number of peripheral nerve endings in the bladder, and even up-regulation of the sacral reflex arc of the pelvic nerves. The physician can suppress the symptoms of IC by addressing this issue, using medications that are known to alter pain or sensory awareness of the bladder fibers, such as tricyclic antidepressants

Figure 9–3

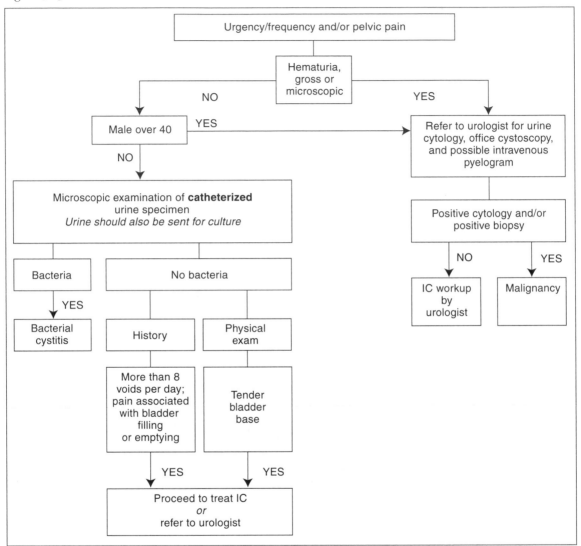

Primary care clinician's algorithm for urgency/frequency and/or pelvic pain.

(e.g., amitriptyline) primarily and antispasmodics (e.g., oxybutynin, tolterodine, or hyocyamine) to a lesser extent.

A third important consideration is that mast cell activation seems to be a prominent feature in many patients with IC. Those with seasonal allergies (in our experience, up to 70% to 75% of patients) should be started on hydroxyzine (Atarax, Vistaril), which is known to be a potent inhibitor of mast cell degranulation and release of hista-

Table 9–5

Therapy Recommendations

Patients with Mild IC

DMSO for 3 months may induce long remission[a]

Pentosanpolysulfate

Patients with Moderate-Severe IC

Antidepressant + pentosanpolysulfate[a]

DMSO

(When improved, slowly taper off heparin)

Patients with Severe IC

Antidepressant + pentosanpolysulfate and/or daily intravesical heparin[a]

DMSO

(When improved, slowly taper off heparin)

[a] Add hydroxyzine if allergies are present.

mine when used chronically. Clinically, IC patients with concomitant inflammatory bowel disease, irritable bowel syndrome, or fibromyalgia may also benefit from hydroxyzine.

Recommendations

Our principal recommendations to meet these goals are to begin all patients with a suspected diagnosis of IC on the oral medication pentosanpolysulfate. In patients with severe disease, intravesical heparin can also be employed; but such patients probably are best referred to a urologist. The minimum effective dosage of pentosanpolysulfate is 100 mg three times a day, but we recommend initiating therapy with at least twice that

Table 9–6

Guide to Heparinoid Therapy for IC

DRUG	DOSE	ROUTE
Heparin	20,000–40,000 units daily	Intravesical and self-administered
Pentosan-polysulfate	100–200 mg tid	Oral

dose, 200 mg three times a day, and in males we routinely recommend the larger dose. For patients who have moderately continuous symptoms with moderate pain, add amitriptyline (Elavil), 25 mg at bedtime, which can help suppress the patient's symptoms through its central down-regulation of pain perception. Amitriptyline also has anticholinergic (antispasmodic) action in the bladder. In patients unable to take amitriptyline, any one of the new selective serotonin reuptake inhibitors (SSRIs) can be substituted and are also of benefit to down-regulate central pain perception.

Dimethylsulfoxide (DMSO) has significant activity in helping patients with mild to moderate disease. It can be used to induce symptomatic remission. In general, the patient undergoing DMSO treatment should be started on pentosanpolysulfate at the same time to achieve chronic control of the problem. DMSO requires bladder instillation through a catheter. Many patients have initial flare-ups after DMSO instillation, and DMSO gives patients a garlic odor to their breath.

Any patient with a history of allergy to pollens and molds should be started on a course of 25 mg of hydroxyzine chronically. This medication, while sedating initially, will lose its sedative effect after 4 to 6 weeks, as it is a tricyclic compound similar to amitriptyline. Hydroxyzine is a potent inhibitor of mast cell degranulation and will help substantially in controlling the allergy flares. Other antihistamines, particularly selective H1 antagonists, do not appear to be as effective as hydroxyzine clinically. Cromolyn likewise is not effective clinically.

Patients who have symptom flares that occur around the menstrual cycle, during the allergy season, or with sexual activity should be given a medication such as phenazopyridine (Pyridium) or phenazopyridine with the antispasmodic hyoscyamine and the sedative butabarbital (Pyridium Plus), along with some sodium bicarbonate tablets several a day (to reduce the amount of urinary potassium) or Polycitra crystals, which can also help in this regard. Such patients should also be given supplementary drugs such as oxybutynin chloride (Ditropan) 5 mg. For allergy season supplementation, they can also be started on non-sedating types of antihistamines, which are also helpful, but the patient must remain on the baseline hydroxyzine to obtain the best relief.

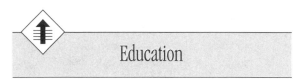

Education

An important point for the primary care clinician to emphasize to the family of an individual with IC is that IC is not a psychological disorder but a physiologic problem. Stress can exacerbate the symptoms of IC, but it does not cause the disease.

The primary care clinician can also help prepare the family to support IC patients in their treatment regimen. The IC patient may need to change his or her diet (to reduce potassium), adhere to a rigorous schedule of self-treatment, or keep detailed records of symptoms and voided volumes. The patient may be placed on medications that cause noticeable changes in the patient's physical and emotional states.

Family Approach

The primary care clinician is in a unique position to recognize when the syndrome of IC exerts significant stresses on an IC patient and members of his or her family. Referring the patient or family members for psychological counseling when necessary is an essential part of the regimen of treatment of IC. The most effective management of IC requires interdisciplinary effort among the family practice physician, the urologist and/or the gynecologist, and the mental health professional.

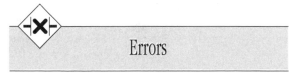

Errors

The errors likely to be made in the diagnosis and treatment of IC owe largely to the fact that the traditional definition of this disorder excludes all but the most advanced cases. In addition, the gradual and variable clinical onset typical of IC makes this disorder difficult to recognize. The most common problems in diagnosis and treatment are described here.

Diagnostic Errors

One of the most common errors in diagnosis is mistaking IC for recurrent urinary tract infection (UTI). As a cause of urgency/frequency and/or pain, bacterial cystitis is probably relatively rare, and early IC the much more common cause. In fact, any patient who has received this diagnosis should be considered to have IC until infection is documented. Early IC tends to respond extremely well to treatment, and it is important to recognize the patient with early-phase disease so that progression to later, more severe stages can be prevented if possible.

Another key diagnostic error is the failure to perform urine analysis and culture on a catheterized specimen when IC is suspected. Because voided volumes in IC are often small, a "clean catch" is impossible; thus, the analysis of a voided specimen will yield unreliable results.

Errors in diagnosis can be minimized if the primary care clinician uses the broad definition of IC presented here, recognizing that IC is a disease frequently in a continuum (Fig. 9–1) and that its symptoms tend to progress slowly in terms of severity, frequency, and duration. This is in contradistinction to the concept that IC is a syndrome of fixed and intense severity.

Treatment Errors

Incorrect oral medication strategies lead to two common errors in the treatment of IC.

The first error is failing to try pentosanpolysulfate (Elmiron) for a period of time that is adequate to determine its efficacy. Because it takes 6 to 12 months to obtain a good response on pentosanpolysulfate, the medication should be tried for at least 12 months before its use is abandoned.

The second error is failing to use a multimodality treatment strategy that addresses all three principles of IC treatment described above. The most common error in this area is the failure to include hydroxyzine (Atarax, Vistaril) in the treatment regimen of IC patients with a history of allergy.

Controversies

Evolving Definition of Interstitial Cystitis

As has been discussed, the traditional definition of IC excludes all but end-stage disease. The diagnosis of IC is made difficult by the lack of an updated, widely accepted set of diagnostic criteria, as well as by the gradual way in which the disorder presents itself clinically. Objective diagnostic tools are few. The controversies concerning the definition of IC are likely to continue as more is learned about this disease.

In evaluating patients with urgency/frequency and/or pain in a primary care setting, it is best to use the broad definition of IC presented in this chapter, taking care to distinguish possible IC from true bacterial cystitis and bearing in mind that "urethral syndrome" is generally early IC. Remember that any patient with urgency/frequency and/or pelvic pain, constant or intermittent, or whose symptoms flare with sex or just before the menstrual cycle has a 90% chance of having IC in the absence of proven urinary infection or endometriosis.

Emerging Concepts

Etiology

The etiology of IC is an area of active debate. In recent years, many investigators have suggested that the permeability of the bladder epithelium is a factor in the etiology of IC, and this is becoming widely accepted. Parsons and coworkers have presented evidence that normal urine contains cations capable of damaging bladder epithelial and smooth muscle cells in culture. These investigators proposed that IC results from a disruption of a delicate balance among bladder surface protective mechanisms and potentially cytotoxic factors in the urine. If this is the case, IC results not from a substance unique to the IC patient's urine, but from the presence of one or more factors that disrupt the healthy balance at the bladder surface.

Further, if normal urine contains substances capable of injuring the bladder surface, healthy individuals must possess urinary defense mechanisms that act to neutralize the potentially injurious urine factors. Parsons and coworkers have proposed that Tamm–Horsfall protein, the most abundant protein in normal urine, may have such an action. Keay and others have published results suggesting that IC patients have altered levels of an epithelial growth factor at the bladder surface. This investigational work raises the possibility that IC results from a disruption in the balance between injury factors and defense mechanisms of the bladder epithelium.

Treatment

An emerging concept in the treatment of IC is the importance of diagnosing and treating individuals who have mild/early-phase disease. Patients who have mild IC, with rare symptom flares, can best be managed with medications such as phenazopyridine (Pyridium) or amitriptyline (Elavil), atropine sulfate and hyoscyamine (Urised), and sodium bicarbonate.

Summary

The majority of patients can now be successfully treated for IC. If the clinician uses a broad definition of IC and recognizes that the disease is significantly underdiagnosed, help can be offered to many patients with milder forms of IC. The best results are obtained when IC is diagnosed early and treatment is initiated before severe bladder damage has occurred. Anyone diagnosed with recurrent bacterial cystitis or urethral syndrome should first be considered to have IC, and should be evaluated and treated as such.

Bibliography

Geist RW, Antolak SJ: Interstitial cycstitis in children. *J Urol* 104:922–925, 1970.

Gillenwater JY, Wein AJ: Summary of the National Institute of Arthritis, Diabetes, Digestive and Kidney Diseases Workshop on Interstitial Cystitis, National Institutes of Health, Bethesda, Maryland, August 28–29, 1987. *J Urol* 140:203–206, 1988.

Hamilton-Miller JMT: The urethral syndrome and its management. *J Antimicrob Chemo* 33(Suppl A): 63–73, 1994.

Hand JR: Interstitial cystitis, a report of 223 cases. *J Urol* 61:291, 1949.

Held PJ, Hanno PM, Pauly MV, et al: Epidemiology of interstitial cystitis. In Hanno PM, Staskin DR, Krane RJ, et al (eds): *Interstitial Cystitis*. London: Springer-Verlag, 1990, pp 29–48.

Holm-Bentzen M, Larsen S, Hainau B, et al: Non-obstructive detrusor myopathy in a group of patients with chronic bacterial cystitis. *Scand J Urol Nephrol* 19:21, 1985.

Jones, CA, Harris M and Nyberg L: Prevalence of interstitial cystitis in the United States. Presented at 89th Annual American Urological Association Meeting, San Francisco, CA. Abstract 781. May 14–19, 1994.

Keay S, Warren JW: A hypothesis for the etiology of IC based upon inhibition of bladder epithelial repair. *Med Hypotheses* 51:79, 1998.

Messing EM, Stamey TA: Interstitial cystitis: Early diagnosis, pathology, and treatment. *Urology* 12:381, 1978.

Nielsen KK, Kromann-Andersen B, Steven K, et al: Failure of combined supratrigonal cystetomy and Mainz ileocecocystoplasty in intractable interstitial cystitis: Is histology and mast cell count a reliable predictor for the outcome of surgery? *J Urol* 144:255–258, 1990.

Nigro DA, Wein AJ, Foy M, et al: Associations among cystoscopic and urodynamic findings for women enrolled in the Interstitial Cystitis Data Base Study. *Urology* 49(suppl 5A):86–92, 1997.

Oravisto KJ: Epidemiology of interstitial cystitis. *Ann Chir Gynaecol Fenn* 64:75–77, 1975.

Parsons CL: Interstitial cystitis: Clinical manifestations and diagnostic criteria in over 200 cases. *Neurourol Urody* 9:241–250, 1990.

Parsons CL, Bautista SL, Stein PC, et al: Cyto-injury factors in urine: A possible mechanism for the development of interstitial cystitis. *J Urol*, in press, 2000.

Parsons CL, Greenberger M, Gabal L, et al: The role of urinary potassium in the pathogenesis and diagnosis of interstitial cystitis. *J Urol* 159:1862–1867, 1998.

Parsons CL, Lilly JD, Stein PC: Epithelial dysfunction in nonbacterial cystitis (interstitial cystitis). *J Urol* 145:732, 1991.

Walsh A: Interstitial cystitis. In Harrison JH, Gittes RF, Perlmutter AD, et al (eds): *Campbell's Urology*, ed 4. Philadelphia, Saunders, 1978.

Tomas L. Griebling

Geriatric Urology

What Is Geriatric Urology?

Geriatric urology is a specialized area of adult urology that concentrates on the evaluation and management of urologic problems in older patients. In particular it is focused on the care of frail, elderly individuals with multiple comorbidities. Although elderly individuals are seen for a wide spectrum of urologic complaints, the two most common disorders seen in this age group are urinary incontinence and urinary tract infections. Other common disorders in this age group include urologic malignancies (particularly prostate and bladder cancer), stone disease, benign prostatic hyperplasia, and erectile dysfunction. These topics are covered in detail elsewhere in this book. This chapter will focus on the evaluation and treatment of elderly patients who present with urinary incontinence and urinary tract infections, as these conditions are commonly seen in geriatric patients, and their management may differ from that of younger patients with similar clinical problems.

Urinary Incontinence

Urinary incontinence is defined as the involuntary or unexpected loss of urine that occurs on a regular basis. Urinary incontinence is common. It is estimated that between 15% and 25% of all adults suffer from regular episodes of urinary incontinence. In those over 65 years of age, the estimated prevalence increases to 30% to 35%. At least 50% of all nursing home residents and 50% to 60% of the homebound elderly have problems with incontinence. In fact, urinary incontinence and behavioral changes related to cognitive impairment and dementia are often cited as the two leading causes of nursing home placement in the United States.

The costs of caring for patients with urinary incontinence are staggering. It is estimated that between $15 and $20 billion is spent annually for continence care in the United States, and one third of this is spent on pads and other absorbent products. Psychosocial costs can also be quite high. It is now recognized that many people with incontinence also suffer from decreased self-esteem and limitations of their desired activities.

Principal Diagnoses and Typical Presentation

There are a variety of causes of urinary incontinence. It is critical that the evaluation be structured to identify the specific type of incontinence, because this will ultimately determine the potential treatments for successful clinical management.

Urinary incontinence can generally be classified into one of five major diagnostic categories: stress incontinence, urge incontinence, mixed incontinence, overflow incontinence, and functional incontinence. Less common types of incontinence include reflex urinary incontinence associated with spinal cord injuries and congenital incontinence caused by an ectopic ureter. It should be remembered that the etiology of incontinence may be multifactorial, particularly in the older adult.

TRANSIENT INCONTINENCE

Sudden or new onset of urinary incontinence in a previously continent older person should raise suspicion about a condition associated with transient incontinence (Table 10–1). These include delirium, urinary tract infections, atrophic urethritis and/or vaginitis, psychologic factors such as psychogenic polydipsia, endocrine disorders such as diabetes mellitus and diabetes insipidus, restricted mobility, and fecal impaction. In addition, some drugs may cause or exacerbate urinary frequency and incontinence (Table 10–2).

Fecal incontinence is a particularly common problem in elderly patients that often coexists with urinary incontinence. Although a discussion of fecal incontinence is beyond the scope of this chapter, it is important to ask patients presenting

Table 10–1

Transient Incontinence Mnemonic "DIAPPERS"

D— Delirium
I— Infection
A— Atrophic vaginitis
P— Pharmacologic
P— Psychological
E— Endocrine
R— Restricted mobility
S— Stool impaction

for evaluation of urinary incontinence about their bowel habits. Fecal impaction and obstipation are often associated with stress urinary incontinence. Patients with urinary urge and urge incontinence may suffer from associated fecal soiling and urgency. Consultation with a gastroenterologist interested in defecation disorders may be quite helpful in this circumstance.

STRESS INCONTINENCE

Stress urinary incontinence is characterized by the loss of urine associated with an increase in intra-abdominal pressure. Patients typically de-

Table 10–2

Medications That May Cause or Exacerbate Urinary Incontinence

Diuretics
Anticholinergics
Antipsychotics
Tricyclic antidepressants
Antispasmodics
Antihistamines
Antiemetics
Drugs for Parkinson's disease (trihexyphenidyl and benztropine mesylate)
Opiates
Adrenergic agents
Sympathomimetics
Sympatholytics
Calcium channel blockers

scribe leakage of urine when they cough, sneeze, laugh, or lift heavy objects. In elderly patients, the symptoms may be most noticeable with transfers in position such as getting up out of bed. Other conditions such as persistent cough or chronic obstructive pulmonary disease may exacerbate stress urinary incontinence symptoms. There is evidence that vaginal delivery and laxity of the pelvic floor support structures are associated with development of stress urinary incontinence, though stress incontinence may occur uncommonly in nulliparous women. In men, the most common causes of stress incontinence are radical prostatectomy for prostate cancer and transurethral resection of the prostate (TURP) for benign prostatic hyperplasia.

URGE INCONTINENCE

In contrast to stress urinary incontinence, urge incontinence (often termed overactive bladder) is characterized by the sudden loss of urine associated with an overwhelming urgency to void. Patients often experience precipitous loss of large volumes of urine with no clear warning signs. Some activities may predispose patients to urge-incontinent episodes. Classic examples include hearing the sound of running water or washing one's hands. Many older people also note that cold weather increases their sense of urinary urgency. Associated neurologic impairments and disorders such as stroke, Parkinson's disease, multiple sclerosis, and back injuries may be associated with urge incontinence.

MIXED INCONTINENCE

Mixed urinary incontinence is the term used to describe subjects who experience symptoms of both stress and urge incontinence. It is common to see mixed incontinence in elderly individuals. Most patients are able to differentiate these symptoms with appropriate questioning during the history. In these cases, initial therapy is usually directed to the predominant component. Once symptoms have stabilized, additional therapy for the secondary component may be necessary.

OVERFLOW INCONTINENCE

Overflow incontinence is generally less common than stress or urge incontinence, although it is more common in older than younger patients. Patients with overflow incontinence typically describe continuous leakage of small volumes of urine. This constant dribbling occurs because the bladder is filled to capacity, and the path of least resistance for the urine is to leak out of the urethra. Most patients with overflow incontinence have an associated neurologic impairment such as neurogenic bladder, diabetes, or another process that impairs bladder sensation. They generally do not feel that their bladder is full. It is not uncommon to see elevated postvoid residual volumes of more than 500 mL in these subjects.

Patients with overflow incontinence may also experience urinary urgency and bladder instability. This has been termed detrusor hyperactivity with impaired contractility (DHIC).

FUNCTIONAL INCONTINENCE

Functional incontinence is a term used to describe those subjects who are incontinent due to nonurologic etiologies. In general, these patients would be continent if they could independently reach toileting facilities in time. Examples include incontinence associated with impaired mobility due to hip fracture, arthritis, or gait disturbances. The urinary incontinence associated with Alzheimer's disease is often considered a form of functional incontinence.

Key History

An accurate history is critical to determine the correct category of incontinence. Major factors to consider in the history include the duration and severity of the urinary incontinence. It is common to see older patients who have suffered from incontinence for months or even years before seeking treatment. Many older individuals also think urinary incontinence is a normal occurrence during old age, and that nothing can be done about it. Older patients may have more difficulty seeking help because urinary and fecal function is often considered a private matter that they are reluctant to discuss. These patients may be too embarrassed to discuss incontinence with their clinician. In this age group, it may be useful to start the history with a nonthreatening statement, such as, "Many older people have difficulty controlling their urine. How would you describe your ability to control your urine?"

Causes of transient incontinence should be elicited, because if discovered, these forms of incontinence are usually addressed easily (Table 10–1). A list of all prescription and nonprescription medications should be reviewed to identify any potential pharmaceuticals that could cause incontinence (Table 10–2). An essential element to history-taking in the elderly is to elicit the timing of incontinence and the timing of taking medications. For example, a diuretic such as furosemide taken at bedtime may produce nocturnal incontinence. Likewise, long-acting hypnotics, typically taken to facilitate sleep, may cause confusion and promote "sundowning." Such patients have pharmacologic and delirium causes of their incontinence.

Further, the addition or cessation of medications should be elicited relative to the onset of incontinence. Many elderly patients have multiple risk factors for incontinence, but do not leak urine until medications are changed. For example, an elderly woman with pelvic floor prolapse may not leak urine until she is given an alpha-antagonist for hypertension. The alpha-antagonist reduces bladder neck tone, which provokes stress incontinence. Some medications listed in Table 10–2 are available in nonprescription (over-the-counter) preparations. For example, antihistamines and alpha-agonists are frequently used for upper respiratory ailments ("cold" compounds). Thus, medication history should elicit all prescription and nonprescription medications.

Severity is most easily measured by determining the number of pads used each day or night. The type of pad and the degree to which it is soaked will indicate the degree of leakage. Activities associated with the incontinence should be identified. For example, some patients only leak urine with strenuous physical activity such as swinging a golf club or dancing, which suggests that significant abdominal pressure (Valsalva) is required to provoke stress incontinence. Other people leak with only minor physical exertion, such as arising from a chair, which suggests a more pronounced stress incontinence.

A self-completed voiding diary that includes the time and amount of both accidents and voids can be quite helpful in the initial review (see Table 8-6). This will help identify patients who may leak due to excessive fluid intake or infrequent voiding. All categories of incontinence may be unmasked or exaggerated by excessive fluid intake or infrequent voiding. Nocturnal polyuria often increases with age. This increase may be due to posture, decreased arginine vasopression, medications, and alcohol and caffeine intake. Thus, the voiding log should include a list of fluid intake, types of fluid the patient drinks, the timing of fluid intake, and the timing of medications.

Additional information to be obtained includes a history of prior pelvic surgery or radiation, spinal or back injuries, or other neurologic disorders. In general, supraspinal neurologic injuries (such as a cerebrovascular accident) produce unstable detrusor contractions (overactive bladder); cervical and thoracic spinal cord lesions (such as spinal cord trauma or cervical stenosis) produce unstable detrusor contractions associated with external sphincter spasticity (detrusor sphincter dyssynergia); and lumbosacral spinal cord lesions (such as trauma or herniated disc) produce detrusor areflexia (no detrusor contractions or overflow incontinence). Radical pelvic surgery (abdominoperineal resection or radical hysterectomy) may interrupt peripheral efferent nerves to the detrusor, producing detrusor areflexia and overflow incontinence. Parkinson's disease may produce variable bladder problems, including overactive bladder and failure of the external sphincter to relax (a form of bladder outlet obstruction). Diabetes mellitus produces a sensory neuropathy to the bladder such that patients void infrequently, which may provoke incontinence of all categories. As diabetes progresses, a motor neuropathy to the bladder occurs such that patients are unable to mount a detrusor contraction, and risk overflow incontinence.

Women should be questioned about their gynecologic and obstetric history. Pelvic floor prolapse and stress incontinence are more likely in women who have had multiple vaginal deliveries or a hysterectomy, or are postmenopausal, and not receiving hormone replacement.

A history of bladder pain or hematuria should raise the suspicion of bladder cancer (or possibly prostate cancer in an elderly male). Fecal dysfunction should be elicited, as bladder dysfunction may be secondary to rectal impaction. Neurogenic bowel and bladder often coexist as they share S2–4 innervation. Finally, it is important to determine what therapies the patient has previously tried to address incontinence.

Physical Examination

The physical examination should focus on genitourinary anatomy, and should also include an examination of other organ systems that may have an influence on incontinence. For example, some patients are incontinent due to severe congestive heart failure that may be manifest by jugular venous distention or lower extremity edema. These patients typically are incontinent more at night when they are recumbent, when third space and lower extremity fluid is returned to their central circulation, and produces a diuresis. Neurologic impairments such as spinal dysraphism or gait abnormalities should also be noted.

Examination of the genitourinary system should include the external genitalia, and an examination of perineal sensation and reflexes including the bulbocavernosus reflex. The presence of a cystocele, rectocele, enterocele, urethral diverticulum, or uterine or vaginal cuff prolapse should be identified. The position and mobility of the urethra at rest and during periods of increased abdominal pressure, such as with cough or strain, should be noted. It is preferable to perform this examination with a full bladder so that loss of urine with cough or the Valsalva maneuver can be observed. A bimanual pelvic examination is performed to identify any vaginal or adnexal mass lesions or abdominal tenderness. Digital rectal examination is used to identify prostate disease or fecal impaction.

Ancillary Tests

Urinalysis should be a routine test in all patients undergoing evaluation for incontinence. This should include both a dipstick and microscopic examination to help prevent false-positive and false-negative results. If the urinalysis is suggestive of a urinary tract infection, the specimen should be sent for culture and antibiotic sensitivities. The presence of hematuria or a urinary tract infection may warrant additional investigation.

Postvoid residual urine volume should be determined to evaluate for possible overflow incontinence. This may be done either by straight catheterization or by use of an ultrasound bladder scanner. The ultrasound offers the advantage of being accurate and noninvasive. However, the device is expensive and may not be available in all offices.

Pad tests may be used to quantify the degree of urinary incontinence. Standardized pad tests have been developed for this purpose. However, patients generally find these time consuming and difficult to complete. This type of testing is often reserved for research purposes, or to evaluate patients before and after surgical intervention.

In complicated cases, in patients with historical risk factors or physical examination findings such as neurologic disease, and when the cause of a patient's incontinence cannot be readily identified or fails to respond to treatment, specialized physiologic tests may be necessary. These include cystometrography, abdominal leak-point pressure measurement, pressure–flow urodynamics, and cystoscopy.

Treatment

The specific choice of therapy is based on the type of urinary incontinence and its etiology. In general, most patients prefer to start with the least invasive form of treatment possible. Therapy is often empiric, and the patient should take an active role in this decision process. Patient motivation and compliance are important issues for most forms of incontinence therapy.

MEDICAL THERAPY

In patients with transient incontinence due to medications, where possible, the medications should be substituted for less problematic medication alternatives. Particularly for diuretics, one option would be to change the timing of diuretics, so that less diuretic is taken before bedtime.

Alpha-agonists may be used to treat patients with minimal stress urinary incontinence. The trigone and bladder neck are richly supplied by alpha$_1$-adrenergic receptors. Stimulation of these receptors causes contraction of smooth muscle that may improve tone at the bladder neck. The most commonly used drug in this class is phenylpropanolamine, 25 to 75 mg bid.

In contrast, alpha-antagonists may be used to relax smooth muscle at the bladder neck. This can be helpful, particularly in men with benign prostatic hyperplasia. Typical medications include doxazosin titrated up to 4 mg qhs or terazosin titrated up to 10 mg qhs. The primary side effects of these medications are orthostatic hypotension and dizziness. Tamsulosin is a more uroselective medication that avoids this central side effect. It does not need to be titrated, and is given 0.4 mg once daily.

Estrogen replacement therapy may be used in the treatment of urinary incontinence, atrophic vaginitis, and urinary tract infection in women. It is most effective given as a topical vaginal preparation. A variety of formulations are available. One-quarter to one-half applicator vaginally three times weekly at bedtime is usually sufficient. A newer formulation is available as a ring impregnated with estrogen that is placed intravaginally and changed every three months. This device releases estrogen slowly over this time period. Care should be taken to assure that patients do not have any contraindications to estrogen use, such as a history of breast or uterine cancer. Estrogens may act synergistically with alpha-agonists in the treatment of stress incontinence.

Anticholinergic medications can be used to relax the detrusor for the treatment of urge incontinence (overactive bladder). The traditional drugs in this class are propantheline bromide (Pro-Banthine) 15 to 30 mg po bid or tid, or oxybutynin chloride given in doses of 2.5 to 10 mg po bid to tid. These anticholinergic drugs may be poorly tolerated in the elderly due to anticholinergic side effects such as dry mouth and constipation. Less commonly, elderly patients suffer confusion or grogginess. Two recent oral anticholinergic drugs with fewer side effects are tolterodine (Detrol) 1 to 2 mg bid, and slow release oxybutynin (Ditropan XL) 5-10 mg qd. Detrol is believed to be more selective for the detrusor over the salivary glands, based on rodent studies. Ditropan XL is unique as a long-acting once-a-day anticholinergic. Due to the sustained release, its pharmacokinetics produce relatively stable serum levels of drug. Thus, side effects may be minimized as few drug peaks occur. And efficacy may be enhanced as therapeutic levels are maintained as few drug valleys occur. Both Detrol and Ditropan XL are effective, and limited uncontrolled data implies that Ditropan XL may have fewer side effects. A clinical trial comparing these two drugs has not been done, however. Tricyclic antidepressants such as imipramine 25 to 100 mg once daily or amitriptyline 25 to 75 mg once daily may also be used for anticholinergic effects. Care should be taken when using any anticholinergic medication due to side effects, primarily dry mouth and constipation. Anticholinergic drugs are contraindicated in patients with narrow-angle glaucoma.

In elderly incontinent patients with nocturnal incontinence related to nocturnal polyuria where diuretics, third-space losses (peripheral edema), or excessive fluid intake or medications do not appear to be causes of nocturnal overproduction of urine, the clinician may presume that reduced argi-

nine vasopression (antidiuretic hormone) may be the cause of incontinence. These patients may be treated with desmopressin 10 to 40 µg intranasally or 0.1 to 0.4 mg orally qhs. Doses may increase every 3 days. Serum electrolytes should be monitored on day 1 of therapy and 1 week after commencing therapy. Side effects may include headache, nausea, vomiting, lightheadedness, and presacral or peripheral edema. These symptoms should be elicited and weight monitored.

BEHAVIORAL THERAPY

A wide variety of behavioral therapies have been developed for the treatment of incontinence. Pelvic floor muscle exercises, also known as Kegel exercises, can help strengthen the muscles and support structures of the pelvic floor. This has been shown effective for both stress and urge symptoms in up to 65% of subjects. Pelvic floor muscle exercises may also be helpful to treat urge incontinence. Biofeedback training, electrical stimulation, and devices such as weighted intravaginal cones have been used to enhance pelvic floor muscle exercises.

The critical factors for success are the identification of the correct muscles and continued performance of the exercises. Discontinuation of the exercises usually results in return of incontinence. If patients do not correctly perform the muscle contractions, they may actually increase intra-abdominal pressure and worsen their incontinence symptoms.

Timed and prompted voiding regimens may be quite effective for people who suffer from functional or overflow incontinence, and for diabetics who do not sense appropriately their bladder filling. Alzheimer's patients are an important example of patients with functional incontinence who benefit from timed voidings. Alzheimer's patients generally sense bladder filling and urge to void correctly, and generally void to completion (unless concomitant urologic problems are present). However, they lack the judgment to withhold micturition until they reach a bathroom. Thus, prompted or timed voidings help to maintain an empty bladder, so they are less likely to have incontinent episodes. Anticholinergic drugs are generally not indicated in these patients. In fact, anticholinergic drugs may make their incontinence worse, as they may induce overflow incontinence, or cloud their sensorium.

Patients with primarily nocturnal incontinence may benefit from behavioral therapy. Specifically, should these patients ingest large volumes of fluid in the evening, they should be instructed to reduce their evening fluid intake. If the patient ingests alcohol or caffeinated drinks in the evening, he or she should be instructed to reduce or eliminate alcohol or caffeine at night.

DEVICES

Pessaries come in a variety of shapes and sizes. These intravaginal devices may increase urethral resistance and reduce cystoceles or other forms of prolapse. Intraurethral plugs or patches that cover the urethra may be useful in patients who suffer from minimal stress incontinence. These devices need to be changed frequently and require adequate hand dexterity. Pessaries may be particularly beneficial in debilitated patients whose pelvic prolapse could not be addressed by pelvic floor exercises or surgery. If the patient lacks the manual dexterity or cognition to change the pessary, the caregiver might be able to assist.

Patients with overflow incontinence may benefit from clean intermittent catheterization to adequately empty their bladders. Intermittent catheterization is preferred over indwelling catheters to minimize the risk of infection and histologic changes in the bladder mucosa.

Neuromodulation is a relatively new technique that may be useful for patients suffering from either urge or overflow incontinence. Stimulation of the S_3 sacral nerve root(s) may reduce detrusor instability while improving functional contractility.

SURGICAL THERAPY

Injection therapy is a minimally invasive technique to treat stress urinary incontinence caused by intrinsic sphincter deficiency. The most com-monly used agent in the United States is gluteraldehyde cross-linked bovine collagen. This is injected submucosally at the level of the bladder neck to increase intraurethral pressure. The overall reported success in women is approximately 80%. It is less effective in women who have received pelvic radiation and men after prostatectomy. It offers the benefit of being performed as an outpatient and it may be repeated.

Bladder neck suspensions such as the Marshall-Marchetti-Krantz, Raz, and Stamey procedures are traditionally used for treatment of stress incontinence caused by urethral hypermobility. More recently, sling cystourethropexy has been advocated for treatment of stress incontinence due to either urethral hypermobility or intrinsic sphincter deficiency. A variety of graft materials may be used to form the suburethral sling including autologous fascia, allograft fascia from cadaver donors, or synthetic material.

The artificial urinary sphincter is a surgically implanted prosthetic device to treat stress incontinence that consists of a urethral cuff that constricts the urethra when inflated, it is controlled by a pump placed in either the scrotum or labia majora. It requires adequate hand dexterity and cognitive function to operate effectively. It is particularly useful in men with post-prostatectomy urinary incontinence, but problems with skin breakdown or infection sometimes occur.

Augmentation cystoplasty may be used for the management of urge incontinence refractory to more conservative treatments. A segment of bowel is used to patch onto the bladder. This serves to increase the bladder capacity and decrease its involuntary contractility. Some patients require intermittent catheterization to adequately empty their augmented bladder. In some patients, supravesical urinary diversion such as an ileal conduit may be required to treat their urge incontinence.

Education

Education of both the public and health care providers is an important aspect of urinary conti-

nence care. Several widely held myths about urinary incontinence should be addressed. Although
urinary incontinence is a common clinical problem that is more prevalent with increasing age, it
is not a normal part of the aging process. Even
very elderly patients should not leak urine. Many
people feel that because they have suffered from
incontinence for a long time, nothing can be done
to help them. In actuality, the etiology of the
incontinence can usually be identified and appropriate therapy initiated. It is also a common
misconception that surgery is the only effective
treatment modality. Continued educational efforts
will help to dispel these misconceptions.

Urinary Tract Infection

Urinary tract infections are a common clinical
problem in elderly patients. Like urinary incontinence, the prevalence of urinary tract infection increases with age, but is not considered a normal
part of aging. Urinary tract infections are traditionally defined by the presence of both significant bacteriuria (more than 10^5 colony-forming
units of bacteria/mL urine) and pyuria on a clean-
catch midstream specimen. More recently, urinary
tract infections have been diagnosed with counts
as low as 10^2 colony-forming units of bacteria/mL
urine in symptomatic patients or when a specimen is obtained from a sterile catheterization.

Isolated bacteriuria, without associated pyuria,
affects an estimated 10% of older men and 20%
of older women and is more common in the institutionalized elderly. The majority of these people have transient or asymptomatic bacteriuria.
Usually, asymptomatic bacteriuria does not require active antibiotic therapy.

A variety of risk factors have been identified
that increase the risk of urinary tract infection in
the elderly. Women are at greater risk than men
due to differences in urethral anatomy. Anatomic
or functional anomalies of the lower urinary tract

such as a urethral diverticulum or incomplete
bladder emptying may predispose patients to urinary tract infection. Functional limitations including impaired mobility and cognitive losses have
also been linked with increased rates of infection
in the elderly. Comorbid diseases such as diabetes, benign prostatic hyperplasia, and urolithiasis are also associated with increased urinary
tract infection risk.

Typical Presentation

In younger patients, the most common signs and
symptoms of urinary tract infection include dysuria, urinary frequency, fever, chills, and cloudy
or foul-smelling urine. In elderly patients, the
presentation may vary due to alterations in the
ability to mount an adequate immune response.
Therefore, leukocytosis may be variable in this
population. Older subjects may demonstrate
lethargy, confusion, anorexia, or new-onset urinary incontinence as the initial presentation of a
urinary tract infection. This is particularly true of
elders who live in nursing care facilities. These
changes may be subtle and detected only by very
close observation.

Patients with pyelonephritis or complex urinary
tract infections may experience flank pain or tenderness in addition to the other signs and symptoms. Severe infections may lead to urosepsis with
associated hemodynamic alterations such as hypotension and tachycardia, nausea or vomiting,
and chills or sweats. Elderly patients with urosepsis may be febrile or hypothermic. The case fatal-
ity rate from urosepsis is approximately 40%.

Ancillary Tests

URINALYSIS

Urinalysis is critical for the diagnosis of urinary tract infection. The most common findings
on dipstick examination include positive leukocyte esterase activity and nitrites. A microscopic

examination of centrifuged urine should also be obtained to help improve diagnostic accuracy. If a large number of epithelial cells are present, the specimen is likely contaminated with skin flora. In these cases, a catheterized specimen should be obtained.

The urine should be sent for culture and antibiotic sensitivity. Traditionally, more than 10^5 colony-forming units of bacteria/mL urine from a clean-catch specimen is considered infected. However, a smaller number of bacteria may be significant if a more sensitive collection technique such as a sterile catheterized specimen is used or the patient is symptomatic. Isolated bacteruria may represent asymptomatic bacteruria or contamination with skin or vaginal flora. Some elderly patients may have a small bladder capacity, or may not understand instructions to give a midstream specimen from a full bladder. In these cases, the small voided volume minimizes accurate midstream collection, and a catheterized specimen should be obtained. Isolated pyuria may be associated with noninfectious inflammatory conditions such as interstitial cystitis. Persistent sterile pyuria should raise the suspicion of possible genitourinary tuberculosis.

IMAGING

Imaging of the upper and lower urinary tract is warranted in elderly women with recurrent infection or complicated infections such as pyelonephritis. All men with urinary infection should be imaged, as men typically have urinary infection from anatomic causes (obstruction or stones). Renal ultrasound is valuable to assess for hydronephrosis and urinary obstruction. Intravenous pyelography is the preferred imaging study to obtain both anatomic and functional information. However, this should be reserved until the acute infection has been cleared, because pyelonephritis adversely affects tubular concentrating ability. Thus, the intravenous contrast is not well concentrated in the kidney. If voiding dysfunction is suspected, formal physiologic evaluation with pressure–flow videourodynamics may be obtained.

Pathophysiology and Bacteriology

A number of theories have been proposed to explain the increased rate of urinary tract infections in elderly patients. There is evidence that aging is associated with a decrease in cell-mediated immunity. There may be alterations in bladder defense mechanisms that increase uroepithelial receptivity for bacteria. Other natural antibacterial factors also change with age. For example, after menopause the normal acidification of vaginal fluid is altered. This causes a reduction in the concentration of lactobacilli in the vagina. As lactobacillus colonization of vaginal and periurethral epithelium decreases, there is increased colonization by more pathogenic enteric bacteria, such as *E. coli*. Changes in lower urinary tract physiology may also predispose older adults to urinary tract infections. Incomplete bladder emptying is the most common finding in these cases. In elderly men, benign prostate hyperplasia (BPH) or prostate cancer may cause bladder outlet obstruction. Bladder outlet obstruction leads to urinary stasis and incomplete bladder emptying.

Gram-negative organisms are the most common source of infection in both younger and older patients. *Escherichia coli* is the most common organism, although its overall prevalence decreases somewhat with age. The rate of infection with other organisms including *Proteus, Klebsiella, Providencia, Pseudomonas*, and *Citrobacter* species increases with age. Gram-positive infections with organisms such as *Enterococcus* are also more common in the elderly and are often associated with concomitant defecation disorders. Infections with urea-splitting organisms such as *Proteus* or *Klebsiella* species may be associated with struvite urolithiasis. Infections with multiple organisms are also more common in the elderly and should not just be assumed to be due to contamination of the specimen.

Treatment

Symptomatic urinary tract infections should be treated with appropriate antibiotics. Typically this may be accomplished with oral antibiotics; however pyelonephritis or other more severe infections typically require intravenous antibiotic coverage. Initial choices of antibiotic therapy are often made empirically based on Gram's stain and urinalysis data. Therapy may be tailored later based on culture and antibiotic sensitivity results. Urosepsis should be managed aggressively with intravenous antibiotics and fluid resuscitation. Any evidence of urinary tract obstruction such as hydronephrosis should be addressed to prevent subsequent development of urosepsis. Indwelling Foley catheterization or intermittent catheterization may be needed to drain the bladder. Ureteral obstruction may require drainage with either an indwelling ureteral stent or percutaneous nephrostomy tube.

In elderly patients, antibiotic toxicity must be carefully considered. Of particular concern are drug–drug interactions in patients who are on multiple other medications. In addition, renal and hepatic dysfunction are more common in the elderly and may necessitate dose adjustment of antibiotics. Peak and trough blood levels should be obtained, particularly for aminoglycosides.

Prevention

Proper hygiene is important in the prevention of urinary tract infections. Frequent urination and adequate hydration should be stressed for all patients. In addition, patients should be advised to void before and after sexual intercourse to prevent bacterial colonization of the urethra that can result in subsequent infection. Women should also be instructed to wipe from anterior to posterior after voiding to avoid fecal contamination of the urethra and perineum.

Prophylactic antibiotics may be used in select patients with recurrent urinary tract infections. Mild antibiotics should be chosen as urinary antiseptics to prevent overgrowth of resistant organisms. Antibiotics commonly used for this purpose include nitrofurantoin 50 mg qhs or trimethoprim-sulfamethoxazole (single strength) one-half tablet qhs. In patients with sulfa allergies, trimethoprim 50 to 100 mg qhs may be used.

Estrogen replacement therapy may be of benefit in elderly women with recurrent urinary tract infections. Application of topical vaginal estrogens leads to acidification of the vaginal fluid that promotes growth of the normal vaginal flora, *Lactobacillus* spp. This helps act as a natural defense mechanism against pathogenic bacteria. Estrogen replacement is somewhat controversial and is generally contraindicated in women who have had breast or uterine cancer.

Dietary modification may also be beneficial in the prevention of urinary tract infections in the elderly. Several studies have demonstrated that daily cranberry juice intake may help lower the incidence of urinary tract infection, particularly in the institutionalized elderly. Cranberry concentrate pills may be substituted for the cranberry juice. This is particularly important in diabetics due to the high glucose and calorie content of cranberry juice. Ingestion of foods rich in *Lactobacillus* spp. such as sweet acidophilus milk or cultured yogurt may also be of some benefit.

The Future of Geriatric Urology

Urologic problems, particularly urinary incontinence and urinary tract infections, are common in the elderly patient population. The need for special understanding of the urologic problems of the aged will continue to increase as the demographics of our society change. The elderly currently comprise 12% of the American population. However, it is estimated that this percentage will increase to 20% by the year 2030. Care of the elderly will occupy an increasing proportion of both primary and specialty care in the future.

Bibliography

Avorn J, Monane M, Gurwitz JH, et al: Reduction of bacteriuria and pyuria after ingestion of cranberry juice. *JAMA* 271:751, 1994.

Brittain KR, Peet SM, Castleden CM: Stroke and incontinence. *Stroke* 29:524, 1998.

Fantl JA, Newman DK, Colling J, et al: Urinary Incontinence in Adults: Acute and Chronic Management. Clinical Practice Guideline, no. 2, 1996 update. Rockville, MD, U.S. Department of Health and Human Services, Public Health Service, Agency for Health Care Policy and Research, March 1996. AHCPR publication no. 96-0682.

Griebling TL, Berman CJ, Kreder KJ: Fascia lata sling cystourethropexy for the management of female urinary incontinence. *Int Urogynecol J Pelvic Floor Dysfunct* 9:165, 1998.

Griebling TL, Nygaard IE: The role of estrogen replacement therapy in the management of urinary incontinence and urinary tract infection in postmenopausal women. *Endocrinol Metab Clin North Am* 26:347, 1997.

Iqbal P, Castleden CM: Management of urinary incontinence in the elderly. *Gerontology* 43:151, 1997.

Johnson TM, Ouslander JG: Urinary incontinence in the older man. *Med Clin North Am* 83:1247, 1999.

Krissovich M: The financial side of continence promotion. *Geriatr Nurs* 19:91, 1998.

Nasr SZ, Ouslander JG: Urinary incontinence in the elderly. Causes and treatment options. *Drugs Aging* 12:349, 1998.

Newman DK: Managing indwelling urethral catheters. *Ostomy Wound Manage* 44:26, 1998.

Nicolle LE, Strausbaugh JG, Garibaldi RA: Infections and antibiotic resistance in nursing homes. *Clin Microbiol Rev* 9:1, 1996.

O'Donnell BF, Drachman DA, Barnes HJ, et al: Incontinence and troublesome behaviors predict institutionalization in dementia. *J Geriatr Psychiatry Neurol* 5:45, 1992.

Ouslander JG, Zarit SH, Orr NK, et al: Incontinence among elderly community-dwelling dementia patients. Characteristics, management, and impact on caregivers. *J Am Geriatr Soc* 38:400, 1990.

Resnick NM: Urinary incontinence in the elderly. *Medical Grand Rounds*, 3: 281–290, 1984.

Resnick NM, Yalla SV: Detrusor hyperactivity with impaired contractile function. An unrecognized but common cause of incontinence in elderly patients. *JAMA* 257:3076, 1987.

Schnelle JF, Ouslander JG: Management of incontinence in long-term care. In O'Donnell PD (ed): *Urinary Incontinence*. St. Louis, Mosby-Year Book, 1997, pp 405–413.

Steeman E, Defever M: Urinary incontinence among elderly persons who live at home: A literature review. *Nurs Clin North Am* 33:441, 1998.

Thom DH, Brown JS: Reproductive and hormonal risk factors for urinary incontinence in later life: A review of the clinical and epidemiological literature. *J Am Geriatr Soc* 46:1411, 1998.

Weiss JP, Blaivas JG: Nocturia. *J Urol* 163:5–12, 2000.

Whishaw M: Urinary incontinence in the elderly. Establishing a cause may allow a cure. *Aust Fam Physician* 27:1087, 1998.

Wood CA, Abrutyn E: Optimal treatment of urinary infections in elderly patients. *Drugs Aging* 9:352, 1996.

Yoshikawa TT, Nicolle LE, Norman DC: Management of complicated urinary tract infection in older patients. *J Am Geriatr Soc* 44:1235, 1996.

Yoshikawa TT, Norman DC: Infection control in long-term care. *Clin Geriatr Med* 11:467, 1995.

Thomas A. Rozanski

Chapter

11

Hematuria

How Common Is Hematuria?

Hematuria (blood in the urine) is a common problem and its presence is usually distressing to both patient and health care provider. The prevalence of hematuria in the general population is 2% to 18%, depending on the methods of collection, preparation, and analysis of urine, population studied, and definition employed.[2,3]

Hematuria may be the first sign of serious disease in the urinary tract, and is the most common presenting sign of urinary tract cancer and parenchymal renal disease. Blood in the urine is a "red flag" that should prompt an appropriate evaluation to rule out or detect disease in otherwise asymptomatic patients. Even a single episode of hematuria should be investigated, as it can signal a problem anywhere along the urinary tract, from kidney to urethra, or a systemic condition.

Defining Hematuria

Hematuria is the presence of an abnormal quantity of red blood cells (RBCs) in the urine. The abnormality may be visible with the naked eye (gross hematuria) or detected only with examination of the urinary sediment (microscopic hematuria). The average adult normally excretes about one million RBCs in the urine every day. The erythrocytes escape through glomerular capillaries into the urine.

The first step in the management of bloody urine is to determine if in fact the patient has significant hematuria. Unfortunately, there is no consensus in the literature among urologists or nephrologists as to what constitutes significant microscopic hematuria. However, this author, and many others in urology and nephrology, con-

siders more than 3 RBCs per high-power field (hpf) in centrifuged urine sediment to be significant. Calculation of confidence levels indicates that over 95% of the normal population has less than 3 erythrocytes per hpf in centrifuged urine.[4]

It is also important to note that not all red urine is due to blood, and not all abnormal urine dipstick readings for blood are true positives on microscopic analysis. Therefore, prior to initiating an evaluation for hematuria, an appropriately performed microscopic examination of urine sediment is mandatory. Many food products, drugs, and chemicals can cause urine to become a red, orange, or red-brown color (Table 11–1). The patient may describe red urine; however, a urinalysis will be negative for RBCs.

Dipstick Urinalysis

Although there is no clear indication for obtaining a urinalysis for screening, screening urine tests are commonly obtained and are the source of detection of many cases of hematuria. Proper urine collection is, therefore, very important. The urine should be a midstream catch after appropriate cleansing of the meatus area. Strenuous activity and urethral manipulation should be avoided for 48 hours before collection, and females should not be menstruating.

Dipstick analysis is based on the peroxidase-like activity of hemoglobin, which catalyzes a reaction resulting in a color change on the stick from orange to green. Green spots indicate intact RBCs, whereas a field change to green can indicate erythrocytes or free hemoglobin and myoglobin.

Urine should be collected in a clean container and tested as soon as possible, preferably within 30 minutes of collection. No centrifugation is required and, in fact, should be avoided prior to dipstick urinalysis. Dipsticks should be stored to prevent exposure to moisture, heat, and light; expiration dates should be recognized; and the bottle recapped immediately in order to prevent false-positive and false-negative reactions.

Table 11–1

Causes of Red, Orange, or Brown Urine without Erythrocytes

Foods	**Drugs**		
Beets	Adriamycin	Metronidazole	Quinine
Berries	Cascara	Nitrofurantoin	Rifampin
Rhubarb	Deferoxamine	Phenazopyridine	Senna
Vegetable dyes	Diphenylhydantoin	Phenindione	Sulfamethoxazole
Food coloring	Ibuprofen	Phenolphthalein	Sulfasalazine
	Levodopa	Phenothiazines	
	Methyldopa	Phenytoin	
Other Causes			
Hemoglobin			
Myoglobin			
Porphyrins			
Urate			
Infection/*Serratia*			

False-positive reactions for blood can occur for a number of reasons (Table 11–2). Microscopic analysis of centrifuged urine may show no RBCs despite a positive dipstick reading for blood in these scenarios. Substances that markedly change urine color may interfere with interpretation of the dipstick (Pyridium, Azo Gantrisin, Azo Gantanol, nitrofurantoin, riboflavin). False-negative reactions for blood can occur with markedly elevated specific gravity, some drugs (captopril), air-exposed dipsticks, and high levels of urinary ascorbic acid. Dipstick analysis for blood is very sensitive (91% to 100%), but the specificity is not as reliable (65% to 99%).[5] Therefore, dipstick urinalysis is an excellent screening tool if negative, but all positive results should be corroborated with microscopic analysis.

Microscopic Urinalysis

The definitive study to identify or confirm the presence or absence of hematuria is microscopic evaluation of the urinary sediment. Proper collection techniques previously described also pertain to specimen collection prior to microscopy. Hospital and regional labs should standardize collection and preparation of urine for analysis. If the procedure is to be done in an office setting, 10 mL of urine should be centrifuged for 5 minutes at 2000 rpm. The supernatant is decanted and one drop of sediment placed on a glass slide with coverslip. Microscopic analysis should include both low (×10) and high (×40) power magnification. Sediment should be examined for cells, casts, crystals, and organisms.

Erythrocyte Morphology

Examination of the urinary sediment is the key to evaluation of hematuria. There are two primary

Table 11–2

False-Positive Dipstick Readings for Blood

Free urine hemoglobin/hemoglobinuria/hemolysis
Free urine myoglobin/myoglobinuria/rhabdomyolysis
Bacterial peroxidase production/infection
Oxidizing contaminants/hypochlorite
Hypotonic urine/specific gravity less than 1.008/hemolysis
Povidine/iodine contamination

categories of hematuria, glomerular and epithelial. Glomerular bleeding suggests renal parenchymal disease and a nephrologic etiology, while epithelial bleeding indicates a urologic source. The basic evaluation differs for each major category. Microscopic urinalysis is critical because information obtained (RBC morphology, casts) will often dictate specifics of patient evaluation.

Glomerular bleeding is suggested by the presence of dysmorphic erythrocytes. The cells are distorted with irregular outlines, heterogeneous in size, and have small protrusions or blebs on the cell membrane (acanthocytes; Fig. 11–1). Phase-contrast microscopy is best suited to identify acanthocytes; however, the characteristic dysmorphic cells can be identified with light microscopy by an experienced examiner. Wright's stain of a dry smear is another method that can detect dysmorphic RBCs.

Erythrocytes of glomerular origin are likely distorted for a variety of reasons: mechanical factors

Figure 11–1

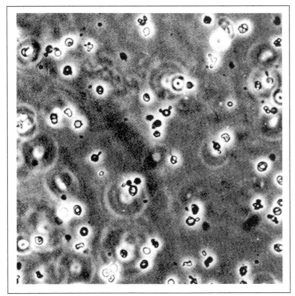

Dysmorphic erythrocytes. (Reproduced with permission from Birch DF, Fairley KF, Whitworth JA, et al: Urinary erythrocyte morphology in the diagnosis of glomerular hematuria. *Clin Nephrol* 20:80, 1983; Dustri-Verlag, Munich-Deisenhofen, Germany.)

as they pass through gaps in the glomerular basement membrane, changes in capillary pressures, tubular enzymes, and possibly by variations in pH and osmotic pressures. In addition, medical renal disease is suggested by RBC casts, marked proteinuria, and smokey, hazy, or reddish-brown colored urine. RBC casts form as erythrocytes are trapped in tubular lumens and gel with proteinaceous substances (Fig. 11–2). Significant proteinuria is greater than 2+ on dipstick analysis or greater than 500 to 1000 mg on a 24-hour urine collection. Ninety-eight percent of patients with all urine erythrocytes being dysmorphic and with RBC casts present were found to have parenchymal (glomerular) bleeding and medical renal disease.[6]

Epithelial bleeding caused by urologic disease is suggested by eumorphic erythrocytes. These cells are regular, smooth, and round and resemble the classic circulating biconcave RBC. Gross hematuria that is bright red or with clots also suggests epithelial bleeding. Once infection has been ruled out, an appropriate evaluation can be initiated based on RBC morphology, presence or absence of protein and casts, and characteristics of the hematuria (Fig. 11–3). If there is any doubt about whether to evaluate for urologic or nephrologic disease, it is safer to perform a complete urologic evaluation to exclude malignancy prior to proceeding with full nephrologic evaluation.

Why Evaluate Hematuria?

The purpose of investigating hematuria is to diagnose and treat lesions that might cause harm to the patient. The yield of diagnosing a life-threatening lesion increases as the degree of hematuria increases. However, there is no safe lower limit of hematuria below which life-threatening disorders do not occur (Table 11–3).[3]

The evaluation of gross hematuria will result in the diagnosis of a life-threatening problem five times more often than evaluations for microscopic

Figure 11–2

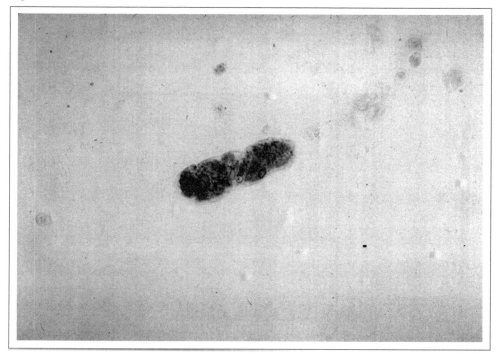

Red blood cell cast.

Figure 11–3

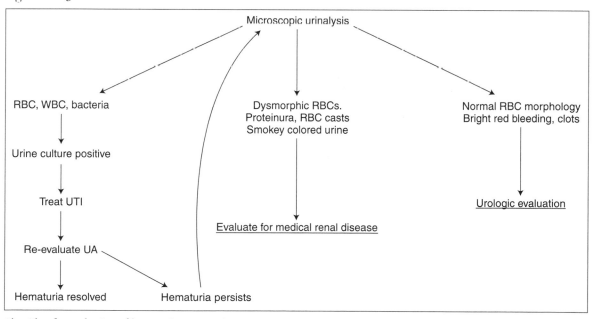

Algorithm for evaluation of hematuria.

Table 11–3

Degree of Hematuria and Detection of Lesions

RBC PER HIGH-POWER FIELD	PATIENTS WITH SIGNIFICANT LESIONS (%)	PATIENTS WITH LIFE-THREATENING LESIONS (%)
0–3	17	0
4–10	12	2.9
11–50	20	3.2
>50	30	8.7
Gross hematuria	58	20.7

Adapted from Mariani AJ, Mariani MC, Macchioni C, et al: The significance of adult hematuria: 1000 hematuria evaluations including a risk-benefit and cost-effectiveness analysis. *J Urol* 141:350, 1989.

hematuria.[3,7] Genitourinary cancers are found in 23% of adults presenting with gross hematuria, and 92% of investigations result in a definitive diagnosis. On the other hand, only 5% of evaluations for microscopic hematuria will lead to a diagnosis of cancer (range, 2% to 15%), and no etiology for the hematuria is found in 43% of these patients.[4] Five percent to 29% of the complete evaluations for microscopic hematuria will lead to a diagnosis that would potentially shorten a patient's lifespan or negatively impact quality of life.[8]

There is no correlation between the degree and persistence of microhematuria and the significance of pathology. Genitourinary cancers (transitional-cell carcinoma and renal-cell carcinoma) bleed on a sporadic basis, not continually. Nineteen percent of patients with life-threatening lesions were found to have at least one normal urinalysis (< 3 RBCs/hpf) within 6 months of diagnosis.[7] Even patients with one episode of microscopic hematuria might harbor a renal-cell carcinoma (RCC) or transitional-cell carcinoma (TCC).

Age and gender are important considerations in a hematuria evaluation. All urinary tract tumors occur more often in adults over age 50, while they are possible but rare in patients under age 40. All genitourinary cancers are more common in men, except for cancer of the urethra, which occurs more frequently in females.

Thorough evaluation of hematuria is cost effective if life-threatening lesions are diagnosed early and can be cured. In a series of 1000 adults evaluated for asymptomatic hematuria, 8.4% were found to have cancer. Of these, 77 (92%) were localized

and potentially curable.[3] The authors determined the cost of screening and evaluation and extrapolated the data. The difference in direct medical costs to diagnose and treat localized cancer versus a delayed presentation with metastases was substantial. If the 77 patients with localized cancer were not diagnosed until a time when the condition was too far advanced to cure, the additional costs would total more than five times the cost of the initial screening of the entire 1000 patients in the study.[3]

In addition to the fiscal justification, other factors are also likely beneficial, though difficult to quantify, such as medicolegal costs, lost patient productivity, and the value of patient reassurance following a thorough evaluation.[3]

Differential Diagnosis

The intent of the hematuria evaluation is to diagnose or exclude life-threatening conditions and significant disorders. The potential etiologies for hematuria are multiple. Table 11–4 lists many of the recognized etiologies for hematuria based on anatomic source of bleeding. Several of the most common, most serious, and interesting diagnoses will be briefly discussed.

In adults, hematuria of any degree should be considered a sign of urologic malignancy until proven otherwise. Tumors of the urinary tract frequently bleed intermittently, which can lead to a

Table 11–4
Differential Diagnosis of Hematuria

Kidney	Ureter	Urethra
Renal-cell carcinoma	Ureteropelvic junction obstruction	Urethritis
TCC of renal pelvis	TCC of the ureter	Prostatitis
Renal cyst	Calculus	BPH
Trauma (contusion, laceration)	Trauma	Stricture
Nephrolithiasis		Foreign body
Pyelonephritis	**Bladder**	Carcinoma
Arteriovenous fistula	TCC	Prostate cancer
Polycystic kidney disease	Infectious cystitis	Urethral prolapse
Medullary sponge kidney	Calculus	Condyloma
Renal artery embolus	Radiation cystitis	Trauma
Renal vein thrombosis	Interstitial cystitis	Caruncle
Loin pain hematuria syndrome	Cystitis cystica	
Papillary necrosis	Bladder neck varicosities	**Other**
Benign/familial/idiopathic hematuria	Hemorrhagic cystitis	Coagulopathy
Alport's syndrome	Endometriosis	Sickle-cell disease
Analgesic nephropathy	Adenocarcinoma	Drugs
Goodpasture's syndrome	Trauma	Renal biopsy
Nutcracker syndrome	Schistosomiasis	Vasculitis
Hypercalciuria	Tuberculosis	Exercise
Berger's disease (IgA nephropathy)	Foreign body	
Hyperuricosuria		
Interstitial nephritis		
Postinfectious glomerulonephritis		
Glomerulonephritis		
Glomerulosclerosis		
Tuberculosis		
Renal infarction		

false sense of security and delayed evaluation. A full evaluation should be pursued for gross or microscopic hematuria, unless a definitive etiology has been determined (documented infection) and the hematuria resolves after treatment. Malignancy is one of the most common causes for adult hematuria (Table 11–5).[9]

Renal-Cell Carcinoma

The most common kidney malignancy is renal-cell carcinoma (RCC), which may present as hematuria or with a wide variety of other symptoms, though it is often found incidentally when CT or ultrasound is obtained for unrelated reasons (Figs. 11–4 and 11–5). At our institution, 221 such tumors were treated over the past 7 years. Average age at presentation was 58, 21% presented with gross hematuria, and 12% presented with microhematuria. There is a three to one male preponderance, and 2% are bilateral (synchronous or asynchronous). Any solid renal mass or complex cystic renal mass on CT scan or ultrasound must be considered RCC until proven otherwise. No specific chemicals or carcinogens have been identified

Table 11–5

Most Common Causes of Hematuria by Age and Gender

0–20 Years
Acute glomerulonephritis
Acute urinary tract infection
Congenital urinary tract anomalies with obstruction

20–40 Years
Acute urinary tract infection
Calculi
Bladder tumor

40–60 Years, Males
Bladder tumor
Calculi
Acute urinary tract infection

40–60 Years, Females
Acute urinary tract infection
Calculi
Bladder tumor

60 Years, Males
Benign prostatic hyperplasia
Bladder tumor
Acute urinary tract infection

60 Years, Females
Bladder tumor
Acute urinary tract infection

Reprinted with permission from Bushman W, Wyker AW: Standard diagnostic considerations. In Gillenwater JY, Grayhack JT, Howards SS, Duckett JW (eds): *Adult and Pediatric Urology*, ed 3. St. Louis, Mosby YearBook, 1996, p. 67.

as causative; however, tobacco use increases the risk of RCC.

The cell of origin for RCC is in the proximal convoluted tubule. Renal-cell carcinoma occurs as one of three histopathologic types (clear cell, granular cell, spindle-shaped cell); clear-cell carcinoma is the most common (80%). Several paraneoplastic syndromes have been described with RCC, including hypertension, hypercalcemia, and erythrocytosis. Stauffer's syndrome is nonmetastatic hepatic dysfunction (abnormal liver function tests) that resolves following nephrectomy.

Figure 11–4

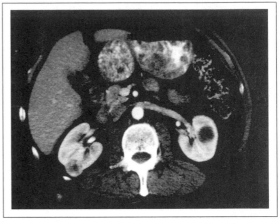

CT scan with small right RCC and benign left renal cyst.

Surgical therapy includes removal of the kidney and tumor, ipsilateral adrenal gland, surrounding perinephric fat, Gerota's fascia, and regional lymph nodes. Small (<4 cm) tumors may be managed by partial nephrectomy. Surgical extirpation of tumors pathologically confined to the kidney results in a greater than 90% 10-year survival. Chemotherapy and radiation therapy have

Figure 11–5

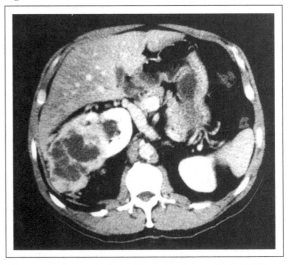

CT scan demonstrating significant local extension of RCC through kidney and into surrounding perinephric fat.

no definitive role in treating RCC. Immunotherapy (interferons, interleukins) has shown a small benefit in metastatic disease. The key to successful treatment is early diagnosis and nephrectomy for organ-confined disease.

Transitional-Cell Carcinoma

The urinary tract is lined by transitional-cell urothelium, and as such, transitional-cell carcinoma (TCC) may develop in the renal pelvis, ureter, bladder, or urethra. The most common cause of gross painless hematuria in patients over age 50 is bladder cancer, which is the most common site of TCC (Fig. 11–6). Ninety percent of bladder cancers are TCC (10% are adenocarcinoma or squamous-cell carcinoma). The majority present with hematuria, though up to 30% have significant irritative voiding symptoms (urgency, frequency, nocturia). Like all genitourinary tumors, bladder cancers may bleed intermittently.

Figure 11–6

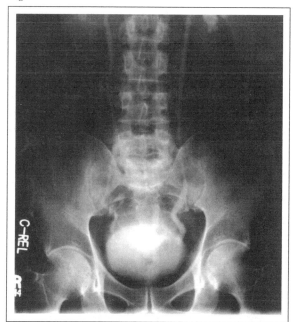

IVP showing filling defect (TCC) in bladder and partial left ureteral obstruction from the tumor.

Bladder cancer is the fourth most common cancer in men and the eighth in women.[10] The incidence has been stable in the past several decades in the United States. Forty-five percent of TCC is attributable to tobacco smoking. Only one in five cases of bladder TCC occurs in females, but it is expected that the percentage will increase as more females smoke cigarettes.[10] Risk factors for TCC are listed in Table 11–6.

Cystoscopy is the gold standard for the diagnosis and management of TCC (Fig. 11–7). The most important issue in local staging is determining the depth of tumor invasion. Superficial TCC can be managed with endoscopic resection, fulguration, and intravesical chemotherapy or immunotherapy agents. The recurrence rate of TCC is very high (>50%) and lifelong surveillance cystoscopies are mandatory. Tumors that invade through the urothelium and into bladder muscle must be managed in a much more aggressive fashion. Cystectomy and urinary diversion is the treatment of choice for invasive lesions. Despite cystectomy, survival rates for muscle invasive TCC are only 50% at 5 years. Multidrug chemotherapy and radiation therapy have limited roles in the management of TCC. The best treatment strategy relies on early diagnosis and treatment, and regular follow-up studies.

Renal Cysts

The regular use of abdominal imaging procedures in all areas of medicine has resulted in increased detection of renal cysts in asymptomatic patients.

Table 11–6

Risk Factors for Bladder Cancer

Smoking
Age > 40 years
Analgesic (NSAID) abuse
Pelvic radiation
Cyclophosphamide
Schistosomiasis
Occupational exposure—chemical, dye, and rubber industries: benzenes and aromatic amines

Figure 11–7

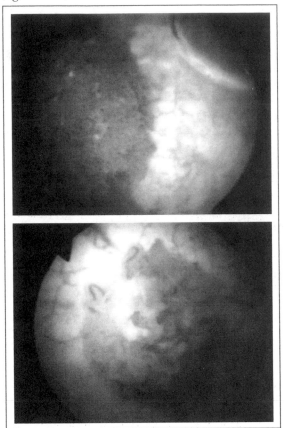

Cystoscopic view of a bladder TCC.

The most common lesions are simple cysts, which are found in 25% to 33% of adults over age 50. The Bosniak classification of renal cysts (based on CT criteria) is used by radiologists and urologists to determine whether a cystic lesion requires fur-

ther diagnostic or treatment measures (Fig. 11–8).[11] The Bosniak grading system uses various aspects of cyst septations, calcifications, and tissue characteristics in order to determine grade. Any suspicious renal cyst or mass on IVP, renal ultrasound, or renal scan should be evaluated with a dedicated renal CT (with and without intravenous contrast, 3- to 5-mm sections). All grade 3 and 4 cysts require urologic referral.

Urolithiasis

Urolithiasis of the urinary tract affects up to 5% of the Western population and up to 20% of patients with hematuria have urinary calculi. The majority of calculi (90%) contain calcium and are therefore visible on plain radiographs.

Typical symptoms include hematuria, and flank and abdominal pain with radiation of pain to the scrotum, labia, or groin. Intravenous pyelography is the classic imaging study used to diagnose and localize the calculus and to determine the degree of obstruction. However, noncontrast, spiral CT scans are considered as sensitive and more specific than intravenous pyelography to evaluate patients with flank or abdominal pain and suspected stone disease.

The three narrow portions of the ureter are natural areas for calculi to lodge and obstruct: the ureteropelvic junction, the point where the iliac vessels cross the ureter, and the ureterovesical junction. Cystine crystals on a urinalysis are indicative of cystinuria and likely cystine calculi. However, other crystals may be found in normal urine and are nondiagnostic (Fig. 11–9). Symptoms

Figure 11–8

Grade	Description	% Malignant
1	Simple cyst	0
2	Mildly complex	0
3	Complicated	50
4	Cystic malignancy	100

Bosniak classification of renal cysts.

Figure 11–9

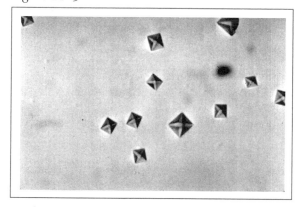

Envelope-shaped calcium oxalate crystals.

are managed acutely with analgesics, and occasionally with a ureteral stent or percutaneous nephrostomy, particularly if the possibility of obstruction and infection coexist. The majority of calculi are less than 7 mm in diameter and will pass spontaneously. A more definitive discussion of urinary calculi appears in Chapter 16.

Infection

Urinary tract infections may account for up to 25% of all episodes of hematuria in a urologist's practice, and well over half of those in primary care practice. Cystitis is the most common infection, and presents as urgency, frequency, dysuria, and suprapubic pain, in addition to microscopic or gross hematuria. When a patient presents with symptoms consistent with cystitis but has a negative urine culture, nonbacterial infection (chlamydia, trichomonas, tuberculosis) and bladder cancer must be considered.

Pyelonephritis usually results from retrograde propagation of infection from the bladder to the kidney. Patients with pyelonephritis usually complain of flank pain and systemic symptoms such as fever, chills, and nausea.

Exercise-Induced Hematuria

Contact and noncontact sporting events both can result in gross or microscopic hematuria. Blood in the urine following strenuous activity is usually benign and occurs on a variable basis depending on the type and duration of exercise and the state of hydration of the athlete.

Hematuria following blunt physical contact is usually due to direct renal trauma. The etiology for hematuria associated with noncontact strenuous exercise is likely multifactorial. Long-distance runners develop bladder ecchymosis and contusions, probably a result of the repetitive up and down motions and contact of a partially filled bladder. These lesions rapidly resolve and exercise-induced hematuria should totally resolve in 24 to 72 hours.

If a pertinent medical history is unremarkable, the incidence of renal or urologic disease is very low, raising the possibility of exercise-induced hematuria, particularly for athletes with microscopic hematuria under age 40. Hematuria following minimally strenuous activity should not be overlooked, however, because congenital abnormalities and tumors tend to bleed with minimal trauma. Medical evaluation is necessary in several clinical situations (Table 11–7). There is no evidence that exercise-induced hematuria leads to renal damage, and it is safe to return to full activity when the urinalysis normalizes.[12]

Benign Prostatic Hyperplasia

The prevalence of benign prostatic hypertrophy is very high in older men. Hematuria may be the first sign or symptom that brings the patient to his health care provider. Prostatic enlargement may

Table 11–7

Indications for Full Evaluation of Exercise Hematuria

Persists >72 hours

Not associated with "strenuous" activity

Recurrent hematuria

Age > 40

Gross hematuria

Significant proteinuria

Presence of RBC casts

result in small mucosal vessel engorgement. These vessels may rupture when the man strains to void, resulting in hematuria. Benign prostatic hypertrophy is discussed in more detail in Chapter 13.

Papillary Necrosis

The papillary tip is the apex of the renal pyramid. Several processes result in ischemic necrosis of the papilla, causing the papilla to slough, leaving a characteristic concavity seen on IVP. Diabetes and analgesic abuse (aspirin, phenacetin, NSAIDs) are the most common predisposing factors. Analgesic abuse also predisposes the patient to TCC and nephropathy. The acronym POSTCARD is a useful means to recall the various causes of papillary necrosis (Fig. 11–10).

Berger's Disease / Immunoglobulin A Nephropathy

Immunoglobulin A (IgA) nephropathy is the most common glomerular disease in the world and the most common cause of glomerular hematuria. Recurrent microscopic or gross hematuria is usually found in young adult men, can be associated with a low-grade fever and erythematous skin rash, and may present following exercise or an upper respiratory tract infection. Diagnosis is made by renal biopsy, where prominent IgA deposits are found in the mesangium by immunofluorescence microscopy. Urinalysis shows a mixed pattern of eumorphic and dysmorphic erythrocytes. This chronic disease has an excellent prognosis. Other glomerulonephritides may cause hematuria. Dysmorphic erythrocytes are typically seen and renal biopsy is generally required for diagnosis.

Hematospermia

Blood in the seminal fluid usually results in prompt self-referral by an anxious patient and partner. The etiology is not known, though is likely due to nonspecific inflammation in younger men, and is seen frequently following prostate biopsy in older men. The condition almost always resolves spontaneously and is rarely associated with any significant pathology.[13] If the bloody ejaculate persists longer than several weeks, urologic referral and a more detailed evaluation is indicated (prostate-specific antigen, prostate ultrasound, cytology, cystoscopy, and so forth), because cancer of the prostate and urethra are possible etiologies.

Hypercalciuria and Hyperuricosuria

Isolated hypercalciuria without calculi is a recognized cause of hematuria in children, and only recently has been shown to be a reversible cause of gross and microscopic hematuria in adults. Patients are usually young adults and many have a family history of kidney stone disease. Etiology of the hematuria is not well defined, though it may be due to small unrecognized microcalculi that result in epithelial or tubular bleeding. A recent study showed that hematuria resolved in 60% of adults with isolated hypercalciuria, hyperuricosuria, or both abnormalities, when urine calcium and uric acid levels were reduced to normal using thiazides and/or allopurinol.[14]

Figure 11–10

P	pyelonephritis
O	obstruction
S	sickle-cell disease
T	tuberculosis
C	cirrhosis
A	analgesic abuse
R	renal vein thrombosis
D	diabetes

POSTCARD: causes of papillary necrosis.

"The cause of hematuria must be determined after a careful history, thorough physical, and complete analysis of the urine."[1] This statement from a 1913 urology textbook remains true today. Unlike medicine in the early 20th century, however, we now have a large armamentarium of studies and tests to help determine the etiology of hematuria. Still, despite the wide array of technology available, there is no substitute for an accurate and detailed history and physical examination.

When a patient presents with hematuria, several key points must be ascertained in the history (Table 11–8). Is the hematuria gross or microscopic? A definitive etiology is found more often with gross hematuria. Is the patient symptomatic or asymptomatic? Painless hematuria suggests cancer or renal parenchymal disease.

Irritative voiding symptoms such as dysuria and frequency suggest infection or inflammation, but carcinoma in situ and TCC can cause similar symptoms and should be considered if the urine culture is negative or the patient smokes cigarettes. Colicky type pain suggests urolithiasis or other causes of ureteral obstruction (e.g., sloughed papilla, clot).

Timing of the hematuria during the urinary stream is significant. Initial hematuria (beginning of stream) suggests urethral bleeding. Terminal hematuria (end of stream) is indicative of bladder neck and prostate bleeding that occurs as the bladder neck contracts at the end of voiding. Blood seen between voids, such as stains on undergarments with clear voided urine, is likely from the meatus or anterior urethra. Total hematuria (throughout the urinary stream) suggests a bladder or more proximal source of bleeding.

The most common cause of gross hematuria in patients older than 50 is a bladder tumor. The presence of blood clots in the urine portends a more significant degree of bleeding and potentially more severe pathology. Amorphous clots suggest bladder and prostate bleeding, while string-like clots usually occur with upper urinary tract bleeding.

Hematuria should be distinguished from hematospermia, blood in the ejaculate, which is usually benign. Cyclic bleeding in females should raise suspicions for endometriosis involving the urinary tract. Trauma, including physical trauma, recent instrumentation (endoscope or catheter), and recent vigorous exercise should be questioned.

Factitious hematuria must be considered in patients suspected of abusing narcotics or having Münchhausen's type personality. Narcotic abusers frequently give a history of uric acid or other radiolucent stones (nonvisible on plain film radiograph), and iodine contrast allergy (unable to obtain contrast study to document obstruction). A family history of diabetes, sickle-cell disease, renal disease, polycystic kidney disease, Alport's syndrome, or urolithiasis is important, because a positive history puts progeny at risk.

Social and travel histories are important. Smoking is a leading cause of TCC. Analgesic abuse (nonsteroids) can lead to papillary necrosis and TCC. Schistosomiasis is a very common cause of hematuria and squamous-cell carcinoma of the bladder around the world, and travel to endemic areas should be explored. Many medications can cause hematuria or renal disease and a complete drug history is important (Table 11–9). Because transitional-cell carcinoma is a common cause of hematuria, risk factors for this disease should be reviewed (Table 11–6). Finally, a thorough review of systems may suggest an etiology for hematuria (Table 11–10).

Table 11–8

Key Points in the History

Gross or microscopic blood
Asymptomatic or symptomatic
Characterize symptoms
Initial, terminal, or total hematuria
Presence of blood clots
Characteristics of clots

Table 11–9

Drugs Associated with Hematuria and Urinary Tract Disease

Interstitial Nephritis	**Papillary Necrosis**	**Loin Pain Hematuria Syndrome**
Allopurinol	Nonsteroidal antiinflammatories (NSAIDs)	Oral contraceptives
Cephalosporins		
Furosemide	**Hemorrhagic Cystitis**	**TCC**
Ibuprofen/NSAIDs	Cyclophosphamide	Cyclophosphamide
Penicillins	Methicillin	
Phenobarbital	Busulfan	
Phenytoin		
Rifampin		
Sulfonamides		
Thiazides		

Physical Examination

Physical examination of the patient with hematuria is somewhat limited and nonspecific, because the majority of the urinary tract is nonvisible and not readily palpable. A flank or abdominal mass may be palpated in a thin individual with renal tumor, polycystic kidney disease, or severe hydronephrosis. A kidney distended by obstruction or inflammation will be tender to palpation or percussion. A distended bladder can be palpated suprapubically and may be tender when due to inflammation, infection, or acute urinary retention. Digital rectal examination can suggest prostate cancer, prostatitis, or benign prostatic hyperplasia. The urethral meatus should be inspected for ulcerations or caruncles. Additional components of a thorough physical and their potential associated etiologies are listed in Table 11–11.

Ancillary Tests

The basic tests available for hematuria include a kidney, ureter, and bladder (KUB) radiograph, an intravenous pyelogram (IVP), urine cytology, and cystoscopy. When a renal mass is suspected (based on physical examination), the IVP may be

Table 11–10

Review of Systems: Etiologies for Hematuria

> Recent upper respiratory tract infection: Poststreptococcal glomerulonephritis, Berger's disease
> Hemoptysis: Goodpasture's syndrome
> Weight loss: Cancer, tuberculosis, vasculitis
> Fever: Infection, cancer, vasculitis
> Joint pain: Lupus nephritis, vasculitis
> Purpura or rash: Henoch–Schönlein purpura (HSP) nephritis
> Hearing loss: Alport's syndrome

Table 11–11

Nongenitourinary Aspect of Physical Examination

> Fever: Pyelonephritis, prostatitis, vasculitis, cancer
> Hypertension: Renal parenchymal disease, renal vascular disease
> Rash and purpura: HSP nephritis, vasculitis
> Deafness: Alport's syndrome
> Arrhythmia: Renal emboli
> Heart murmur: Endocarditis
> Renal bruit: Arteriovenous fistula
> Peripheral edema: Renal parenchymal disease

replaced with a CT scan. Ultrasound should not be the initial imaging study in hematuria as it is not sensitive enough to exclude transitional-cell carcinoma, and generally is not capable of imaging the ureters. Regardless of whether the clinician images first with IVP or CT scan, other imaging studies may be indicated based on the results of the initial imaging study.

All patients with hematuria should have a basic laboratory evaluation including urinalysis, urine culture, serum chemistries, and creatinine. If the clinical situation warrants, evaluation for coagu-lopathy should be pursued, and a hemoglobin electrophoresis should be considered in blacks to rule out sickle-cell disease. Findings on urinalysis will guide further workup (Fig. 11–11). If a nephrologic or renal parenchymal disease is suspected, further laboratory testing should be pursued as indicated, along with a plain film radiograph of the abdomen (KUB) to evaluate for calcifications in the urinary tract, and a renal ultrasound to assess the renal parenchyma. A consultation with a nephrologist may be indicated to consider renal biopsy.

Figure 11–11

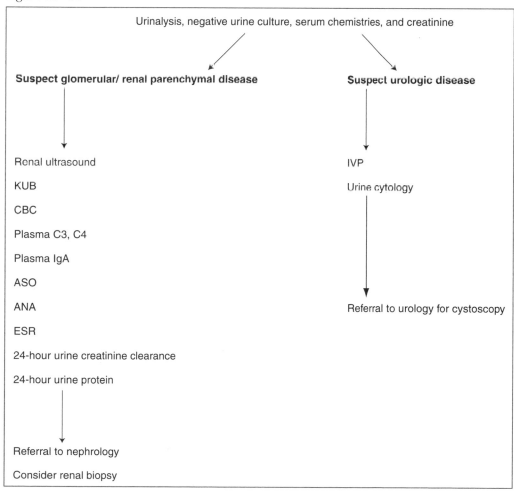

Algorithm for nephrologic and urologic evaluation.

As mentioned previously, if there is doubt as to whether the source of bleeding is glomerular (nephrologic) or epithelial (urologic), a urologic evaluation should be performed to rule out malignancy, obstruction, and urolithiasis. Following a negative evaluation, renal parenchymal disease should be investigated.

The majority of patients with hematuria will require a urologic evaluation, which is primarily anatomic. The IVP is the standard first procedure obtained, because it evaluates the renal parenchyma and upper tract urothelium. If the patient has a contraindication to intravenous iodine contrast agents, a renal ultrasound should be obtained and retrograde injection of contrast to evaluate the ureters and collecting system can be performed at the time of cystoscopy. A voided urine specimen should be sent for cytologic evaluation. Referral to a urologist is indicated for cystoscopy, because radiographs do not adequately evaluate the bladder.

Plain Film Radiograph/ Kidney-Ureter-Bladder

The primary value of the kidney, ureter, and bladder (KUB) radiograph is to detect calcifications in the urinary tract. The majority of renal calculi contain calcium and are visible on plain film radiographs. Nephrocalcinosis may suggest medullary sponge kidney, renal tubular acidosis, or hyperparathyroidism. Up to 10% of tumors of the urinary tract may have associated calcium deposits. Unusual infections of the urinary tract such as tuberculosis and schistosomiasis have characteristic calcifications.

Intravenous Pyelogram

The intravenous pyelogram (IVP) is the classic study used to evaluate the urinary tract and is the accepted and proven first step in the evaluation of hematuria when a urologic abnormality is suspected. The study is dependent on normal renal function (generally a creatinine value less than 2.0 mg% or less than 1.7 mg% in diabetics); the renal parenchyma and outlines, intrarenal collecting system, ureters, and bladder are visualized as intravenous iodine contrast is filtered and concentrated in the urinary tract. The IVP should be performed prior to cystoscopy; if visualization of the urothelium is suboptimal, retrograde studies can be performed at the time of endoscopy.

The two adverse events that might occur with intravenous iodine use are nephrotoxicity and anaphylaxis. Fortunately, nephrotoxicity is avoidable if risks are identified before the study, and anaphylaxis is very rare.

The most important risk factor for nephrotoxicity is preexisting renal insufficiency. A normal serum creatinine value should be obtained prior to ordering a study that uses intravenous iodine contrast agents. Other risk factors for renal failure are diabetes, severe congestive heart failure, and a markedly elevated serum uric acid level. Risk factors that double the risk of an anaphylactic-like reaction are a history of multiple drug allergies, shellfish and seafood allergy, and reactive airway disease. The history of a prior iodine contrast reaction is not a guarantee that anaphylaxis will recur, though it does increase that risk three to fourfold. The usual intravenous agent used for an IVP is high osmolar, ionic, iodine contrast media. In the last decade, newer agents that are nonionic and low osmolar have been developed and used extensively. These two properties only slightly decrease the risk of nephrotoxicity; however, they markedly lower (by 80%) the incidence of anaphylactic-like reactions. Unfortunately, the newer nonionic, low osmolar agents are very expensive (six to ten times the cost of routine contrast media) and their use should be limited to high-risk patients. Other options for patients at risk for anaphylaxis include utilizing studies that avoid intravenous iodine agents (ultrasound, MRI, nuclear scans, CT without contrast), or pretreatment with steroids and antihistamines prior to intravenous contrast administration.

Ultrasound

The kidney is well visualized with ultrasound. The parenchyma may be adequately assessed, most obstruction detected or ruled out, and sound waves are an excellent means to characterize a renal mass as cystic or solid. Ultrasound is portable, safe, and utilizes no ionizing radiation or intravenous contrast agent. Small renal lesions, however, may not be visualized. Renal ultrasonography is not a reliable modality to detect TCC of the urinary tract.

Computed Tomography

Renal lesions found on IVP or solid masses on ultrasound are definitively evaluated with a dedicated renal CT (scans with and without intravenous contrast, 3 to 5-mm sections). CT scan should be the imaging study of choice when a renal mass is suspected (e.g., abdominal mass on physical exam with hematuria). The CT scan provides excellent visualization of the abdominal contents and retroperitoneum. Intravenous and oral contrast agents are usually employed. Computerized tomography is more sensitive than a KUB for the presence of calcium (Fig. 11–12), and the study is an excellent staging tool for ma-

lignancies of the upper and lower urinary tract (Figs. 11–13 and 11–14).

A recent technical advance in CT is spiral or helical scanning, which allows full abdominal imaging in about 1 minute. Spiral CT scanning is becoming the preferred modality to screen for urolithiasis for flank pain or renal colic in the emergency department setting.

Magnetic Resonance Imaging

The MRI scan avoids ionizing radiation, can use non-nephrotoxic contrast agents (gadolinium), and new-generation machines and coils scan rapidly with improved resolution. At the present time, however, MRI scans have no definitive role in the routine assessment of a patient with hematuria.

Cystogram

Cystography (retrograde instillation of contrast material into the bladder) can determine bladder capacity, the presence of vesicoureteral reflux, and a voiding film will demonstrate urethral anatomy and postvoid residual volume. Unfortunately, the cystogram is inadequate to assess the bladder for small or moderate-sized tumors, and therefore has

Figure 11–12

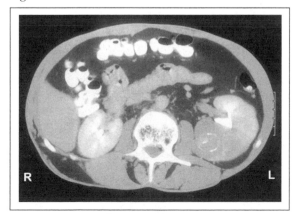

Calcified left renal-cell carcinoma.

Figure 11–13

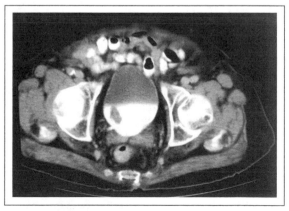

CT scan of superficial, non-invasive bladder tumor.

Figure 11–14

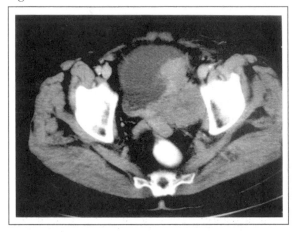

CT scan showing extensive TCC through bladder wall into adjacent pelvic structures.

no regular role in the evaluation of adults with hematuria.

Cystoscopy

Direct endoscopic visualization of the bladder epithelium is the gold standard lower urinary tract study for hematuria. The primary function of cystoscopy is to rule out TCC or carcinoma-in-situ, though visual inspection will detect all other lower urinary tract pathology. Cystoscopy is best performed following an IVP and while the patient is actually bleeding, so that the source of hematuria can be localized.

Suboptimal IVP or other upper tract study, or bloody efflux from a ureteral orifice, should prompt the urologist to perform a retrograde pyelogram during cystoscopy. Retrograde instillation of contrast directly into the ureter and collecting system under low pressure is safe in patients with significant risks for intravenous iodine contrast exposure, because the contrast agent stays in the urinary tract and does not enter the vascular system.

Cystoscopy should never be performed in the presence of acute infection, as high vesical pressures may result in dissemination of infection, pyelonephritis, or sepsis. Cystoscopy is an invasive and often uncomfortable procedure, though the routine use of flexible endoscopy has virtually eliminated the need for anesthesia and can be performed rapidly and with minimal discomfort in an office setting.

Urine Cytology

The potential to sample the entire urothelium for malignancy is accomplished with urine cytology. A voided urine specimen placed into preservative is examined microscopically by a cytologist/pathologist for malignant and benign transitional cells. Specificity exceeds 95%, though overall sensitivity is only 35% to 50%. Sensitivity increases with higher-grade tumors; the sensitivity of cytology for high-grade, poorly differentiated TCC is 70% to 100%.

Renal Biopsy

Percutaneous renal biopsy is an outpatient procedure routinely performed by nephrologists. For high-risk patients (solitary kidney, coagulopathy), open biopsy can be performed by a urologist in the operating room. Percutaneous renal biopsy is a widely used procedure, very safe in the properly selected patient, and provides definitive histologic information about renal parenchymal/glomerular disease. Biopsy is performed at the discretion of the nephrologist, and is often reserved for those patients with a negative urologic workup, significant proteinuria, and renal insufficiency.

Nuclear Renal Scans

Nuclear scans are an excellent means to assess for differential renal function and functional obstruction of the ureteropelvic junction or ureter. Renal scans may help to clarify the nature of a potential renal mass or pseudotumor, but they have a limited role in the evaluation of hematuria.

Algorithm

An algorithm for evaluating hematuria is outlined in Figure 11–11. The essential feature is to exclude urologic disease, because life-threatening diseases may be heralded early by hematuria, as mentioned. An essential feature of the algorithm is that virtually all patients with hematuria require evaluation.

Special Considerations

Trauma

Hematuria is an important nonspecific indicator of genitourinary trauma, but the degree of hematuria does not correlate with the degree of injury. Multiple studies have shown that very few significant injuries are found in patients with blunt trauma, microhematuria, and no evidence of shock; evaluation in this scenario is not mandatory. All areas of the urinary tract are susceptible to injury with penetrating or blunt trauma to the flank, abdomen, or pelvis. Renal injuries are graded on a 1 to 5 scale (Table 11–12). Depending on the overall status of the patient and associated injuries, grades 1 to 3 are usually managed conservatively. Grade 4 and 5 injuries often require surgical intervention.

Absolute indications for urologic evaluation following trauma include penetrating injury with either microscopic or gross hematuria, blunt renal trauma with gross hematuria, blunt hematuria with microhematuria and shock (systolic pressure less than 90 mm Hg), and rapid deceleration accident. Computed tomography should be performed unless the victim is unstable and requires immediate surgical exploration, in which case a one-shot IVP will suffice (2 mL intravenous contrast per kg body weight, KUB at 10 minutes).[15]

If urethral injury is suspected, a retrograde urethrogram should be performed prior to catheterization. Blood at the urethral meatus, high-riding prostate on rectal exam, inability to void, perineal or genital injury, and pelvic fracture are all associated with urethral injury. Cystography is the procedure of choice to rule out bladder injury.

Patients on Anticoagulants

The current recommended doses of anticoagulant medications do not predispose patients to hematuria. The prevalence of hematuria in patients using anticoagulants is the same as control groups, and there is no correlation between the degree of anticoagulation and incidence of microscopic hematuria.[16] Therefore, patients who develop hematuria while on anticoagulants should be evaluated for urinary tract abnormality.[17] No degree of hematuria can be attributed to anticoagulant therapy.

Severe, Acute Hematuria

The source of sudden, severe hematuria is usually the bladder and likely due to TCC, or to hemorrhagic cystitis secondary to radiation or chemotherapy effects. Immediate treatment should be insertion of a large catheter (22 to 26 Fr) and irrigation with normal saline solution via a syringe. A

Table 11–12

Grading System for Traumatic Renal Injuries

Grade 1: Renal contusion
Grade 2: Superficial (cortical) laceration
Grade 3: Deep (medullary) laceration
Grade 4: Laceration with contrast extravasation (collecting system injury) or thrombosis of a segmental renal artery
Grade 5: Renal pedicle injury or shattered kidney

three-way catheter can be placed for continuous irrigation once the blood clots have been evacuated.

Urology consultation is indicated because cystoscopy is often required to evacuate organized clots and fulgurate bleeding vessels. Once the bladder is free of clots, various intravesical solutions can be instilled to facilitate hemostasis. Uncontrollable hemorrhage may require drastic measures such as embolization of the vesical arteries, or cystectomy.

Controversial Issues

Screening

At the present time, routine screening is not recommended to detect hematuria. However, screening is feasible, inexpensive, easy, and may result in reduced morbidity and mortality of disease by way of early detection of life-threatening disorders, primarily malignancies. In unselected, community-based screening programs where patients tested themselves at home daily for 2 weeks, 20% of asymptomatic participants over age 50 years were found to have at least one positive test. Of these subjects evaluated, 8.3% were found to have a urologic cancer and 24% had other diagnoses requiring treatment (stones, stricture, obstruction, infection, nephropathy).[18] Screening programs may have a role in the overall evaluation of the asymptomatic population.

Recurrent Unexplained Hematuria

No standard evaluation is universally accepted for patients who had a completely negative evaluation and have persistent hematuria. Approximately 20% of patients who undergo thorough evaluation for hematuria will have no etiology determined. Approximately 1% to 3% with persistent microscopic hematuria will eventually be diagnosed with a urologic malignancy, while 18% with re-

current gross hematuria will have a cancer on subsequent evaluation.[4,19]

Patients with persistent microhematuria are at low risk for significant disease and can probably be followed with urinalysis, urine cytology, and renal ultrasound every 6 to 12 months until resolution or up to 3 years. Patients with recurrent gross hematuria are much more likely to harbor a malignancy and should undergo complete evaluation. In addition, patients who have a significant increase in microhematuria (>50 RBCs/hpf) or new onset of irritative voiding symptoms with negative urine cultures should be considered for complete evaluation. Unexplained recurrent hematuria in young adults should be considered for nephrologic referral and renal biopsy to rule out glomerular disease.

Minimal Evaluation for Low-Risk Patients

The risk for life-threatening disease is age dependent. The incidence of significant disease in adult females under age 40 with microscopic hematuria is very low (Table 11–13).[7] Although gross hematuria must be evaluated in all patients, some would propose minimal evaluation for women under age 40 who have microscopic hematuria and no significant risk factors for TCC (Table 11–6). Renal ultrasound and urine cytology are rapid, safe, and simple, and may screen this population with acceptable risk. Although ultrasound will miss many renal pelvic and ureteral tumors, both are rare in women under 40. Ultrasound may

Table 11–13

Microhematuria: Risk of Significant Disease by Age and Gender

Female >50 6.0%	Males >50 7.0%
Female >40 1.7%	Males >40 6.6%
All females 1.5%	All males 6.0%

Adapted from Mariani AJ, Mariani MC, Macchioni C, et al: The significance of adult hematuria: 1000 hematuria evaluations including a risk–benefit and cost-effectiveness analysis. *J Urol* 141:350, 1989.

miss some small calculi, so a KUB may be beneficial study.

This evaluation would avoid the risks, costs, and discomfort associated with IVP and cystoscopy, with little loss of accuracy. At Brooke Army Medical Center in San Antonio, Texas, 267 patients with bladder tumors were treated over a 10-year period; only 4 were under age 40 at presentation (1.5%). During the same time period, 165 renal tumors were treated; 13 patients were under age 40 (8%). The patient and health care provider must understand and accept the limitations of a partial or minimal evaluation for hematuria.

Emerging Concepts

Several new concepts may influence the way we evaluate hematuria. Rapid advances in technology, large cohort studies, accurate risk–benefit analyses, and new treatment modalities may alter the diagnosis and/or treatment regimens for urologic and nephrologic diseases.

New Scans

Rapid advances in CT and MRI technology are making these scans faster, shorter, and safer. The costs of these modalities will likely decrease in the future, and as they approach the cost of an IVP, they may become first-line imaging studies for hematuria. The current cost of nonionic, low-osmolar iodine contrast agents prohibits their use in all patients. As the relative costs of the safer agents decrease, they may be used on a routine basis in patients who require intravenous contrast.

Bladder Tumor Markers

Very recently, three bladder tumor markers were approved by the U.S. Food and Drug Administration for use in the follow-up of patients

with known TCC. The tests detect basement membrane complexes, nuclear matrix proteins, or fibrinogen degradation products in the urine. The tests are noninvasive and are performed on voided urine specimens. Some are more sensitive than urine cytology (especially for low-grade TCC), though specificity is not as good as cytology. As this type of test becomes more sensitive and specific for TCC, the tests may have applicability as a screening test or in the evaluation of hematuria in place of cystoscopy.

Commercial Cytodiagnostic Assays

Several comprehensive and refined urine cytodiagnostic assays have been reported. The assays combine multiparameter reagent strip chemical tests and enhanced cytologic and microscopic techniques to assess urine and urine sediment. The studies quantify and characterize erythrocytes, and report the presence of mucus, fibrin, crystals, bacteria, yeast, casts, WBCs, and malignant cells.[6,8] Improved techniques of urinalysis yield better cell recovery, microscopic visualization, and quantitative analysis. Turnaround time for assays is rapid, cost is reasonable, and the report generated may emphasize the likely site of origin of the hematuria.[6] Long-term follow-up and large control groups are lacking; however, this type of expanded urinalysis may play a central role in future hematuria evaluations.

Best Practice Policy Panel

A microscopic hematuria best practice policy (MHBPP) panel is currently working on a multidisciplinary report (urology, nephrology, radiology, family practice) that should be available through the American Urological Association in October 2000.[20] The MHBPP panel report will address problem definition, evaluation, follow-up, and technologies best suited for the suspected diagnosis. This consensus-based policy recommendation should assist all medical disciplines to better deal with the patient with microscopic hematuria.

Note: The author is a full-time federal employee. This work is in the public domain. The views expressed are those of the author, and are not to be construed as official or as reflecting those of the Department of Defense, the Army Medical Department or the U.S. Air Force.

References

1. Guiteras R: Special urinary symptoms. In Guiteras R (ed): *Urology. The Diseases of the Urinary Tract in Men and Women.* New York, D. Appleton, 1913, pp 277–279.
2. Rockall AG, Newman-Sanders APG, Al-Kutoubi MA, et al: Haematuria. *Postgrad Med J* 73:129, 1997.
3. Mariani AJ: The evaluation of adult hematuria: A clinical update. *AUA Update Series* 17:186, 1998.
4. Sutton JM: Evaluation of hematuria in adults. *JAMA* 263:2475, 1990.
5. Pels RJ, Bor DH, Woolhandler S, et al: Dipstick urinalysis screening of asymptomatic adults for urinary tract disorders. *JAMA* 262:1214, 1989.
6. Fracchia JA, Motta J, Miller LS, et al: Evaluation of asymptomatic microhematuria. *Urology* 46:484, 1995.
7. Mariani AJ, Mariani MC, Macchioni C, et al: The significance of adult hematuria: 1000 hematuria evaluations including a risk–benefit and cost-effectiveness analysis. *J Urol* 141:350, 1989.
8. Fracchia JA: My approach to the patient with asymptomatic microhematuria. *Contemp Urol* 9:74, 1997.
9. Bushman W, Wyker AW: Standard diagnostic considerations. In Gillenwater JY, Grayhack JT, Howards SS, Duckett JW (eds): *Adult and Pediatric Urology,* ed 3. St. Louis, Mosby YearBook, 1996, p 67.
10. Landis SH, Murray T, Bolden S, et al: Cancer statistics, 1999. *CA Cancer J Clin* 49:8, 1999.
11. Bosniak MA: The use of the Bosniak classification system for renal cysts and cystic tumors. *J Urol* 157:1852, 1997.
12. Gambrell RC, Blount BW: Exercise-induced hematuria. *Am Fam Physician* 53:905, 1996.
13. Mulhall JP, Albertsen PC: Hemospermia: Diagnosis and management. *Urology* 46:463, 1995.
14. Andres A, Praga M, Bello I, et al: Hematuria due to hypercalciuria and hyperuricosuria in adult patients. *Kidney Int* 36:96, 1989.
15. Ahn JH, Morey AF, McAninch JW: Workup and management of traumatic hematuria. *Emerg Med Clin North Am* 16:145, 1998.
16. Culclasure TF, Bray VJ, Hasbargen JA: The significance of hematuria in the anticoagulated patient. *Arch Intern Med* 154:649, 1994.
17. Van Savage JG, Fried FA: Anticoagulant associated hematuria: A prospective study. *J Urol* 153:1594, 1995.
18. Messing EM, Young TB, Hunt VB, et al: Home screening for hematuria: Results of a multi-clinic study. *J Urol* 148:289, 1992.
19. Ahmed Z, Lee J: Asymptomatic urinary abnormalities. *Med Clin North Am* 81:641, 1997.
20. Schwartz CR: Microscopic hematuria best practice policy panel meets. *AUA Health Policy Brief* 9:5, 1999.

Ian M. Thompson
Dean Troyer

Prostate Cancer Screening

How Common Is Prostate Cancer?

Prostate cancer is the most common cancer in U.S. men, both in clinical incidence (with 185,000 new cases in 1998) and in histologic prevalence.[1] The time-worn adage that "if you live long enough, you'll get it" is true for prostate cancer, but insufficiently emphasizes that it is a disease of young men as well. Sakr and associates, in a unique partnership with the Medical Examiner's officer in Detroit, has examined the prostates removed at autopsy of men below the age of 50.[2] Distressingly, he has found histopathologic evidence of prostate cancer in 34% of men in their fifth decade of life. Overall, the lifetime risk of prostate cancer is approximately 15%.

Prostate Anatomy and Histology

To understand prostate cancer, one must first examine the gland and its histology. The prostate is an epithelial gland of multiple ducts lined by epithelial cells (Fig. 12–1). The prostate forms in utero under the influence of androgens. The fetal testis secretes testosterone (T) that diffuses into the primordial prostatic cells, where it is acted upon by the enzyme 5-alpha reductase (5AR), forming dihydrotestosterone (DHT). DHT is the principal androgen in the prostate cell, having a 10 to 20-fold increased affinity for the androgen receptor (AR). It is thus DHT that leads to the development of the prostate cell.

Throughout life, androgens continue to affect the prostate. At puberty, a surge in luteinizing hormone (LH) increases androgen secretion, leading to further prostatic growth. Continued androgen exposure maintains cell proliferation throughout the remainder of life.

Figure 12–1

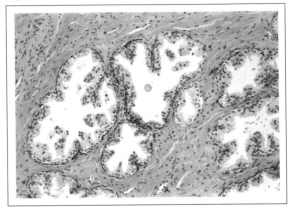

Benign prostatic hyperplasia.

Risk Factors

Two factors are critical in the development of prostate cancer: (1) an intact hormonal axis and (2) aging. With reference to the first, it is known that boys born with a deficiency of 5AR (unable to efficiently produce DHT, the primary androgen in the prostate) do not develop BPH or prostate cancer or produce PSA. With reference to the second, Fig. 12–2 shows the relationship between age and prostate cancer found at autopsy. Risk of clinical disease (disease that has been detected during life) only begins to become significant in men over the age of 50.

Other groups of men are at a higher risk of disease. Most notable are African Americans who develop the disease at a younger age, overall have a higher PSA, and are more likely to die from the disease. Potential sites of genes associated with the disease have been identified: chromosome 1 and the X chromosome. An additional risk factor may be PSA itself, as it has been clearly demonstrated that men with a PSA level below 1.0 ng/mL are at a lower risk for subsequent diagnosis of prostate cancer, while those with the

Figure 12–2

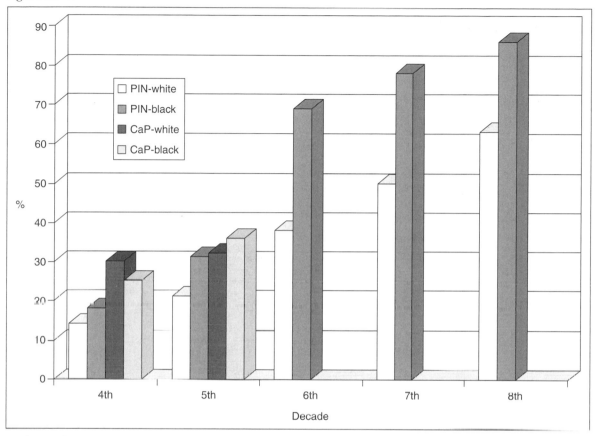

Incidence of prostate cancer at autopsy by age. PIN: prostatic intraepithelial neoplasia; CAP: prostate cancer. (Data from references 18 and 19.)

"high-normal" range (e.g., 3 to 4 ng/mL) are at a significantly higher risk.

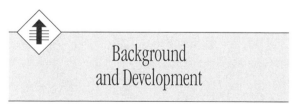

Background and Development

For reasons that are not completely clear, changes can occur over time in the prostatic epithelium. Although atypical epithelial changes are frequently seen, the lesion most commonly recognized as premalignant is high-grade prostatic intraepithelial neoplasia (PIN) (Fig. 12–3). This lesion, first noted by Bostwick and Brawer, is generally felt to be a precursor of moderately differentiated prostate cancer for several reasons: (1) 30% to 70% of patients with high-grade PIN will subsequently be proven to have prostate cancer on biopsy, (2) high-grade PIN is cytologically similar to moderately differentiated prostate cancer, (3) a number of cellular changes associated with prostate cancer are seen in high-grade PIN, and (4) high-grade PIN is found in similar frequency in men at autopsy, generally preceding prostate cancer by 5 to 10 years.[3] It is generally felt that the result of this carcinogenesis process is invasive prostate cancer.

Figure 12–3

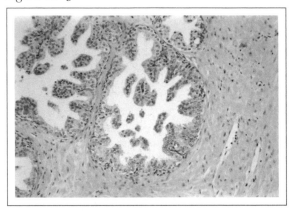

Prostatic intraepithelial neoplasia. Note the proliferation of cells with hyperchromatic nuclei and nucleoli. Despite cellular changes, lesion remains confined to the prostatic gland without stromal invasion.

Natural History

Prostate cancer follows an unpredictable course. This is not only because some indolent tumors can grow slowly but also because prostate cancer occurs most commonly in elderly men who are at risk of death due to other causes. As such, if a tumor progresses at a moderate pace but the patient dies from a myocardial infarction before the development of metastatic disease, the view of many physicians might be of a tumor best characterized as a "toothless lion." That same tumor, however, occurring in a man 5 years younger, may be not just his cause of death but the cause of considerable morbidity, anxiety, and costly and painful interventions. Perhaps the best estimates of the progression rates of untreated prostate cancer were published by Albertsen and associates, who studied 767 men with untreated prostate cancer from the Connecticut tumor registry.[4] As shown in Fig. 12–4, the risk of dying from prostate cancer is directly related to age at diagnosis, in addition to tumor grade.

Clinical Presentation

A truism of prostate cancer is that, although localized to the prostate, it is almost always asymptomatic. Although symptoms of benign prostatic hyperplasia (BPH) can be associated, they are not due to prostate cancer but to BPH and do not make a diagnosis of prostate cancer more likely. Conversely, if symptoms of prostate cancer are present, in over 95% of patients, the disease is outside the prostate and probably not curable.

Progression of Disease

Once invasive prostate cancer develops, although the duration is variable, much is known about the method of spread. Hematogenous spread is possible (and may be supported by the recognition of prostatic cells in the circulation), but most authorities suggest that lymphatic spread is the most common, with prostate cancer cells exiting the gland often via perineural spread. Although pelvic lymph node involvement was seen in 25% to 30% of patients in the early 1980s, it is seen in only about 5% of patients at this time—probably due to the phenomenon of PSA screening, detecting earlier-stage and lower-grade tumors than were detected in the past. The next most common site of metastasis is bone.

Diagnosis: Prostate Biopsy

The only method available to definitively diagnose prostate cancer is a prostate biopsy. We

Figure 12–4

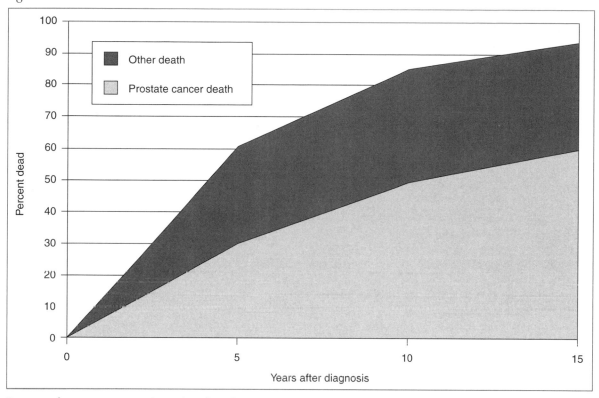

Outcome of prostate cancer patient cohort from the Connecticut tumor registry managed without treatment.

and others have demonstrated that enhanced diagnostic sensitivity can be achieved using ultrasound guidance. Modern transrectal transducers allow real-time imaging of the prostate during biopsy, assuring biopsy of any hypoechoic regions and systematic sextant (or random) biopsies in all regions of the gland. As the procedure is accomplished using an automated biopsy "gun" and a small 18G needle, it can be performed in the outpatient setting without anesthesia. Although it has been traditional to obtain 6 "cores" (biopsies) of the gland, evidence is accumulating that an additional number of cores (as many as a total of 15 to 18) will yield an additional 30% to 40% more tumors. For the patient in whom there is a high index of suspicion and in whom a prior biopsy was negative, we

frequently will perform more than 6 (e.g., 12) cores to minimize the risk of missing significant disease.

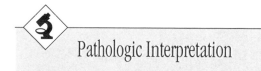

Pathologic Interpretation

Essential to the diagnosis of prostate cancer is expert pathologic interpretation. With the significant increase in the number of cases diagnosed, the majority of pathologic laboratories have considerable experience in diagnosis and grading of prostate cancer. Integral to this process is the recognition of prostatic intraepithelial neoplasia (PIN) as the most probable premalignant lesion in the prostate. Historically, the entity of low-grade PIN was recognized, but it is currently felt that this lesion is *not* associated with prostate cancer and therefore should not be acted upon. High-grade PIN (called PIN hereafter), however, is highly associated with prostate cancer. On re-biopsy of a patient whose initial biopsy shows PIN, between 30% to 50% will be found to have prostate cancer. It is for this reason that a re-biopsy is in order. To minimize the risk of sampling error, it is reasonable to perform additional biopsies (12 to 15) in this case. The patient with PIN and two negative biopsies must be monitored carefully, and a repeat biopsy will probably be necessary with further follow-up. However, PIN—at this time—is not an indication for treatment, because as many as 30% of patients with PIN will not have prostate cancer on complete examination of the prostate.

Fig. 12–5 shows a moderately differentiated prostate cancer while Fig. 12–6 shows a poorly differentiated tumor. These tumors are usually graded using the Gleason system, which assigns a score of 1 (well differentiated) to 5 (poorly differentiated) to the most common tumor pattern as well as a score of 1 to 5 for the second most common pattern. The result is a sum of 2 to 10 (1+1 to 5+5), with 2 to 4 representing a well-

Figure 12–5

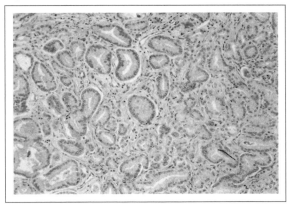

Moderately differentiated prostate cancer, Gleason grade 2+3. Malignant cells have invaded the prostatic stroma while recapitulating the glandular characteristics.

Figure 12–6

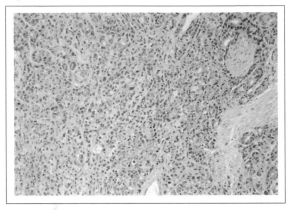

Poorly differentiated prostate cancer, Gleason grade 5+5. Sheets of malignant cells are seen throughout the section and surrounding a nerve on the top right of the figure.

differentiated tumor, 5 to 7 representing moderately differentiated disease, and 8 to 10 poorly differentiated disease. (Some authors suggest that a Gleason score of 7 should be included in poorly differentiated disease as it "behaves" more like such tumors.) This grading system is extremely useful, as the tumor grade is closely associated with biologic activity (rate of growth) and likelihood of metastases.

Staging

It is imperative to conduct a thorough evaluation of the tumor to determine if and to what degree extraglandular spread has occurred, because this information guides treatment options. In prostate cancer, although the TNM staging system is used, one can conceptualize stages into four categories: locally confined (T1 to T2NXM0), locally advanced (T3 to T4NXM0), nodal involvement (TXN1M0), and metastatic disease (TXNXM1). Staging patients can then be conceptualized simply, as can be seen in Fig. 12–7.

Figure 12–7

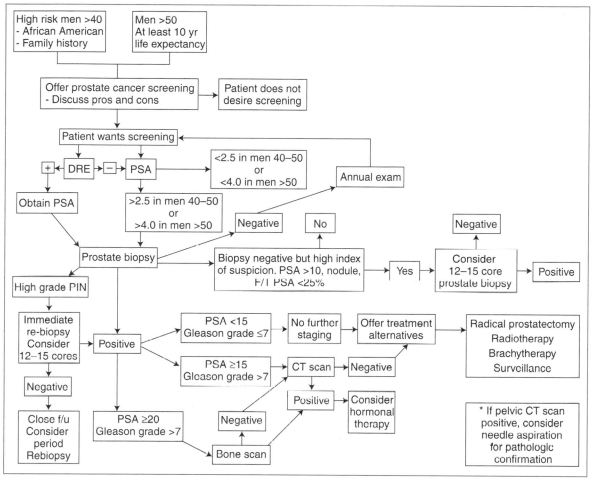

Diagnosis, staging, and therapeutic algorithm for carcinoma of the prostate. DRE: digital rectal exam; PSA: prostate specific antigen; PIN: prostatic intraepithelial neoplasia.

Staging in prostate cancer is further assisted by a number of predictors that allow the physician to tailor the testing to minimize cost and risk of false-positive examinations as well as maximize the likelihood of identifying patients with extraprostatic disease. With regard to the diagnosis of metastatic disease with bone scan, it has been determined by a number of authors that in the absence of symptoms of new-onset, continuous bone pain *or* a PSA above 20 ng/mL *or* a Gleason score of 8 or above, a bone scan is probably unnecessary, as fewer than 1% of patients will truly have metastatic disease at the time of diagnosis and the risk of false-positive scans is then far in excess of the likelihood of a true-positive scan.

There are nomograms that provide predictive values of the likelihood of positive lymph nodes. These nomograms allow subsequent determinations of the margin value of lymph node dissection for staging. In general, we do not recommend staging of pelvic lymph nodes unless the PSA level exceeds 15 ng/mL or the Gleason score is 8 or above. If staging is pursued, a CT scan is most preferable to evaluate for enlarged lymph nodes; and if they are encountered, a fine-needle aspiration is usually performed.

The optimal evaluation of local-stage prostate cancer is poorly understood. Although digital rectal examination (DRE), transrectal ultrasound (TRUS), CT, MRI, and endorectal MRI have been used, both CT and MRI have proven to be poorly associated with T3 to T4 disease. Endorectal MRI has had variable outcomes in different studies and is not generally performed due the uncertain added value and the substantial cost. DRE and TRUS have recently been compared in a head-to-head multi-institutional study. The investigators found that the performance characteristics of TRUS were no better than DRE alone. For this reason, we generally recommend using DRE alone, and any observations from TRUS performed at the time of biopsy can be used in the evaluation process.

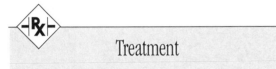

Treatment

Locally Confined Disease

Above all, treatment is tailored to the patient, his tumor, and his personal wishes and priorities. The four most commonly employed treatments for clinically locally confined prostate cancer are surveillance, radical prostatectomy, external-beam radiotherapy, and brachytherapy.

SURVEILLANCE

An option for all patients, surveillance is generally reserved for patients with limited life expectancy or with small, very well-differentiated tumors. Patients should be provided with estimates of their risk of progression without treatment. The best estimates were published by Albertsen and associates.[4] Although an advantage

of observation for patients is a lack of side effects of treatment, the risk of disease progression, especially without significant change in PSA or DRE, is a major disadvantage. Patients are generally monitored every 6 months with PSA and DRE. An increase in PSA is anticipated in all patients so they must be apprised of this in advance and a method to manage this must be understood and agreed upon in advance.

RADIATION THERAPY

External-beam radiotherapy, especially with new high-energy linear accelerators, results in excellent long-term survival of patients with locally confined disease. Survival and progression-free survival of patients with more locally advanced disease can be improved with the addition of hormonal therapy, which is generally begun before and continued during radiation therapy. Radiotherapy is generally given for a period of 6 to 7 weeks, 5 days per week. It is possible to increase the dose to the prostate using advanced targeting techniques (conformal therapy), but the effect of these increased doses on survival or progression-free survival is unknown. Outcomes of radiotherapy for localized prostate cancer are excellent, with survivals of treated patients quite similar to those of the normal population. For patients with locally advanced disease (T3 to T4), the addition of the LHRH-agonist goserelin (Zoladex) has been demonstrated to increase both disease-free as well as overall survival.[5]

The primary advantage of radiotherapy for prostate cancer is its simplicity of administration and the long track record of results. Disadvantages include the risk of local progression or recurrence (as the glandular epithelium remains in place and as there is an increasing risk of positive repeat biopsies over time), the cost, and the risk of complications. Complications are generally due to the unavoidable receipt of radiation by normal tissues including the bowel and bladder. These side effects include impotence, incontinence, cystitis, and proctitis.

BRACHYTHERAPY

The concept of placing radioactive sources directly into the prostate is not new but has had a renaissance, primarily due to the availability of perineal placement under transrectal ultrasound guidance. This procedure can be done as same day surgery. If the implanted "seeds" achieve a homogeneous dose to the prostate, it is likely that the cancer control will be similar to radiotherapy. Long-term results are not available. However, advantages are the ease of placement and relatively short duration of therapy. Disadvantages include cost, impotence, disease recurrence (in the same fashion as external radiotherapy, discussed earlier), incontinence (seen most commonly in men who have had prior resection of the prostate), and seed migration (into the bladder or the circulation, including migration to the lung). In 1998, the longest follow-up in treatment series was approaching 6 to 7 years. At 2 to 3 years of follow-up, metastasis-free survival rates of 95% to 98% have been reported.[6] Unfortunately, it is only with 10 to 15 years of follow-up that the efficacy of treatment for localized prostate cancer can be assessed. It will thus be in 2005 to 2008 that such data become available.

RADICAL PROSTATECTOMY

The oldest form of treatment for prostate cancer, radical prostatectomy has undergone many advances in the past two decades. The principle of the procedure is that if the disease is confined to the prostate and the prostate and seminal vesicles are removed, the patient should be cured. In practice, this is accomplished in the majority of patients as manifested by excellent long-term, PSA-free survival. (PSA after radical prostatectomy should be undetectable, as it is effectively only made by prostate cells.) The procedure can be performed either retropubically (through the lower abdominal wall) or perineally (through an incision between the scrotum and anus). The primary advantage of the perineal approach is a shorter hospital stay, lower risk of blood loss,

and less pain. The principal advantage of the retropubic approach is the opportunity to simultaneously sample lymph nodes during the prostatectomy. In our hands, we generally reserve retropubic prostatectomy for patients who are at the highest risk of nodal involvement while those with a less than 5% risk of nodal disease undergo perineal prostatectomy.

The primary advantage of radical prostatectomy is that it not only removes all tumor confined to the prostate and seminal vesicles but also precludes the *development* of new cancer as all epithelium has been removed. Disadvantages include the risk of impotence and incontinence as well as the more general surgical risks including bleeding and infection.

Krongrad and colleagues analyzed outcomes of radical prostatectomy among patients in the surveillance, epidemiology, and end results database (SEER).[7] For men under age 65, disease-specific survival 10 years after radical prostatectomy for patients with well or moderately differentiated tumors with negative lymph nodes and no extraprostatic spread is 97%. Extraprostatic extension reduces disease-specific survival to 85%, and the combination of positive lymph nodes and extraprostatic extension further reduces 10-year disease-specific survival to 75%. For men over age 65, these rates fall to 95%, 95%, and 82%, respectively. At 10 years of follow-up in a series of 955 men undergoing radical retropubic prostatectomy at Johns Hopkins University, the likelihood of PSA failure was 30%, the risk of distant metastasis 7%, and the likelihood of local recurrence 4%.[8] These data provide a strong argument for the ability of radical prostatectomy to provide long-term disease control in localized prostate cancer.

Lymph Node–Positive Disease

The best management of node-positive prostate cancer is unknown. However, it must be emphasized that whatever treatment is chosen, the patient must be advised that the disease is probably systemic and that the vast majority of patients treated only locally will fail in a short period of time. Options include hormonal therapy, radiotherapy, or in *very* select cases, radical prostatectomy and hormonal therapy. Certainly, the backbone of therapy is systemic, of which hormonal therapy is the most frequent choice.

Metastatic Disease

In general, as is illustrated in Figure 12–7, patients with bony metastases are best managed with hormonal therapy. Options in this case include immediate, intermittent, or deferred (wait until symptoms develop) treatment. Deferred treatment may be considered for the sexually active male without clinical symptoms and with low-volume disease. It must be recalled, however, that this group of men also has the best response to hormonal therapy.

Prevention

A number of potential opportunities to prevent prostate cancer have emerged over the past several years. Principal among these is the concept that hormonal manipulation may reduce prostate cancer risk. Both prostate cancer and benign prostatic hyperplasia require long-term androgen stimulation of the gland. In addition, in those conditions in which androgen action is reduced (e.g., intersex states such as that seen in children born with congenital 5AR deficiency), prostate cancer does not develop. Thus, it is hypothesized that reducing cumulative androgen exposure of the prostatic epithelium may reduce the risk of developing prostate cancer; such androgen manipulation may offer a unique manner to reduce prostate cancer risk. As traditional hormonal therapy (e.g., orchiectomy, LHRH-agonist therapy, or antiandrogens) is associated with significant and lifestyle-altering side effects, a more

suitable alternative is the use of a 5AR inhibitor such as finasteride. It is this hypothesis that is currently undergoing testing in the 18,884-patient prostate cancer prevention trial (PCPT). The PCPT is a 7-year randomized trial of finasteride versus placebo that is designed to determine whether finasteride administration can reduce the incidence of prostate cancer detected during the course of the study. Results are anticipated in 2004.

Other possible methods to prevent the development of prostate cancer have been suggested by two studies of antioxidants—vitamin E and selenium—tested in randomized trials that analyzed other endpoints. In the ATBC trial, conducted in Finland, male smokers were randomized in a 2 × 2 manner to alpha-tocopherol or beta-carotene. (Each man received two pills, one either alpha-tocopherol or placebo and the other either beta-carotene or placebo.) Although the study was designed to determine if alpha-tocopherol could reduce the risk of lung cancer, an unanticipated finding was a 30% reduction in prostate cancer incidence among men who received alpha-tocopherol.[9] Similar research, studying the hypothesis that selenium could reduce the risk of skin cancer, found that selenium supplementation in a population with low dietary selenium intake reduced prostate cancer risk by two-thirds.[10] Both substances may function as antioxidants, a potential explanation for these findings.

Controversies

Early Detection

A major series of discussions has ensued as a result of efforts at early detection of prostate cancer in the United States. To understand the issues, it is necessary to first describe the criteria for effective and appropriate disease screening and to examine how prostate cancer "fits" these criteria.

1. The disease must have a high prevalence.
2. The disease must be associated with either high morbidity or mortality.
3. It either must be possible to predict who will develop disease morbidity or mortality, or all patients with the disease must develop this condition.
4. There must be a test that effectively detects disease early.
5. There must be an effective treatment.
6. Screening and treatment must be accomplished at an acceptable cost.

Assessment of Criteria

Both pro-screening and con-screening groups generally concur that prostate cancer meets both criteria 1 and 2, although to different degrees. Certainly, the incidence of the disease of over 180,000 per year constitutes a significant number, but some will contend that many men with insignificant disease are diagnosed with screening. Certainly too, both groups will concur that 1 death every 13 minutes from the disease in the United States constitutes unacceptably high mortality, and the associated morbidity (pain, bleeding, renal obstruction, need for hormonal therapy, and its attendant morbidity) is deserving of prevention.

The two sides of the argument frequently enter into major disagreement relating to criterion 3. The "con" group will contend that with the increased number of biopsies, small, insignificant tumors may be detected frequently. They then point to the multiple publications that attest to the frequently indolent behavior of the disease.[11–13] Advocates of screening, however, will point out that in excess of 90% of all tumors detected are of clinical significance as manifested by the tumor volume and grade. They will frequently cite comparisons between screening-detected tumors (moderate to high grade and high volume) and

the type of tumors detected at autopsy (low grade, low volume). It appears for the comparison that the small amount of the prostate sampled during biopsy is inadequate to frequently detect such small "autopsy" tumors. Additional evidence from more contemporary studies (e.g., Albertsen and associates[4]) demonstrates compellingly that given 10 to 15 years without treatment, these tumors pose a serious threat to the patient's well-being.

An entire body of literature exists regarding the potential flaws in the application of screening for cancer. Two of these biases are potentially operational in prostate cancer screening. The first of these is *lead time bias*. Fig. 12–8 displays this concept. As prostate cancer is usually associated with no symptoms in the absence of screening, a prolonged presymptom disease period exists, and the time from diagnosis to death may be a relatively short period, let us say for example, 2 years. It is possible to diagnose the disease considerably earlier with screening. However, if local or metastatic spread has already occurred at the time of the earlier diagnosis, the patient may only appear to have a prolonged period with disease but will ultimately die of the disease at the same time as he would have without screening. In Figure 12–8, if it is assumed that the PSA-driven diagnosis was 6 years earlier, the patient's cancer survival increased from 2 to 8 years with PSA screening. However, the patient's life expectancy was not affected by screening, but he did receive treatment with its attendant costs and morbidity. This same concept would hold true for the patient who was destined *not* to die of his disease as well. In this case, treatment would lead to a prolonged disease-free interval and the patient would appear to have been cured of his disease.

Length time bias reflects the observation that screening is most likely to diagnose more slowly growing tumors. Fig. 12–9 shows this phenomenon. If we presume that prostate cancer develops and grows in an orderly fashion, then the y-axis of the figure reflects this pattern: from PIN to a small collection of tumor cells, to local invasion, to further growth in volume, to penetration of the

Figure 12–8

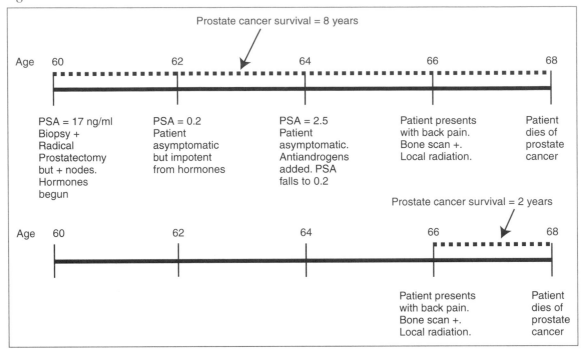

Lead time bias.

Figure 12–9

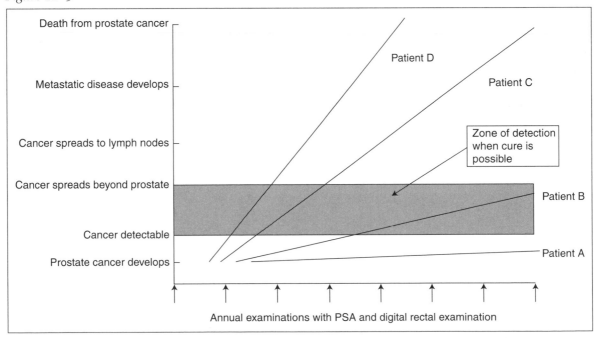

Length time bias.

prostatic capsule, to nodal spread, to metastases and subsequent death. For screening to be effective, either PSA or DRE must detect the disease before disease is outside the prostate.

If we assume that the patient is evaluated with PSA annually, there are four different scenarios whereby disease may be detected. Curve A illustrates the patient with occult, slow-growing prostate cancer who never develops an abnormal PSA or DRE and dies a natural death years later. Curve B illustrates a patient with a more rapidly growing tumor, but one that does not escape the prostate nor cause symptoms during his lifetime. However, in this man's case, annual screening detects this slow-growing tumor, treatment is initiated, and he lives the remainder of his life without disease. (For this man, treatment was successful but unnecessary.) A third patient, patient C, has a more rapidly growing tumor that if left untreated is destined to cause his death. Annual screening detects the tumor before it spreads, and after treatment, he is cured. (In this case, treatment was both necessary and successful.) The final patient, patient D, has a poorly differentiated, rapidly growing tumor. After his third visit shows a normal PSA, he returns for a fourth visit. The PSA is elevated and his tumor is detected, but staging reveals metastatic disease and the patient ultimately dies of his disease. In this particular case, treatment was necessary but unsuccessful.

As can be seen from this theoretical graph, only in patient C was screening beneficial. In both patients A and B, treatment was unnecessary, and in patient D, it was ineffective in preventing the disease. How often does theoretical patient B occur? The answer is unknown, as it is impossible to predict the natural history of the disease. However, using frequently employed definitions of "significant" and "insignificant" disease, a number of authors have estimated rates between 5% and 15%.[14] With the publication of the data of Albertsen and associates,[4] and the better understanding that the risk of prostate cancer death increases dramatically with time and with tumor grade, an insignificant tumor in a 70-year-old man

may truly be life threatening in a 50-year-old. As such, it appears that the patient B scenario is relatively uncommon. Similarly, patient D is probably uncommon as well, because with serial screening, there are few patients with metastatic disease. However, from time to time patients will present with a rapid increase in their PSA and will be found to have advanced disease.

There is some disagreement on criterion 4. On one hand, the evidence is compelling that serial screening with PSA and DRE finds significantly more tumors than with DRE alone, that this screening finds significant disease, and that the majority of tumors are organ-confined and therefore curable. However, even with serial exams, some patients will be found to have extraprostatic disease (positive surgical margins or seminal vesicle invasion) that puts them at risk of disease relapse. An additional subset of some 10% or so of patients who have pathologically organ-confined disease at radical prostatectomy (margins, capsule, seminal vesicles, and lymph nodes all negative for disease) will have a PSA recurrence (generally heralding disease recurrence) at 10 years of follow-up. Thus, the "con" screening faction will point out that the test may not be sufficiently sensitive. In rebuttal, the proponents of screening will point out that it is possible to lower the PSA threshold value (e.g., decrease the upper limit of normal of PSA from 4.0 ng/mL to 2.5 ng/mL) and thereby increase the likelihood that all tumors will be organ-confined. Unfortunately, if one does decrease the PSA threshold, it decreases the test specificity, thereby increasing the number of men without prostate cancer who have an abnormal result and therefore require biopsy.

Criterion 5 is frequently disputed for many of the same reasons. Screening advocates will point out the very low cancer mortality rates among men screened, as well as the decrease in prostate cancer deaths in the United States beginning in 1994, about 4 to 5 years after the initiation of widespread screening. Their adversaries in the "con" camp point to the high risk of secondary treatments in the Medicare population as well as the relatively high (10% to 25%) PSA failure rates after radical prostatectomy or radiotherapy.

The final issue is cost. The "con" group will often cite data to suggest that the overall cost of mounting a screening program nationwide would be between $10 and $25 billion.[15] However, using some middle-of-the-road assumptions regarding treatment efficacy, it is possible that the cost per quality-adjusted-life-year gained may be quite comparable to other commonly used prevention and wellness activities.[16]

Two major trials are currently underway to determine in a randomized, controlled, and prospective fashion whether screening for prostate cancer will improve survival. The first of these is the prostate, lung, colorectal, and ovarian cancer trial of the National Cancer Institute. This study is randomizing patients to either screening or usual clinical care using DRE and PSA for prostate cancer. A similar study is currently ongoing in the Netherlands and is solely a study of prostate cancer screening.

A much-discussed third study was reported in 1998 at a meeting of the American Society of Clinical Oncology.[17] In this study, 46,289 men were randomized in a 2:1 fashion to screening or usual community care. The authors reported at the meeting and in abstract form that a 2.7-fold advantage was noted in prostate cancer deaths in the group of screened patients. Unfortunately, a substantial number of men initially assigned to the control arm of the study were screened, and an even greater number (7,155 out of 30,956) assigned to be screened opted not to be examined. Using what is a generally accepted analysis technique (called "intent-to-treat analysis," a method to reduce the bias inherent in patient decisions after randomization is completed), prostate cancer deaths in the no-screen arm were 45 of 15,237 patients compared to 97 of 30,956 patients in the screening arm of the study, a difference that was not statistically significant. It will thus be necessary to await the results of the Netherlands and PLCO studies to have better evidence to determine the impact of prostate cancer screening on population survival.

Screening Guidelines

Although population screening for prostate cancer (with all men obtaining screening tests) is not practiced in any location in the United States, screening of individual patients is quite common. It is the generally accepted consensus that if screening is to be performed, it should begin at approximately age 50 (as cancer detection in younger men is quite uncommon), but that men at a high risk—African Americans or men with a strong family history of prostate cancer—should begin earlier, perhaps at age 40. At some later age, screening should probably be discontinued. Much discussion on this subject has not led to a definitive age, but a more flexible (or vague) time to stop screening is commonly accepted: Screening should not be offered to men when their estimated life expectancy is less than 10 years.

There is some consensus that if screening is to be performed, both a DRE and PSA should be included. Although the performance characteristics (sensitivity, specificity, positive predictive value) of PSA are much better than DRE, fully one quarter to one third of all newly diagnosed prostate tumors will *have a normal PSA.* The examining physician should be alert not just to nodules in the gland but also to subtle changes that may herald the presence of cancer such as asymmetry or induration. We generally use a diagram as shown in Fig. 12–10 to record these changes in the patient's medical chart.

A few comments are needed in relation to PSA normal values. Although an upper limit of normal of PSA of 4.0 ng/mL has served quite well, the astute clinician quickly realizes that it indicates a spectrum of risk. For example, a PSA value between 4 and 10 ng/mL indicates a prostate cancer risk of about 25%, while a PSA value greater than 10 ng/mL is associated with a 50% to 60% risk of disease. It has also been recognized that PSA rises with increasing age. As

Figure 12–10

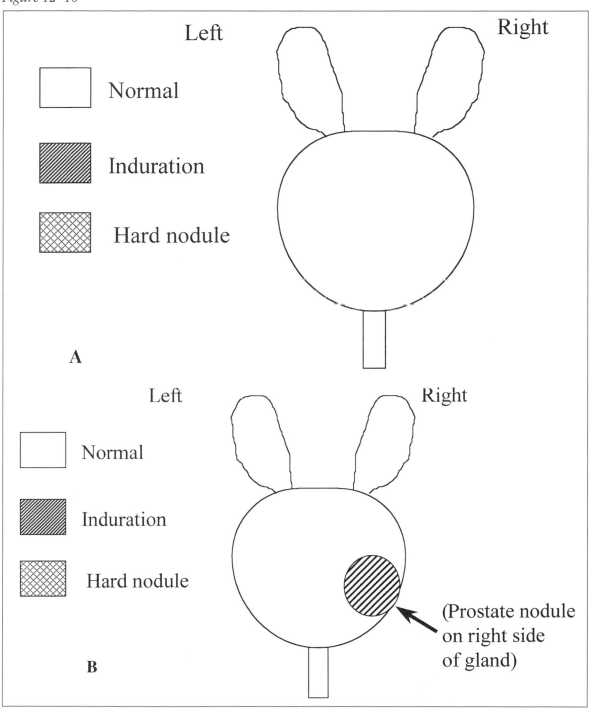

A. Digital rectal examination diagram. **B.** Digital rectal examination diagram for patient with prostate nodule.

such, although a normal PSA for a 60-year-old man may be below 4.0 ng/mL, a normal value for a 40-year-old man should be below 2.5 ng/mL. Table 12–1 displays commonly accepted age-adjusted normal values of PSA. Some authors have generally accepted these values, but we have applied them cautiously and in a manner to improve test sensitivity. As such, even for a man in his late 60s, we will be suspicious of a PSA of 4.1 ng/mL.

Recent evidence has demonstrated that PSA circulates in two primary forms in the blood: unbound (free) and complex to a variety of substances including alpha-1-antichymotripsin and other plasma proteins. For reasons that are not clear, men with prostate cancer have a lower percent of PSA in the free form. A number of studies have documented that in men with a PSA value between 4 and 10, using a cutoff of between 20% to 25% and only performing a biopsy on those men with a value less than the cutoff, a substantial number of biopsies can be avoided—thereby improving test specificity—while only slightly decreasing sensitivity. In general, as shown in Figure 12–7, we have not applied a free/total PSA ratio to men with a PSA value between 4 and 10 ng/mL initially, as doing so will certainly cause some men with disease to go unrecognized. However, if a man undergoes a prostate biopsy for a PSA level between 4 and 10 ng/mL and the biopsy is negative, before a second biopsy is contemplated it is reasonable to perform a free/total PSA test and if the value exceeds 25%, to consider observing without a repeat biopsy.

Table 12–1

Age Range	Median Value (ng/mL)	Normal Reference Range (ng/mL)
40–49	0.7	0–2.5
50–59	1.0	0–3.5
60–69	1.4	0–4.5
70–79	2.0	0–6.5

Patient Education

There are a number of resources to assist clinicians in counseling patients with regard to prostate cancer evaluation and treatment. These resources include booklets and handouts from the American Cancer Society and the American Urological Association. Especially helpful to many patients has been the *Patient's Guide* for patients with newly diagnosed prostate cancer, prepared by the American Urological Association and available from their offices. An additional excellent resource is the Physician's Data Query (or PDQ), which is available online. The PDQ statements included summaries for prostate cancer prevention, prostate cancer screening, and treatment.

Emerging Concepts

Prostate cancer research and knowledge is expanding rapidly in a wide variety of areas, thanks to the efforts in a number of sectors. In the basic sciences, new efforts are afoot to identify those genes that place individuals at a higher risk for prostate cancer and thereby to target early detection for those at the highest risk. Similar efforts are ongoing to use biologic markers to determine the risk from individual prostate cancers; as we know that some cancers are relatively indolent while others will kill the patient, we very much need to know *in the individual patient* which tumor requires treatment. Features such as p53 or bcl-2 expression have been identified as characteristics of more aggressive tumors.

In the area of prevention of prostate cancer, the field is expanding exponentially. Following close behind the prostate cancer prevention trial will be the SELECT study (selenium vitamin E chemoprevention trial), a study of alpha-tocopherol and selenium in 32,000 men. Smaller studies will be investigating the role of retinoids (vitamin A-like substances), cyclooxygenase inhibitors (similar to aspirin or NSAIDs), flavenoids (components of a number of foods), and dietary interventions.

Diet seems to play a major role in the development of prostate cancer. A number of studies have found that high-fat diets, especially those rich in animal fat, place men at a much higher risk of disease. The mechanism of action of dietary fat is unknown but may modulate prostate cancer risk in a manner similar to male hormones. Studies of healthy volunteers have found that a reduction in dietary fat reduces serum and urinary androgen levels. Additional components in fat seem to function as inhibitors of testosterone action, functioning as weak estrogens. These isoflavenoids, including genestein and daidzen, are found in a number of foods but are notably rich in soy-based products.

A number of other large clinical trials are currently ongoing and will address major issues with regard to the treatment of prostate cancer. The almost 150,000-patient PLCO (prostate, lung, colorectal, and ovarian) cancer screening study is enrolling patients into a study that randomizes them into screening or observation and is designed to answer the question whether prostate cancer screening reduces mortality from the disease. The 1000-patient PIVOT (prostatectomy intervention versus observation trial) has almost reached its halfway mark of enrolling patients into a study randomizing men with localized prostate cancer to either observation or surgery. This study is designed to determine the extent to which treatment affects survival in men with clinically localized prostate cancer. Other ongoing studies are addressing the importance of adjuvant radiotherapy for locally advanced prostate cancer and are determining the optimal method of hormonal therapy for advanced prostate cancer.

Major advances can be expected additionally in the area of new agents for the management of advanced disease. Although cytotoxic chemotherapy has been demonstrated to significantly reduce pain in men with metastatic disease, no chemotherapeutic agent has been demonstrated to improve survival. New opportunities will include the use of vaccine therapy, the introduction of genes that lead cancer cells to autodestruct (apoptosis-inducers), agents that strip the tumor's ability to recruit new blood vessels, and drugs that infect and destroy only those cells that express abnormal genes (e.g., p53).

It will be essential for all physicians who manage men over the age of 40 to pay close attention to the prostate cancer medical literature over the next decade to enable them to offer the very best of preventive and therapeutic care for diseases of prostate. It can be anticipated that not only will survival be enhanced but that we will witness improvements in quality of life as well.

Conclusions

Prostate cancer remains one of the most important tumors in U.S. males. Emerging data supports the concept that screening for prostate cancer is successful using both digital rectal examination and serum PSA. When applied to an appropriate population of men at high risk, usually due to their age and life expectancy, there is a high likelihood of diagnosis and subsequent treatment of clinically significant disease. Future randomized, phase-III studies will definitively answer the question (regarding the effect of screening on prostate cancer mortality), but it must remain the responsibility of all physicians to provide information regarding prostate cancer screening and potential benefits of early diagnosis and treatment.

References

1. Landis SH, Murray T, Bolden S, Wingo PA: Cancer statistics 1998. *CA Cancer J Clin* 48:6–29, 1998.
2. Sakr WA, Haas GP, Cassin BF, et al: The frequency of carcinoma and intraepithelial neoplasia of the prostate in young male patients. *J Urol* 150:379, 1993.

3. Sakr WA, Grignon DJ, Haas GP, et al: Age and racial distribution of prostatic intraepithelial neoplasia. *Eur Urol* 30:138–144, 1996.

4. Albertsen PC, Hanley JA, Gleason DF, Barry MJ: Competing risk analysis of men aged 55 to 74 years at diagnosis managed conservatively for clinically localized prostate cancer. *JAMA* 280:975–980, 1998.

5. Bolla M, Gonzalez D, Warde P, et al: Improved survival in patients with locally advanced prostate cancer treated with radiotherapy and goserelin. *N Engl J Med* 337:295, 1997.

6. Blasko JC, Ragde H, Luse RW, et al: Should brachytherapy be considered a therapeutic option in localized prostate cancer? *Urol Clin North Am* 23: 633–650, 1996.

7. Krongrad A, Lai H, Lai S: Survival after radical prostatectomy. *JAMA* 278:44–46, 1997.

8. Walsh PC, Partin AW, Epstein JI: Cancer control and quality of life following anatomical radical retropubic prostatectomy: Results at 10 years. *J Urol* 152:1831–1836, 1994.

9. Alpha-tocopherol, beta carotene cancer prevention study group: The effect of vitamin E and beta carotene on the incidence of lung cancer and other cancers in male smokers. *N Engl J Med* 330: 1029–1035, 1994.

10. Clark LC, Combs GF, Turnbull BW, et al: Effects of selenium supplementation for cancer prevention in patients with carcinoma of the skin. *JAMA* 276: 1957–1963, 1996.

11. Hugosson J, Aus G, Bergdahl C, Bergdahl S: Prostate cancer mortality in patients surviving more than 10 years after diagnosis. *J Urol* 154:2115–2117, 1995.

12. Whitmore WF Jr, Warner JA, Thompson IM Jr: Expectant management of localized prostate cancer. *Cancer* 67:1091–1096, 1991.

13. Adolfsson J, Steineck G, Hedlund PO: Deferred treatment of clinically localized low-grade prostate cancer: Actual 10-year and projected 15-year follow-up of the Karolinska series. *Urology* 50:722–726, 1997.

14. Dugan JA, Bostwick DG, Myers RP, et al: The definition and preoperative prediction of clinically significant prostate cancer. *JAMA* 275:288–294, 1996.

15. Lubke W, Thompson IM, Optenberg S: The economic impact of prostate cancer screening. *J Natl Cancer Inst* 86:1790, 1994.

16. Thompson IM, Optenberg SA: An overview cost–utility analysis of prostate cancer screening. *Oncology* 9(suppl):141, 1995.

17. Labrie F, Dupont A, Candas, B, et al: Decrease of prostate cancer death by screening: First data from the Quebec prospective and randomized study. *Proceedings ASCO* 17:2A, 1998.

18. Sakr WA, Haas GP, Cassin BF, et al: The frequency of carcinoma and intraepithelial neoplasia of the prostate in young male patients. *J Urol* 150:379–385, 1993.

19. Sakr WA, Grignon DJ, Haas GP, et al: Epidemiology of high grade prostatic intraepithelial neoplasia. *Pathol Res Pract* 191:838–841, 1995.

Ryan F. Paterson
S. Larry Goldenberg

Benign Prostatic Hyperplasia (BPH)

Definitions

Benign prostatic hyperplasia (BPH) is a histo-logic condition encountered in most aging men. "Prostatism" has traditionally been used to describe a constellation of symptoms attributable to BPH. However, it has become apparent that these symptoms are not specific to BPH and can occur in a multitude of lower urinary tract disorders in both men and women. These symptoms have been labeled LUTS (lower urinary tract symptoms), and consist of the irritative symptoms of dysuria, frequency, urgency, and nocturia; and the obstructive voiding symptoms of slow stream, hesitancy, intermittency, straining to void, sense of incomplete emptying, and terminal and postvoid dribbling.

Over time, BPH can progress to benign prostatic enlargement (BPE), benign prostatic obstruction (BPO), and lower urinary tract symptoms (LUTS).

Epidemiology

BPH is the most common benign neoplasm in the aging male. Growth of the prostate tissue is age dependent, with the fastest replication occurring in middle age.[1] There is little geographic or racial variation in the prevalence of BPH. Fifty percent of 50-year-olds and 80% to 90% of 80-year-olds will have a histologic diagnosis of BPH. The clinical prevalence of BPH increases from 10% in the fourth decade to approximately 40% after age 70.

Surgical treatment of BPH is the second most common operative procedure in the Medicare population, with an estimated one in every four men in the United States treated for the relief of symptomatic BPH by age 80.[2]

Etiology

Aging and androgens remain the only established etiologic factors for BPH. It is well accepted that development of BPH is an androgen-dependent process. Eunuchs and patients with congenital 5-alpha-reductase (5AR) deficiency do not develop BPH.

Growth of BPH involves a balance between cell proliferation and programmed cell death (apoptosis), with androgens both increasing cell proliferation and inhibiting apoptosis. Testosterone is converted to dihydrotestosterone (DHT) in the prostate cell by the enzyme 5AR. The DHT then binds to the androgen receptor and enters the nucleus, where the DHT–receptor complex activates DNA transcription of androgen-dependent genes.

Estrogen; growth factors such as basic fibroblast growth factor, epithelial growth factor, and transforming growth factor; and stromal–epithelial interactions also play a large part in prostate growth. These factors are currently under study.

Diets high in butter, margarine, and seed oils and low in fruit content and zinc may predispose to the development of symptomatic BPH, but it is not clear if these dietary factors are etiologic. Genetic factors currently being investigated likely play a significant role as patients with a positive family history, especially those whose relative required treatment before age 60, have at least a 50% chance of requiring therapy (autosomal dominant inheritance) in their lifetime. No association of BPH with obesity, alcohol, or vasectomy has been established, though there may be a slightly increased extent of prostate growth in nonsmokers. No association with prostate cancer has been found.[1]

Pathophysiology

BPH arises from the periurethral glands in the proximal and midprostatic urethra ("transition zone"; Fig. 13–1). The growth begins as spherical nodules composed of prostatic glands and ducts, smooth muscle (up to 40% of the enlarged prostate), and fibrous tissue whose external growth is limited by the prostatic true capsule. As these nodules coalesce to form discrete lobes, varying degrees of bladder outlet obstruction result. Smooth muscle in the bladder neck, prostate, and prostate capsule is richly innervated with alpha-adrenergic receptors, and may play a critical role in the development of LUTS, particularly in men with smaller glands.

The symptoms experienced by the patient are a result of the combination of static and dynamic factors, and the bladder's response to obstruction. Other factors that may contribute to an in-dividual's clinical profile include changes in the detrusor muscle function, urethral disease, neurologic disorders, metabolic abnormalities, and prostatic infection or infarction. The variability of symptoms that occurs with stress, cold temperatures, and sympathomimetic drugs is related to the adrenergic activity at the level of the prostate and anticholinergic activity in the bladder. The presence of infection, prostatic infarction, systemic illness, urethral disease, and neurologic lesions will all contribute to bladder outlet obstruction.

There is little correlation between the physical size of the prostate and the degree of bladder outlet obstruction. Hyperplasia of the middle lobe can result in the same degree of bladder outlet obstruction as markedly enlarged lateral lobes due to its strategic location at the bladder neck. Also, smaller glands contain a higher proportion of stroma (mostly smooth muscle with $alpha_{1a}$-adrenergic innervation), while larger glands are predominantly epithelial. Symptomatology cannot differentiate these different histologic and pathophysiologic conditions, yet the most appropriate and optimal management would differ for each situation.

The common initial complaints of nocturia, frequency, and postvoid dribbling result from the development of bladder irritability and early detrusor smooth-muscle fatigue. With ongoing obstruction, the bladder wall thickens with hypertrophy of its muscle fibers to allow generation of high-pressure voiding and compensate for the obstructed outlet. This bladder compensation may be sufficient to delay the onset of symptoms. Unrelieved obstruction, however, will result in the progression of symptoms, with eventual bladder decompensation, retention of urine, development of bladder diverticula, decreased tone and sensation, and in the most severe situation, hydroureteronephrosis and azotemia. Superimposed urinary tract infections, episodes of gross hematuria, and bladder stones are not uncommon.

Figure 13–1

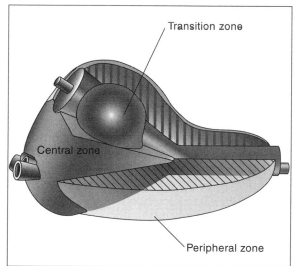

Anatomy of BPH.

Diagnosis

The initial evaluation in all patients with symptoms of prostatism should include a voiding history, physical examination, urinalysis, serum creatinine measurement, and for most cases, a serum prostate-specific antigen (PSA) test to screen for prostate cancer. Other investigations made as necessary include diagnostic imaging, cystoscopy, uroflowmetry, postvoid residual urine measurement, and pressure–flow studies.

History

The primary care clinician should ask for obstructive and irritative voiding symptoms. The typical patient initially complains of postvoid dribbling, slow urinary stream, and nocturia. As the obstruction progresses, the patient notes increasing hesitancy, daytime urinary frequency, urgency, a sense of incomplete emptying, abdominal straining to void, and urinary intermittency.

Symptom evaluation may be facilitated with the use of a semiquantitative and reasonably objective scoring system such as the International Prostate Symptom Score and Quality of Life Scale (I-PSS + QOL). This scoring system of seven items has a total score range of 0 to 35 (Table 13–1). In validation studies, almost all men with scores of 0 to 7 were not bothered more than "a little" by their symptoms and were considered the mild symptom group. Most of the men with scores from 20 to 35 were bothered a lot and were considered to have severe symptoms. All of those with scores of 8 to 19 were labeled as having moderate symptoms. The I-PSS is useful to determine disease severity, document symptom progression over time, evaluate the response to therapy, and compare the effectiveness of various interventions. The Quality of Life Scale, by quantifying the degree of bother of the symptoms to the patient, is an added tool in decision making. The I-PSS +

QOL is internally consistent (Cronbach's alpha = 0.85), reliable (test–retest correlation 0.93), and strongly correlates with the patient's global rating of symptoms.

Additional historical items of importance include episodes of urinary incontinence, urinary retention, dysuria, hematuria, urinary tract infections, stones/gravel passed in urine, and erectile/ejaculatory dysfunction.

As similar symptoms can be caused by other lower urinary tract disorders, it is important to inquire about a history of previous lower urinary tract surgery, catheterizations, urethral strictures, or risk factors for stricture disease (urethral or pelvic trauma, sexually transmitted diseases). Bladder function can be impaired by diabetes, neurologic disease, and previous pelvic surgery.

A review of the patient's medications is important, as many prescription and over-the-counter medications have anticholinergic (e.g., tricyclic antidepressants) or sympathomimetic (e.g., phenylephrine found in cold medications) side effects. Other factors that may contribute to symptoms include fluid intake (especially caffeine and aspartame), alcohol, stress, and cold temperature. For some patients, a voiding diary may help in determining the frequency and nature of their complaints.

Physical Examination

Examine the abdomen for the presence of a palpable or a percussible bladder suggesting urinary retention. Meatal stenosis and urethral masses are sometimes encountered on genital exam. A focused neurologic exam of S2,3,4 innervation (an indirect assessment of bladder innervation) should be performed. This consists of perianal sensation, anal tone, and the bulbocavernosus reflex (a gentle squeeze of the glans penis results in a reflex contraction of the anal sphincter). Inguinal hernias are often encountered in severely symptomatic men who chronically strain to void.

The digital rectal exam should determine the size, shape, symmetry, and consistency of the pros-

Table 13–1

International Prostate Symptom Score and Quality of Life Scale

TIME: DATE:

	NOT AT ALL	LESS THAN 1 TIME IN 5	LESS THAN HALF THE TIME	ABOUT HALF THE TIME	MORE THAN HALF THE TIME	ALMOST ALWAYS	YOUR SCORE
1. Incomplete emptying Over the last month, how often have you had a sensation of not emptying your bladder completely after you finish urinating?	0	1	2	3	4	5	
2. Frequency Over the last month, how often have you had to urinate again less than 2 hours after you finished urinating?	0	1	2	3	4	5	
3. Intermittency Over the last month, how often have you found you stopped and started again several times when you urinated?	0	1	2	3	4	5	
4. Urgency Over the last month, how often have you found it difficult to postpone urination?	0	1	2	3	4	5	
5. Weak stream Over the last month, how often have you had a weak urinary stream?	0	1	2	3	4	5	
6. Straining Over the last month, how often have you had to push or strain to begin urination?	0	1	2	3	4	5	

	NONE	1 TIME	2 TIMES	3 TIMES	4 TIMES	5 OR MORE TIMES	YOUR SCORE
7. Nocturia Over the last month, how many times did you most typically get up to urinate from the time you went to bed at night until the time you got up in the morning?	0	1	2	3	4	5	

Total I-PSS Score =

	DELIGHTED	PLEASED	MOSTLY SATISFIED	MIXED	MOSTLY DISSATISFIED	UNHAPPY	TERRIBLE
Quality of life due to urinary symptoms If you were to spend the rest of your life with your urinary condition just the way it is now, how would you feel about that?	0	1	2	3	4	5	6

tate. Any abnormalities warrant further investigation to exclude prostate cancer. The size of the prostate on DRE does not correlate with symptom severity, degree of urodynamic obstruction, or treatment outcome and should not be considered in deciding whether active treatment is required.[3]

Urinalysis

Urinalysis, either by dipstick or by examination of the spun urinary sediment, needs to be done to rule out microhematuria, glucosuria, and urinary tract infection. The positive predictive value of hematuria for cancer or other urologic disease ranges from 4% to 26%.[3]

Serum Creatinine

The incidence of renal insufficiency in this patient population is approximately 10% with a small percentage of patients (<2%) presenting with minimal symptoms and renal insufficiency ("silent prostatism"). An increased serum creatinine level is an indication for upper urinary tract imaging (renal ultrasound) to determine if hydronephrosis is present.

Prostate-Specific Antigen

As a screening test, the PSA test is best used in asymptomatic men younger than 72 years of age with a life expectancy greater than 10 years (please see Chapter 12). However, in a male with voiding symptoms, "case-finding" requires that serum PSA be monitored to rule out the possibility of malignancy. Abnormal findings on DRE such as asymmetry of the gland, induration, or discrete hard nodules also necessitate PSA measurement. PSA may be elevated in the presence of infection or after lower urinary tract surgery/prostate biopsy. The DRE does not have a clinically significant effect on serum PSA concentration. A biopsy (usually a transrectal

ultrasound-guided sextant biopsy) is recommended to rule out prostate cancer prior to any BPH-specific treatment.

BPH is known to elevate the PSA by 0.3 ng/mL per g tissue, and approximately 28% of men with histologically proven BPH have an elevated PSA above 4.0 ng/mL. Also, up to 20% of prostate cancer patients present with a normal PSA, highlighting the importance of combining the PSA with a DRE to maximize cancer detection.[3]

Diagnostic Imaging

There are several indications for evaluating the upper urinary tract with diagnostic imaging. Approximately one third of BPH patients will have one or more of the following indications: hematuria, urinary tract infections, renal insufficiency, history of urolithiasis, or prior genitourinary surgery.

The preferred examination is ultrasound, as it is noninvasive and has no significant adverse effects. In large screening studies of this population, 70% to 75% of exams were normal, and a change in management occurred in only a small portion (10% to 25%) of patients with abnormal imaging.

Cystoscopy

Cystoscopy is indicated for several reasons (Table 13–2). Cystoscopy may help determine the optimal technique of surgical intervention when surgery is indicated, especially with new minimally invasive treatment options.

Uroflowmetry

This optional test is commonly used as a noninvasive tool to objectively quantify the degree of bladder outlet obstruction, follow progression over time, and monitor response to therapy. Uroflowmetry requires that the patient have a full

Table 13–2

Indications for Cystoscopy

Microscopic or gross hematuria
History of urethral stricture
Risk factors for urethral stricture (prior gonorrhea, urethral trauma)
Prior recurrent urinary tract infections
Prior bladder cancer
Moderate or severe symptoms, when surgical intervention is contemplated

bladder and void into a uroflowmeter that measures the volume voided, maximum flow rate (Q_{max}), average flow rate (Q_{avg}), flow time, and voiding pattern.

Although flow measurements are useful to document the presence or absence of an impairment of the urinary stream, they cannot differentiate between obstruction and decreased bladder contractility. Uroflowmetry also cannot differentiate between causes of obstruction (e.g., BPH versus urethral stricture), and threshold values have not been established to determine the appropriateness of intervention.

Very low flow rates do not necessarily predict a poor treatment outcome and there is no minimal threshold of Q_{max} that can reliably diagnose detrusor failure or predict a poor surgical outcome. In fact, low flow rates may portend ultimate success for patients to undergo transurethral resection of the prostate (TURP), because these patients tend to notice the improved urinary flow most. Uroflow measurements do not correlate well with symptom scores.

Postvoid Residual Urine Measurement

Postvoid residual (PVR) measurement does not predict outcome. A normal PVR is less than 50 mL. Large residual volumes may predict a slightly higher failure rate in patients being treated conservatively. However, it is uncertain

what threshold volume defines a poor outcome. A high PVR does not predict bladder or renal damage, nor an increased risk of complications of BPH such as infections or bladder calculi.[3]

PVR is usually obtained using a portable ultrasound scanner, which correlates well with PVR measured by catheterization. However, PVR measurements have poor test–retest reliability and cannot be determined reliably from a single measurement. There is also intraindividual variation with this measurement, and poor correlation between PVR and symptom scores, flow rates, or urodynamic measures of obstruction. Anxiety and concurrent medications contribute to false-positive results, and abdominal straining can result in a false-negative result.

Pressure–Flow Studies

The optional, invasive, urodynamic pressure–flow study measures pressure in the bladder during voiding with recording devices placed transurethrally and transrectally. It may differentiate between patients with a low maximum flow rate (Q_{max}) secondary to bladder outlet obstruction and those whose low Q_{max} may be caused by a decompensated or neurogenic bladder. Patients with a history of neurologic diseases known to affect bladder or sphincteric function, as well as patients with normal flow rates (Q_{max} >15 mL/sec) but bothersome symptoms, should be evaluated by pressure–flow study, certainly prior to any meaningful therapeutic intervention.

The role of pressure–flow determination is not universally accepted in the evaluation of BPH or LUTS patients, and as a result there has been little standardization in the interpretation of pressure–flow plots or the determination of cutoff values for defining obstruction. In the otherwise uncomplicated situation, it appears that pressure–flow studies may slightly decrease the surgical failure rate. However, the evidence is not strong enough to mandate the universal use of this study. It is a concern that some patients who are excluded from surgery based on pressure–flow testing may actually benefit from intervention.

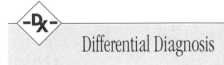

Differential Diagnosis

Lower urinary tract symptoms common to BPH may result from urethral strictures, bladder neck contractures (primary or secondary to prior prostate surgery), meatal stenosis, advanced prostate cancer, bladder stones, and bladder cancer. Urinary frequency and urgency can result from urinary tract infections, diabetes, excessive caffeine, diuretic medication, or alcohol intake.

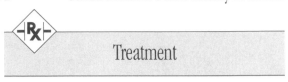

Treatment

In general, BPH is not a life-threatening disorder but one that primarily affects the patient's quality of life. The treatment of prostatism is dependent on a number of factors including the International Prostate Symptom Score and Quality of Life Scale, personal biases, sexual function, age, occupation, social situation, comorbidity, and potential adverse effects of treatment. This is the classic situation where appropriate treatment depends on the shared decision process between patient and physician (Fig. 13–2). There are only a few, but definite, absolute indications for surgical intervention, such as transurethral resection, laser

Figure 13–2

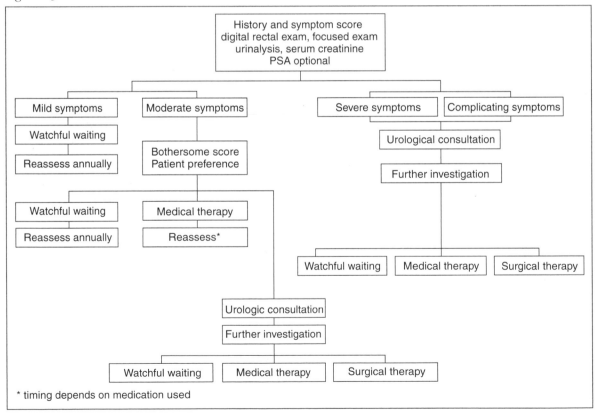

BPH treatment algorithm.

prostatectomy, minimally invasive techniques, or open prostatectomy. These are refractory urinary retention (patients who have failed medical management after urinary retention and require repeat catheter placement), recurrent urinary tract infections, recurrent gross hematuria, bladder stones, renal insufficiency, or large bladder diverticula.

Over the last decade new medications and minimally invasive procedures have been developed in an attempt to replace the TURP, considered the "gold standard" of treatment of BPH. Many of these therapies showed initial promise but failed in their reproducibility, durability, and cost-effectiveness.

Noninvasive therapies commonly used for BPH are shown in Table 13–3 and Fig. 13–3. Invasive therapies with acceptable results (reproductibility, durability, minimal adverse effects, cost-effectiveness) are shown in Table 13–4.

Table 13–3
Noninvasive Therapies for BPH

THERAPY	EXAMPLES
Watchful waiting	—
Phytotherapy	Saw palmetto
α_1-adrenergic antagonists	Terazosin
	Doxazosin
	Tamsulosin
Hormonal	Finasteride

Watchful Waiting

Voiding symptoms, particularly in patients with minimal symptoms (I-PSS ≤7), usually wax and wane over time. Symptoms may be exaggerated in cold weather or during times of physical or emo-

Figure 13–3

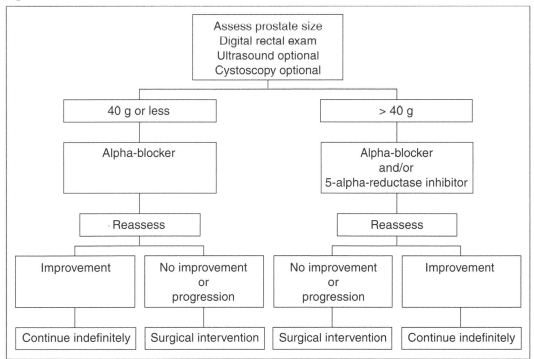

Medical therapy algorithm.

Table 13–4

Invasive Therapies for BPH

> Transurethral resection of the prostate (TURP)
> Open prostatectomy
> Transurethral electrovaporization of the prostate
> Transurethral laser prostatectomy
> Transurethral incision of the prostate
> Transurethral microwave thermotherapy
> Transurethral needle ablation

tional stress. Some patients are reassured by this knowledge alone and may feel little need for intervention. These men often benefit from dietary and lifestyle adjustments such as restricting evening fluid consumption, decreasing intake of caffeine (coffee, tea, chocolate) and artificial sweeteners, avoiding spicy or acidic foods, taking diuretics during the day rather than at night, stopping smoking, and using a timed voiding schedule. They can be monitored over time for improvement or progression using the I-PSS and QOL questionnaire.

Medical Management

PHYTOTHERAPY

Increasing interest in the use of alternative and complementary medicines has resulted in the emergence of agents such as saw palmetto (+/− zinc), African pygeum, *Serenoa repens* (sago palm), and *Hypoxis rooperi* (South African star grass). Most clinical studies of these products

have been nonrandomized, non-placebo controlled, and of short-duration follow-up. Their mode of action may result from antiandrogenic or antiestrogenic effects, inhibition of growth factors, or an antiinflammatory effect. It is possible that these agents may be powerful placebos. Nevertheless, in light of their minimal side effects, they should not be discouraged in the man with mild to moderate symptoms who declines standard drug therapy.

ALPHA-ADRENERGIC BLOCKADE

For men with bothersome symptoms impacting their activities of daily living, pharmacotherapy has become the first line of therapy. Alpha-adrenergic blockade is the most widely used approach (Table 13–5). Up to 40% of the volume of BPH is composed of smooth-muscle fibers. The bladder neck, prostatic stroma, and prostate capsule are richly innervated with $alpha_{1a}$-adrenergic receptors that are responsible for smooth-muscle contraction. Alpha-blockers relax prostatic smooth muscle and thereby decrease outflow resistance.

Currently, the long-acting $alpha_1$-selective antagonists terazosin and doxazosin, and the newer $alpha_{1a}$-selective adrenoceptor antagonist tamsulosin, are used. The long half-life of these drugs allows for once-a-day dosing. Although side effects vary, claims of superiority of one agent over another are unwarranted as there has never been a comparative, randomized clinical trial. These agents have shown statistically significant and durable improvements in symptom scores and

Table 13–5

Medication Dose and Efficacy

MEDICATION	DOSAGE	% IMPROVEMENT IN SYMPTOM SCORE	% LIKELIHOOD OF SYMPTOM IMPROVEMENT FOR ≥1 YEAR
Finasteride	5 mg	25–30	50–70
Terazosin	2–10 mg	32–44	60–85
Doxazosin	1–8 mg	15–40	60–70
Tamsulosin	0.4 mg	35–36	66

urinary flow rates without any changes in prostate volume or PSA level.

Primary care clinicians should record patient blood pressure prior to initiating therapy, because postural hypotension may occur. Most patients will sense a clinical improvement in urinary symptoms within a 2-week period. Terazosin is initially started at a dose of 1 mg at bedtime and titrated over 1 to 2-week periods to 2, 5, and 10 mg. Occasionally, the dose may be increased to 20 mg or may be administered in divided doses to allow for better tolerability. Doxazosin is similarly titrated from 1 mg to 2, 4, and 8 mg. Because of its uroselectivity, tamsulosin is administered at its optimal dose of 0.4 mg without titration, though if the patient fails to respond to the 0.4-mg dose, this can be increased to 0.8 mg. However, side effects increase substantially at this higher dose.

The major side effects of alpha-blockers relate to the cardiovascular system, particularly postural hypotension, though no clinically significant drops in blood pressure have been encountered in normotensive men (Table 13–6). Other documented adverse effects include fatigue/asthenia, dizziness, syncope, headaches, rhinitis, nasal congestion, nausea, and abnormal ejaculation (with tamsulosin).

Contraindications to alpha-blockade include a history of orthostatic hypotension (terazosin and doxazosin) and concurrent use of verapamil (terazosin).

5-ALPHA-REDUCTASE INHIBITOR

A competitive inhibitor of the enzyme, type-II 5AR blocks the reduction of serum testosterone to the more active dihydrotestosterone. As a result, intraprostatic dihydrotestosterone levels decrease by 80% to 90%, causing a reduction of prostate volume (approximately 30%), a decrease in the "static" component of bladder outlet obstruction, and an average 50% decrease in PSA. These effects may take up to 6 months to occur. Serum testosterone does not change. Finasteride is well absorbed after oral administration and is metabolized by the liver with no significant drug–drug interactions reported. The 5 mg/day dose does not require adjustment in the elderly or in the presence of renal failure.

The adverse effects of finasteride include decreased libido (4%), decreased ejaculate volume (3%), and impotence (2% to 4%). This drug should be avoided in males wishing to initiate a pregnancy due to the theoretical risk of inhibiting masculinization of a male fetus.

The best results with finasteride occur in men with large prostates (≥ 40 g), with improvements in flow rates and symptom scores that may be durable. Unfortunately, finasteride offers minimal to no advantage over placebo in the majority of patients and no advantage in combination with an alpha-blocker. The role of this agent will likely be limited to those men with large prostates who fail to respond to an initial trial of an alpha-blocker.

Surgical Treatment

Transurethral prostatic resection (TURP) remains the gold standard surgical treatment of obstructing BPH. Over the past decade, new "less-invasive" technologies have emerged in attempts to reduce

Table 13–6

Side Effects of Alpha-Adrenergic Blockers

MEDICATION	POSTURAL HYPOTENSION (%)	ASTHENIA (%)	DIZZINESS (%)	FLU SYNDROME (%)	HEADACHE (%)
Terazosin	6–8	6–10	5–10	6	6
Doxazosin	8	12	24	—	12
Tamsulosin	0	1	3	2	2

the complications of therapy while achieving similar results to TURP. Many of these have come and gone (for example, balloon dilatation). However, the following options remain potentially important in the urologist's armamentarium.

TRANSURETHRAL RESECTION OF THE PROSTATE

Transurethral resection of the prostate (TURP) is performed under a spinal or general anesthetic. A resectoscope is placed transurethrally and the obstructing lobes of the prostate are removed as chips of tissue that are submitted for pathologic analysis. At the end of the procedure a catheter is placed per urethra for 1 to 3 days with irrigation of the bladder until bleeding has stopped. The outcome for 80% to 90% of patients is excellent with marked improvements in symptoms and flow rates.

The mortality rate of 0.2% is probably no different than age-matched controls. However, the morbidity rate may be high and includes failure to void (6.5%), bleeding requiring transfusion (3.9%), clot retention (3.3%), dilutional hyponatremia (2%), capsular perforation (2%), retrograde ejaculation (50% to 95%), bladder neck contracture (1% to 2%), and urethral stricture (3%). The need for reoperation occurs in 5% to 15% of men by 10 years after the initial procedure.

OPEN PROSTATECTOMY

In men with very large glands (>100 mL volume), TURP may require a prolonged resection time and a potential increase in complications such as fluid absorption from bladder irrigation, along with bleeding and stricture. An open operation through the retropubic space is a safe, fast, and effective alternate treatment with slightly better results than TURP and a lower incidence of most long-term complications. The major disadvantages are the requirement for longer catheter drainage, increased hospitalization time, and slightly more bladder neck contractures.

ELECTROVAPORIZATION OF THE PROSTATE

This transurethral technique uses a standard resectoscope with a roller electrode to desiccate and vaporize obstructing prostate tissue. It is carried out under a spinal or general anesthetic. Results approach those achieved with TURP with fewer complications, particularly intraoperative blood loss. Most patients have their catheters removed in less than 24 hours and the procedure can be performed on an outpatient basis. This technique cannot be used if tissue is required for histologic analysis.

LASER PROSTATECTOMY

Many laser techniques have been developed to treat bladder outlet obstruction from BPH. Most notable are visual laser ablation of the prostate (VLAP) utilizing the neodymium:yttrium-aluminum-garnet (Nd:YAG) laser and the holmium laser resection/enucleation of the prostate (HoLRP). VLAP is primarily a noncontact technique that ablates tissue by coagulation necrosis and has resulted in outcomes similar to TURP, at least in the short term, with minimal complications. However, concerns over prolonged postop retention (urethral catheterization up to 2 to 4 weeks) and significant postoperative irritative voiding symptoms, as well as questionable long-term durability, have precluded widespread acceptance.

The holmium laser, which uses direct contact ablation of tissue, can be used to enucleate large lobes of the prostate. To date, this technique is the only minimally invasive option proven to approach the results of TURP, at least with follow-up to 1 year. Long-term follow-up is still lacking.

TRANSURETHRAL INCISION OF THE PROSTATE

Transurethral incision of the prostate (TUIP) remains an effective treatment for the younger patient with a small gland (<30 g), especially when bladder neck hyperplasia (median bar) is the cause of obstruction. This procedure, usually performed on an outpatient basis, involves making incisions at the 5 and 7-o'clock positions with a cutting electrode or laser fiber, across the bladder neck and prostatic urethra to the verumontanum. As the incisions are deepened, the bladder neck and prostatic urethra spring open to relieve the bladder-outlet obstruction. The results in properly selected patients are similar to TURP, with minimal complications and no difference in re-operation rates at 10 years follow-up.

TRANSURETHRAL MICROWAVE THERMOTHERAPY

Transurethral microwave thermotherapy involves the delivery of microwave frequencies to the prostate through a transurethral probe that increases intraprostatic temperatures to 45°C to 70°C. These temperatures cause coagulation necrosis and subsequent cavity formation within the prostate. A change in the alpha-adrenergic tone of the capsular smooth muscle from destruction of neuroreceptors also contributes to improved micturition. Short- and moderate-term results have shown acceptable improvements in symptom scores and flow rates with minimal morbidity. Transurethral surface cooling of the urethra prevents damage to the urothelium, but postoperative retention requiring catheterization occurs in as many as 80% of patients.

TRANSURETHRAL NEEDLE ABLATION OF THE PROSTATE

Transurethral needle ablation of the prostate utilizes interstitial radiofrequency needles guided through the urethra under cystoscopic control into the lateral lobes to cause coagulation necrosis. The obstructing tissue is heated to approximately 100°C with cavities of ≥1 cm. These cavities eventually coalesce, creating a defect in the prostate. The urethra is shielded, so the patient experiences minimal postoperative morbidity. Performed with local anesthetic and IV or oral sedation and a procedure time of 30 minutes, it is an outpatient procedure in the urologist's office. Although most studies are short term, acceptable improvements in symptom scores and flow rates

are achieved. Advantages include little pain, early return to work and activity, no retrograde ejaculation, and no sexual dysfunction. Hematuria and dysuria last less than a week, but 25% of patients develop urinary retention. At present the long-term durability remains unclear.

Summary

The *clinical* prevalence of BPH increases from 10% in the fourth decade to approximately 40% after age 70. In 25% of men over the age of 50, lower urinary tract symptoms are bothersome enough to cause the individual to seek medical or alternative therapies.

Almost 80% of men over the age of 70 have at least *histologic* evidence of BPH. Multiple factors are involved in the progression of BPH from a microscopic disease to a pathologically enlarged prostate gland. Understanding the factors for bladder outlet obstruction will help develop effective policies of prevention and treatment in the future. The mechanical or static component of bladder neck obstruction is secondary to the growth of the BPH nodules within the gland. The dynamic or neural component is related to the tone of smooth muscle in the bladder neck, prostate, and prostate capsule. Most clinicians recognize the discordance between the size of the gland and the degree of symptoms in a given individual. The variability of symptoms that occurs with stress, cold temperatures, and sympathomimetic drugs is related to the adrenergic activity at the level of the prostate as well as to anticholinergic activity in the bladder. The presence of infection, prostatic infarction, systemic illness, urethral disease, and neurologic lesions will all contribute to the often-complex picture of bladder outlet obstruction. Current selection of treatment for a given individual will depend on the severity of symptoms, objective changes in urodynamic characteristics, presence or absence of complications, comorbidity, sexual function, physician experience and biases, patient biases, and the availability and cost of less invasive devices.

References

1. Walsh PC, Retick AB, Vaughan D Jr, Wein AJ (eds): *Campbell's Urology*, ed 7. Philadelphia, Saunders, 1998.

2. Barry MJ, Fowler FJ Jr, O'Leary MP, et al: The American Urological Association symptom index for benign prostatic hyperplasia. *J Urol* 148:1549–1557, 1992.

3. McConnell JD, Barry MJ, Bruskewitz RC, et al: Benign Prostatic Hyperplasia: Diagnosis and Treatment. Clinical Practice Guideline no. 8. Agency for Healthcare Policy and Research, Public Health Service, U.S. Department of Health and Human Services, Rockville, MD, February 1994. AHC PR publication no. 94-0582.

Joseph Chin

Chapter

Scrotal Mass and Pain

How Common Is the Problem?

With the long list of differential diagnoses, it is impossible to provide a comprehensive estimate of the prevalence of scrotal masses. For certain individual disorders, however, there is documentation of their prevalence. For example, testicular torsion, which is a very painful scrotal disorder, affects 1 in 4000 males under 25 years of age. Acute epididymitis is one of the leading of causes of disability of men in the military, and in the past was one of the leading urologic diagnoses requiring hospitalization.

Inguinal hernias affect approximately 1% to 4% of the general population, and hydroceles have been found in about 6% of full-term male babies. Varicoceles are rare before puberty but affect 15% of the adult population.

The most accurate statistics are documented for testicular tumors. The annual incidence is estimated at 3 to 4.5 in 100,000 adult North American males, although recent studies suggest an increase in Northern European and North American countries. The lifelong probability of developing a testicular tumor is estimated at 0.2%. Testicular tumors in childhood comprise from 0.5% to 1% of all childhood malignancies. Of all testicular tumors, 2% are seen in children.

Thus, some of the possible diagnoses for scrotal masses are fairly common (for example, epididymitis, hydroceles), whereas others are relatively uncommon (for example, testicular tumors). The implications of many of these conditions are immense, as young men in the productive years of life are afflicted.

History

The diagnosis of problems relating to the scrotum relies heavily on careful history and physical ex-

amination, because the proper diagnosis can often be determined without the need for extensive invasive investigations. Dermatologic conditions of the scrotum can often be diagnosed on visual appearance (please see Chapter 15). Scrotal masses can often be diagnosed by history and physical examination. These masses may or may not be painful, and include hydrocele, hernia, spermatocele, varicocele, tumors, and hematocele. Two scrotal conditions that are usually painful are epididymitis/orchitis and torsion of the testis and spermatic cord (Table 14–1).

With a complaint of a scrotal mass, relevant history includes the onset and any associated signs and symptoms. The patient may have been totally asymptomatic and the abnormality noted on routine self-examination. Presence or absence of pain is an important feature. Any complaint of scrotal pain should be characterized further by clarifying whether there are any possible aggravating and relieving factors.

The important associated signs and symptoms include dysuria, hematuria, and urethral discharge. An infective cause such as epididymo-orchitis would be more likely if associated with these symptoms.

Sudden onset of severe pain would suggest possible torsion of the spermatic cord or "testicular torsion." The history of strenuous activity might be associated with a hernia. Any history of trauma should be elicited from the patient.

Constitutional signs and symptoms such as weight loss, fever, and change in energy level or appetite should also be elicited, as these symp-

Table 14–1

Scrotal Lesions

Hydrocele
Hernia
Varicocele
Hematocele
Epididymitis
Testicular torsion
Testicular tumors

toms might suggest metastatic testis tumor. Referred pain—pain originating from other organs or sites radiating to the scrotal area (e.g., kidney stones)—should be kept in mind.

Physical Examination

Physical examination should be conducted in a warm room and should include inspection and palpation of the scrotal area and inguinal region, both with the patient standing and supine. Any skin abnormality should be noted, as dermatologic conditions may be responsible for the symptom. Attention should be paid to the size of any mass, its location, and its relationship to the normal anatomic structures (testis, epididymis, and spermatic cord). Attention should also be paid to the general examination including possible lymphadenopathy in the cervical and supraclavicular area as well as abdominal examination for possible abdominal mass such as a renal tumor and retroperitoneal lymphadenopathy. Note should be made of the size, shape, and consistency of the testis on palpation. The orientation or "lie" is of importance. The contralateral testis should also be carefully examined, and comparison with the symptomatic side should be made.

Varicocele

A varicocele is the dilation of the pampiniform plexus of the spermatic veins above the testis. Varicoceles occur in up to 15% of men and are usually asymptomatic. Occasionally, however, they are painful, presumably due to venous congestion. Some patients complain of a "dragging sensation."

The typical appearance and palpatory sensation is that of a "bag of worms" on the superior aspect of the scrotum. The testis may be atrophic.

It is extremely important to examine the patient in the standing and supine positions. Although a very large varicocele may be evident in the supine position, the more subtle cases can only be elicited by having the patient stand and by increasing his intra-abdominal pressure by performing a Valsalva maneuver.

Commonly, there is valvular incompetence within the internal spermatic venous system on the left side. In contrast, on the right side, the right gonadal vein drains obliquely into the inferior vena cava. This junction itself may well serve as a "natural valve" and valvular failure causing stasis and pooling of blood is much less common in the testis area on the right side compared with the left side. Presence of a right varicocele, however, should increase the suspicion of some form of compromise or obstruction of the intra-abdominal venous drainage including retroperitoneal lymphadenopathy from lymphoma and testicular cancer. A fairly rapid development of a right varicocele may also be due to obstruction by tumor thrombus within the vena cava itself, most commonly from renal-cell carcinoma.

A varicocele may be associated with a low sperm count and has been implicated as a male factor in some cases of infertility. Atrophy of the ipsilateral testis is suggestive of an infertility problem. The proposed etiology includes endocrinopathy, abnormal efflux of adrenal metabolites, venous congestion, and unfavorable local environment for spermatogenesis because of the higher testicular temperature. It should be noted that some patients with large varicoceles have no trouble with infertility, and conversely, an infertile or subfertile male does not necessarily have a varicocele.

If the varicocele is discovered in the infertility workup, correction of the problem may result in improvement in semen analysis in approximately 60% of cases. Options include open surgical ligation of the internal spermatic veins (to decrease backflow and to decrease the venous pressure) and percutaneous venous occlusion or embolization (with gelfoam and/or metal coils). Of those patients who show an improvement in the semen analysis picture (approximately 60% of the cases), up to 60% of the couples will have success with pregnancies. Occasionally varicocele surgery may also be indicated as a result of severe discomfort, presumably from severe venous congestion in the testis. A more detailed discussion of varicocele appears in Chapter 18A.

Hematocele

Hematoceles (blood in the scrotum) usually result from trauma, often blunt trauma due to sports injuries or other physical contact. There typically is severe discomfort with an expanding mass along with ecchymosis and severe diffuse swelling plus possible bleeding from scrotal skin violation.

The main concern is testicular rupture from high-energy impact due to the injury, but rupture can be difficult to detect because the testis is often nonpalpable and obscured by hematoma formation. Attempt at transillumination is usually unsuccessful because of the presence of dark blood that may have clotted, but scrotal ultrasound is extremely helpful in making the diagnosis. Clinical progression and expansion of the scrotal swelling suggests the need for prompt surgical exploration.

In general, disruption of testicular tunica albuginea or extensive hematoma are best treated by surgical exploration. Penetrating trauma to the scrotum should be managed with surgical exploration, debridement of necrotic and nonviable tissue, and evacuation of hematoma as well as repair of the lacerated structures.

Hydrocele

A hydrocele is a collection of fluid between the visceral and parietal layers of the tunica vaginalis. The usual history is that of gradual scrotal enlargement. The cause of a hydrocele is usually "idiopathic," but may be due to an infection or inflammation as well as possible malignancy. Rapid enlargement would suggest one of these underlying causes, such as testis cancer or epididymitis.

A hydrocele usually covers the anterior surface of the testis and may extend up into the spermatic cord area. However, the examiner's fingers should still be able to reach above the swelling, as opposed to a hernia where the swelling continues up along the spermatic cord. Careful palpation of the testis and epididymis are of paramount importance, because these structures may be responsible for some significant underlying conditions.

Transillumination of the scrotal mass should be performed to assess and confirm a hydrocele by the clear nature of its fluid. A flashlight should be placed under the scrotal sac with the room lights turned off, and a pinkish glow should appear if indeed the fluid is clear. If the swelling is tense enough to preclude adequate examination of the testis and epididymis, scrotal ultrasound examination should be performed, to exclude a testis mass.

Previously, aspiration of the fluid was recommended to allow adequate palpation of the testis. However, there is a risk of bleeding and infection as well as possible tumor spillage with violation of the testis, and thus aspiration of the hydrocele for diagnostic purposes is definitely not recommended.

If the scrotal ultrasound shows an underlying condition (either testicular tumor or epididymitis), it should be treated accordingly. With an asymptomatic hydrocele that is not associated with any underlying conditions, it can be safely observed. In symptomatic cases, transcutaneous needle aspiration is usually associated with a high recurrence rate and may also be complicated by bleeding and infection, and thus is not generally recommended. Definitive treatment, if necessary, should be by open surgery.

In an infant or child, hydroceles usually have a different presentation and significance. They usually indicate patency of the processus vaginalis with communication of the scrotal sac with the peritoneal cavity. The defect is also associated with an indirect inguinal hernia. Typically the hydrocele varies in size, increasing in the later part of the day, and the parents may notice a sudden increase in tenseness of the scrotal swelling when the child cries. If the communication has not closed by 1 year of age, surgical repair is recommended.

Inguinal Hernia

Indirect inguinal hernias are among the most common scrotal masses in adults. Sometimes, a hernia may be difficult to distinguish from a hydrocele or other scrotal mass. A hernia is usually reducible, although it may be incarcerated or strangulated. Another distinguishing feature may be the presence of bowel sounds on auscultation in the hernia if there are bowel contents. However, this finding is not always reliable. The most reliable distinguishing maneuver is with the examining fingers being able to go above a hydrocele sac, but not above a hernia.

Spermatocele

A spermatocele is usually a painless spherical cystic mass that is separate from the testis and that is distinct from, but associated with, the spermatic cord or epididymis. It arises from the area between the rete testis and the head or the upper pole of the epididymis. It is filled with sperm and seminal fluid. Occasionally a spermatocele can become extremely large and can be mistaken for a hydrocele. However, hydroceles usually cover the entire testicular surface, whereas the spermatocele should be separable from the testis. A large spermatocele may also impinge on the inguinal canal; to distinguish that from a hernia, the examining fingers can pass superiorly to the spermatocele but cannot encircle a hernia. Transillumination of the spermatocele reveals whitish fluid. Surgical excision can be undertaken if the lesion has become large and causes limitation to physical activities.

Painful Scrotal Masses

The main differential diagnoses of a painful scrotal lesion are testicular torsion and epididymo-orchitis.

Testis Torsion

Torsion of the testis or spermatic cord is a painful lesion, usually with extremely abrupt onset. The patients are typically prepubescent boys or adolescents, although adults may sometimes be afflicted. The patients may have had previous torsion episodes that may have resolved spontaneously.

Often the patients are awakened from sleep or there may have been some definite precipitating event. The child may have had a similar history in the past, and he may have had spontaneous pain relief previously. However, some younger patients are unreliable in their history.

The defect is caused by congenital underdevelopment of the gubernaculum with a horizontal lie of the testis, instead of the normal vertical lie and secure anchoring of the testis towards the inferior portion of the scrotum. The resultant "free-hanging" testis suspended from a spermatic cord has a horizontal lie and a "bell-clapper" deformity. The defect is often bilateral. The testis is prone to turn on its axis, either spontaneously or with some provocation.

With torsion of the testis on the cord, there is a shortening of the cord and elevation of the testis. Initially the venous blood flow is obstructed, and with ongoing arterial inflow, the testis becomes congested and engorged, and hard in consistency. As the situation progresses, arterial flow is eventually impaired. Testicular infarction results if the torsion is not corrected and blood flow reestablished within 6 to 8 hours.

On examination the patient is usually in a fair amount of distress, with a "high-riding" or retracted testis that is very firm. It usually has an unusual "lie" as described previously. The contralateral testis should be examined, and typically will have a rather mobile transverse lie as well.

The pain may be accentuated by lifting the testis up above the symphysis, as this may aggravate the "kinking" of the spermatic cord. This so-called Prehn's sign, however, is not reliable. In contrast, the presence of the cremasteric reflex more reliably indicates that there is *no* torsion.

The diagnostic challenge with a painful testis is to distinguish between testicular torsion and epididymitis. Distinguishing clinical signs and symptoms are discussed in the next section. Further, a testicular tumor, because of its "unbalanced" configuration, is more prone to testicular torsion, and that fact should be kept in mind when therapy is being planned.

If testicular torsion is suspected based on the clinical presentation, urgent exploration and correction of the torsion are imperative. No diagnostic studies are necessary. Testis viability is significantly decreased with greater than 6 to 8 hours of ischemia. Thus, it is imperative that once the diagnosis is suspected that surgical exploration be expedited.

In equivocal cases where the primary care clinician doubts that torsion is present, but wants to exclude the diagnosis, some form of imaging (scrotal colored Doppler ultrasound or nuclear scan, if available) would be recommended. If confirmatory imaging studies are not available in such doubtful cases, surgical exploration is indicated to salvage the testicle, which otherwise might be lost if an erroneous diagnosis of epididymitis were made.

In the case of torsion, one may attempt manual detorsion prior to formal surgical exploration. With the patient supine and the examiner standing on the patient's right side facing the patient's head, the left testis should be manually turned clockwise while the right testis is turned counterclockwise.

Often, however, the patient is in severe distress with exquisite pain, rendering the attempt at manual detorsion inadvisable or impossible. Even with successful detorsion, the patient needs to be treated definitively at some point with formal orchiopexy to prevent future recurrences. The contralateral testis should be surgically fixed because there is an increased likelihood of torsion on the contralateral testis.

Epididymo-orchitis and Epididymitis

Epididymitis and orchitis are painful, and the main challenge is to distinguish them from testicular torsion. The history is extremely helpful in making this distinction. Age is one important factor. In epididymo-orchitis there is usually a bimodal distribution, with sexually active young men as one group and older men with prostatic urinary obstruction as the other. In contrast, torsion more commonly occurs in adolescence. However, there is overlap between the age distributions of the two entities.

Epididymitis usually causes pain with a more gradual onset, and often with no clear precipitating events. However, history of timing of onset can be notoriously unreliable, especially in younger individuals.

Patients with epididymitis are often sexually active, and sexual history including details of possible sexually transmitted diseases should be sought. In epididymitis, there may be associated urinary tract symptoms including dysuria, frequency, and possibly urethral discharge, fevers, and chills.

On examination there may be a variable degree of swelling in the scrotal area. The epididymis may be clearly palpable as a separate structure from the testicle, with induration and severe tenderness in the upper or lower pole. The testis itself may be palpable separately and is nontender, and there may be a reactive hydrocele.

In more severe cases, the epididymis may be extremely swollen to the point of almost obscuring the testicle with the whole testis and epididymis complex exquisitely tender. Most often, one can still differentiate the most tender area in the lower pole, and less commonly in the upper pole. In torsion, by contrast, tenderness is often in the center portion of the testis. In torsion, the testis also has a "rock hard" consistency and has a horizontal lie.

Urinalysis (for leukocytes and bacteria) and smear of urethral discharge are useful diagnostically, because evidence of infection suggests epididymitis. If one cannot clinically differentiate with reasonable certainty whether the problem is epididymitis or testicular torsion, open surgical exploration should be considered. If epididymitis seems more likely, however, and the clinician wants confirmation that torsion is not present, then Doppler scrotal ultrasound is useful in establishing the diagnosis. In testicular torsion, there should be no flow in the affected testis compared to the normal testis. In epididymo-orchitis, there is hyperemia from inflammation and high flow should be detected. One should be aware that occasionally in the delayed torsion phase, there may be reactive hyperemia that might be detected as increased blood flow, and this could be a source of error. Nuclear scintigraphy of the scrotal area is an alternative in assessing the blood flow of the scrotum, although this is more cumbersome and labor intensive and is possibly somewhat less accurate than scrotal Doppler ultrasound for this purpose.

Because testicular torsion is a genuine urologic emergency, definitive treatment is imperative within 6 to 8 hours from the onset of pain. In the case where one cannot be certain based on clinical grounds whether it is torsion or epididymitis, one should assume and treat for torsion. The patient should undergo exploration of the testis with correction of the torsion on an emergency basis.

If one is certain that the diagnosis is epididymitis, the recommended treatment includes antibiotics and bedrest with icepacks applied to the scrotum and avoidance of strenuous physical activities. The choice of antibiotic depends on the likely organism. For epididymitis associated with urinary tract infections (or at least, the presence of leukocytes and bacteria in the urine), a broad-spectrum antibacterial agent such as sulfonamide

(trimethoprim-sulfamethoxasole) may be used. Alternatively, in more severe cases, a quinolone should be the first choice. With severe infection, intravenous antibiotics (for example, aminoglycoside) are recommended along with strict bedrest. For the younger sexually active patient, where sexually transmitted urethritis is the likely causative factor with organisms such as *Neisseria gonorrhoeae* or *Chlamydia trachomatis,* the patients should be treated with single-dose parenteral ceftriaxone followed by oral tetracycline for a few weeks.

The patient should be warned that one of the most serious consequences may be scrotal abscess leading to loss of the testis, especially if he maintains or prematurely returns to strenuous physical activities. Oral antibiotic therapy should be maintained for a minimum of 3 weeks.

Torsion of Testicular Appendages

One other less common painful lesion is torsion of one of the appendages of the testis or the epididymis. The vestigial remnants of both Wolffian and Müllerian ducts may suddenly infarct with torsion. These structures include the appendix testis (hydatid of Morgagni), appendix epididymis, and paradidymis. In a child who presents with sudden testicular pain, this condition should be kept in mind along with torsion of the testis and epididymitis. On physical examination these lesions have a discrete tenderness, and typically in a younger child who has fairly thin skin a "blue dot" can be seen underneath the scrotal skin from the hemorrhage and vascular engorgement of the lesion. The blue dot sign is reliable as a diagnostic criterion. Often, as inflammation progresses, the blue dot sign is not present, and the entire testis is tender to palpation, mimicking testis torsion. Torsion of a testicular appendage can often be treated conservatively with analgesics but may require several days of analgesics. If the clinician is not certain of the diagnosis, then surgical exploration is mandatory to ensure that testicular torsion has not been missed. If at surgical exploration one of the appendages has been found to be in-farcted, these can be managed by simple excision of the small lesion.

Neoplasms

Testicular Tumors

The diagnosis that has the most important clinical consequence is that of a testicular cancer. This comprises only 1% of all malignancies in males, but because it affects primarily young men in their prime of life, the impact on human productivity is disproportionally immense. The peak age is between 20 and 35. Testicular cancers are, in fact, the second most common form of malignancy in men at that age group (second to lymphoma).

GERM-CELL TUMORS

The most common form of testicular cancer is germ-cell tumor, which accounts for 90% to 95% of all testis tumors; non-germ-cell tumors account for 5% to 10%. Germ-cell tumors can be broadly subdivided into seminomas and nonseminomas (Table 14–2). The most common predisposing factor for germ-cell tumors is cryptorchidism. Other predisposing factors include dysgenesis of the testis, which usually presents clinically as a

Table 14–2

Germ-Cell Tumors: Relative Frequency

GERM-CELL TUMOR HISTOLOGY	RELATIVE FREQUENCY (%)
Seminoma	40
Nonseminomatous germ-cell tumors	60
Embryonal	20–25
Teratocarcinoma	25–30
Teratoma	5–10
Choriocarcinoma	1

small atrophic testis and maternal exposure to es-trogens during pregnancy. A history of a testicu-lar tumor on the contralateral testis is associated with a higher incidence of testicular cancer in the remaining testis. There is no evidence to support trauma or infection as causal factors in testicular cancers. Not infrequently, young men discover a testicular mass after they have suffered some form of trauma to the genitalia area, which eventually leads to a diagnosis of testicular tumor. However, the trauma itself is not the cause but has simply drawn attention to the testis itself.

CLINICAL PRESENTATION   The most common pre-sentation is an asymptomatic painless testicular mass discovered by the patient or sexual partner. Occasionally, however, a testis tumor may pre-sent as acute pain from intratesticular hemorrhage or from torsion.

Occasionally the initial presentation is a mani-festation of metastatic disease. The first echelon of lymph node involvement from testicular cancer is the retroperitoneal periaortic and pericaval area at the level of the renal hilium (L1 level). The first sign of lymph node involvement is, therefore, often retroperitoneal lymph node enlargement. Subsequent spread in the lymphatic system in-cludes lymph nodes along the great vessels, either cephalad or caudally, as well as iliac, mediastinal, supraclavicular, and cervical nodes. The cancer also disseminates hematogenously and commonly involves the lungs. Less commonly, other organs such as liver and brain are involved.

Thus, patients who present first with metasta-tic disease may have pulmonary symptoms and signs such as dyspnea (from malignant pleural effusion and extensive lung parenchymal in-volvement), hemoptysis, cough, or an abnormal chest x-ray with lung lesions ("cannonballs"). The patients may also present with a large pal-pable abdominal mass from retroperitoneal lym-phadenopathy.

PHYSICAL EXAMINATION   The most common physi-cal finding on examination is a hard, painless, ir-regular mass felt within the testis. Both testes should be examined carefully, keeping in mind potential ectopic locations. In the presence of a hydrocele, which precludes adequate examination of the testis, scrotal ultrasound examination should be performed rather than needle aspiration of the fluid collection. Areas of potential lymphadenopathy should be examined along with the chest and abdomen.

INVESTIGATIONS Initial investigations should include baseline blood serum markers (alphafetoprotein and beta human chorionic gonadotropins). Elevation of these markers would strongly suggest a diagnosis of a germ-cell tumor. However, a significant proportion of men with germ-cell tumors will have normal markers, which naturally does not preclude the possibility of a germ-cell tumor, because in general seminomas are not associated with an elevation of alpha-fetoprotein. Serum markers are invaluable for monitoring the progress and the course of disease and response to treatment. Other useful markers for following progress include lactate dehydrogenase (LDH), placental alkaline phosphatase, and gamma glutamyltranspeptidase. The chest x-ray is included in the initial evaluation.

MANAGEMENT Any suspicious testicular masses should be explored through a high inguinal incision to control the spermatic cord early on in the procedure to minimize possible dissemination of tumor cells. Radical orchiectomy involves dividing the spermatic cord high at the internal inguinal ring area. Subsequent management is determined by (1) tumor cell type and (2) stage of disease. Detailed discussion of the treatment options for the various stages is beyond the scope of this chapter.

PROGNOSIS The prognosis for germ-cell tumors is very favorable, with expected survival of 99% for tumors confined to the testis, 95% for tumors that have metastasized to the retroperitoneal lymph nodes, and 75% to 80% for high-spread distant metastatic disease. The patients are young and can withstand vigorous aggressive therapy. The main challenge facing the physician is to mini-

mize the treatment-related morbidity while maintaining the efficacy of treatment.

An important point for clinicians is that many young men with a testis tumor may not be compliant. A clinical scenario seen occasionally is the young man with a painless testis mass discovered on physical examination who is permitted to come back later for follow-up or for scheduled radical orchiectomy. Unfortunately, some young men deny they have a life-threatening lesion, and are reluctant to undergo orchiectomy. Because germ-cell tumors grow rapidly, these men often return with higher-stage disease than had they been treated with radical orchiectomy as soon as the mass was discovered. Cure rates for localized disease are excellent. Morbidity and mortality increase for metastatic disease. Thus, any man with a testis mass should undergo prompt radical orchiectomy.

NON-GERM-CELL TUMORS

Non-germ-cell tumors constitute 5% to 10% of adult testicular tumors. Excluding germ-cell tumors, the most common tumor found in the testis is lymphoma, either as a primary extranodal tumor or as a manifestation of widespread lymphoma. Lymphoma is the most common testis tumor in men over 50 years of age. Malignant infiltration by leukemia should also be kept in mind, although the diagnosis should be evident from the history of such malignancies. As a "sanctuary site" due to the "blood–testicular barrier," patients with lymphoma or leukemia may harbor residual malignant cells in the testis even after demonstrating response to systemic treatment in other sites. Other secondary testis tumors include reticuloendothelial tumors and metastases from other solid malignancies such as the prostate, lung, gastrointestinal tract, kidney, adrenal gland, and melanoma.

Uncommon primary testis tumors of non-germ-cell origin include Leydig-cell tumors and Sertoli-cell tumors. They present as intratesticular lesions usually without manifestations of metastatic disease. Leydig-cell tumors in adults may be associated with endocrine manifestations. A triad of precocious puberty, testicular mass, and elevated plasma 17-ketosteroid levels is highly diagnostic of a Leydig-cell tumor. Some manifestations include accelerated somatic growth, gynecomastia, more advanced bone age, and penile enlargement. Radical orchiectomy suffices. Sertoli-cell tumors, in contrast, are rare and do not have endocrine manifestations.

TESTICULAR TUMORS IN CHILDREN

Testicular tumors in children comprise only 1% of childhood tumors. The majority occur in children under 2 1/2 years of age. The majority (60% to 70%) are germ-cell tumors, but stromal tumors, gonadoblastoma, leukemia, and lymphoma infiltrates and stromal tissue tumors make up a high percentage. Choriocarcinoma has not been reported in children. Leydig-cell tumors are relatively common, and children usually present with precocious puberty and gynecomastia; these features when associated with a testicular mass should lead to the diagnosis. Radical orchiectomy is the preferred treatment. In more advanced cases, chemotherapy, radiation, and retroperitoneal lymph node dissection are also done.

Paratesticular Tumors

A solid nontender mass in the epididymis suggests a neoplastic process when epididymitis has been ruled out.

Adenomatoid Tumors

Adenomatoid tumors are the most common paratesticular tumor, usually affecting the lower pole of the epididymis. They are most prevalent in ages 30 to 40 and are solid, smooth, spheroid masses that are usually asymptomatic. Confirmation of the epididymal location can be made on ultrasound examination. Treatment is by local excision (epididymectomy). These tumors are histologically benign. If the diagnosis is uncertain, exploration and radical orchiectomy would be indicated.

Papillary Cystadenoma

Another epididymal tumor is papillary cystadenoma. This is associated with Von Hippel–Lindau syndrome, a condition where patients commonly have renal-cell carcinomas and some have pheochromocytomas. It is important to recognize this association. The actual cystadenoma in the epididymis has a benign and indolent course.

Sarcomas

Paratesticular sarcomas sometimes occur, and these include rhabdomyosarcomas, fibrosarcomas, leiomyosarcoma, and liposarcomas. In children, rhabdomyosarcomas are the most common. In older individuals, benign lipomas are the most common. Inguinal exploration and excision are the preferred management.

Referred Scrotal Pain

Patients with renal colic may have pain radiating into the scrotal area. A careful history and physical examination revealing no scrotal or testicular pathology should suggest the diagnosis with referred pain to the genitalia. Occasionally, irritation or entrapment of nerves such as the genitofemoral nerve and ilioinguinal nerve will present as pain or irritation in the scrotal area. The correct diagnosis requires a high index of suspicion and exclusion of all scrotal pathology.

Algorithm

Algorithms for scrotal pain and scrotal masses are shown in Figs. 14–1 to 14–3. Figure 14–1 shows how the clinician must assume testis torsion is present in the setting of scrotal pain when torsion

Figure 14–1

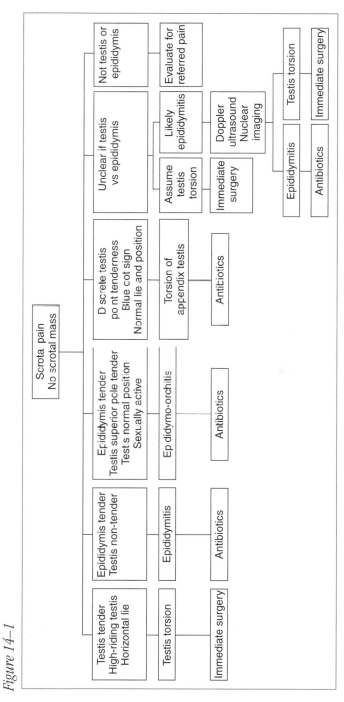

Algorithm for scrotal pain.

Figure 14-2

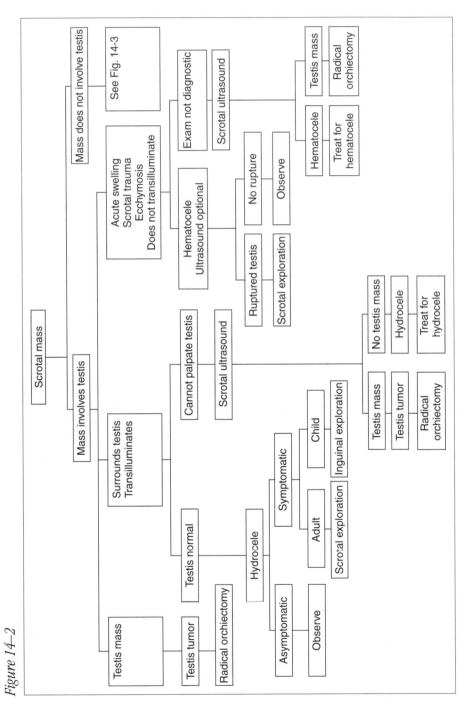

Algorithm for scrotal mass involving testis.

Figure 14–3

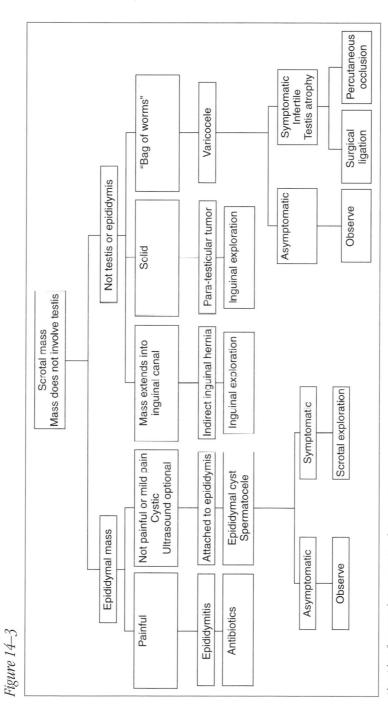

Algorithm for scrotal mass not involving testis.

cannot be excluded. Figure 14–2 shows how the clinician must assume a testis tumor is present in the setting of a testis mass, unless the mass can be clearly demonstrated to be entirely from either a hydrocele or a hematocele.

References

Berger, RE: Sexually transmitted diseases: The classic diseases. In Walsh, Retik, Vaughan, Wein (eds): *Campbell's Urology,* ed 7. Philadelphia, Saunders, 1998.

Berger RE, Kessler D, Holmes KK: The etiology and manifestations of epididymitis in young men: Correlation with sexual orientation: *J Infect Dis* 155:1341, 1987.

Bomalaski DM, Garver K, Bloom DA: Assessment of testicular torsion. In Resnick M (ed): *Topics in Clinical Urology: New Diagnostic Tests.* New York, Igaku-Shoin Medical Publishers, 1995.

Caesar RE, Caplan GW: Incidence of the valve clapper deformity in an autopsy series. *Urology* 44:114–116, 1994.

Campbell HE: The incidence of malignant growth of the undescended testicle: A reply and re-evaluation. *Urology* 81:664, 1959.

Dresner M: Torsed appendage: Blue dot sign. *Urology* 1:63–64, 1973.

Mostafi FK: Testicular tumors: Epidemiologic, etiologic and pathologic features. *Cancer* 32:1186, 1973.

Dirk M. Elston
Richard Laws
Joseph Wilde
George Keough

Chapter
15

Genital Skin Rash

Penile Lesions

Lichen Sclerosus et Atrophicus

Lichen sclerosus (balanitis xerotica obliterans) is a chronic, progressive, sclerosing, inflammatory dermatosis of unclear etiology.[1] Many cases go unreported, and its prevalence is probably much greater than Wallace's[2] estimate of 1 in 300 to 1 in 1000.[3] Lichen sclerosus (LS) may occur on any area of the body; however, the majority of reported cases involve the genitalia.

LS of the penis begins as discrete, single or multiple erythematous macules or papules that progress with coalescence to atrophic or sclerotic white, ivory, or bluish plaques (Fig. 15–1).[1] Lesions will most commonly involve the glans and prepuce, although the frenulum, urethral meatus, fossa navicularis, penile shaft, and perianal area may be involved.[4,5] Erosions, fissures, bullae, telangectases, atrophy, and petechiae of the glans may also occur (Fig. 15–2). With disease progression, the prepuce may become adherent to the glans. Phimosis is common (Fig. 15–3). Stenosis of the urethral meatus may occur.[6,7] Associated signs and symptoms include pruritus, paresthesia, painful erection, dysuria, and urethritis. There have

Figure 15–2

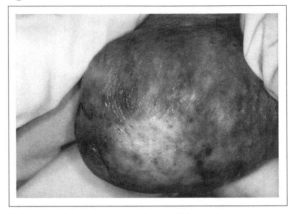

Deformity of the glans secondary to lichen sclerosus. (See also color plates.)

been rare reports of squamous cell carcinoma arising in male genital LS.

Although the etiology of genital LS is unknown, there has been no shortage of theories regarding its pathogenesis.[1] An androgen deficiency has been postulated, but there is generally little therapeutic response to topical testosterone. Recently, the presence of human papilloma virus has been detected in some cases of childhood penile lichen sclerosus.[8]

Treatment of male genital LS may be challenging. When involvement is limited to the prepuce,

Figure 15–1

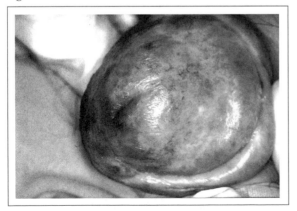

Lichen sclerosus. (See also color plates.)

Figure 15–3

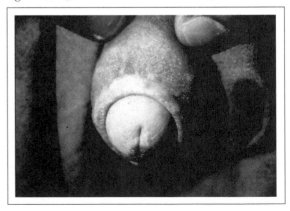

Phimosis secondary to lichen sclerosus.

therapeutic circumcision is often successful. Most patients with genital lichen sclerosus respond well to moderate-strength or potent topical corticosteroids (Table 15–1). Refractory cases generally respond to ultrapotent topical corticosteroids. Atrophy is a potential complication of topical corticosteroid therapy, but the disease process itself commonly results in marked atrophy, and properly used corticosteroid therapy can reverse much of the atrophy caused by the disease. Fluorinated topical corticosteroids should be applied daily for no longer than 2 weeks to avoid tissue atrophy and other steroid side effects. Close monitoring for atrophy and therapeutic response is essential. With appropriate monitoring, pulse application of a potent or ultrapotent corticosteroid on weekends often proves suitable for long-term therapy. Other treatment modalities include intralesional corticosteroids, oral retinoids, and laser therapy.[3]

Papulosquamous Disorders

PSORIASIS

Genital psoriasis usually presents as a chronic red scaly patch on the glans penis (Fig. 15–4). Patients may also have psoriatic plaques on the elbows, knees, scalp, or cleft of the buttocks. Nail pitting may be present. The lesions generally respond to a mild or mid-strength topical steroid such as desonide. Some patients benefit from the addition of a topical antifungal such as clotrimazole cream applied bid.

LICHEN PLANUS

The appearance of genital lichen planus differs in circumcised and uncircumcised patients. Uncircumcised patients are more likely to pre-

Table 15–1

Ranking of Commonly Used Topical Steroid Creams and Ointments by Potency (applied once or twice daily)

Ultrapotent
Betamethasone dipropionate ointment
Clobetasol propionate cream and ointment
Diflorasone diacetate ointment
Halobetasol propionate cream and ointment

Very Potent
Amcinonide ointment
Halcinonide cream
Fluocinonide cream and ointment
Mometasone ointment

Potent
Desoximetasone cream
Diflorasone cream
Fluticasone propionate ointment
Triamcinolone acetonide ointment

Moderately Potent
Flucinolone acetonide cream and ointment
Hydrocortisone butyrate cream
Hydrocortisone valerate cream and ointment
Mometasone cream
Triamcinolone acetonide cream

Mild
Aclometasone dipropionate cream and ointment
Desonide cream and ointment

Very Mild
Hydrocortisone

Figure 15–4

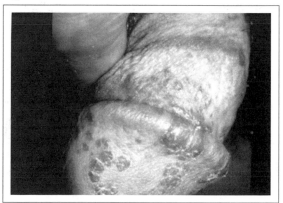

Penile psoriasis. (See also color plates.)

Figure 15–5

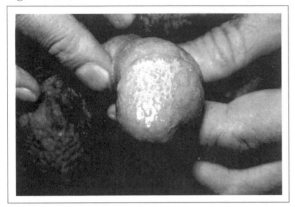

Lichen planus in an uncircumcised male. (See also color plates.)

sent with a reticulated white to violaceous pattern on an erythematous background (Fig. 15–5). Circumcised patients are more likely to present with flat-topped polygonal papules that may have an adherent scale (Fig. 15–6). Lichen planus may involve the foreskin or penile shaft (Fig. 15–7). Black patients are more likely to present with annular (ring-like) and hyperpigmented lesions. Annular lesions are also common in secondary syphilis, so appropriate serologic testing should be performed if the diagnosis is in question.

Figure 15–6

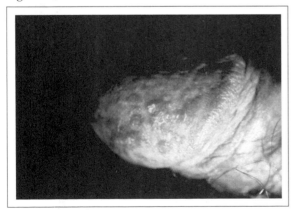

Lichen planus in a circumcised male. (See also color plates.)

Figure 15–7

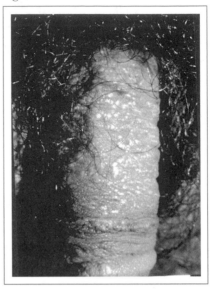

Lichen planus affecting the shaft. (See also color plates.)

Initial treatment generally consists of a midpotency to potent topical corticosteroid preparation applied daily. Patients should be monitored for atrophy. Ultrapotent corticosteroid preparations used only on weekends are effective in some cases. Refractory cases should be referred to a dermatologist.

PITYRIASIS ROSEA

Pityriasis rosea can present with prominent genital involvement (Fig. 15–8). Sometimes genital and flexural involvement predominates (inverse pityriasis rosea). Associated typical lesions on the trunk, a herald patch, and negative serologic testing for syphilis help to confirm the diagnosis. Pityriasis rosea is a self-limited disease. Symptoms generally respond to mild or midstrength corticosteroid preparations, applied bid.

LICHEN NITIDUS

Lichen nitidus presents with many tiny, asymptomatic hypopigmented papules. The lesions are

Figure 15–8

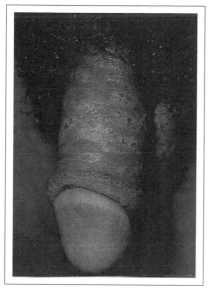

Penile pityriasis rosea. (See also color plates.)

Figure 15–9

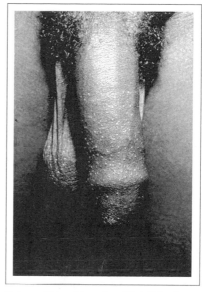

Lichen nitidus. (See also color plates.)

commonly grouped. Penile involvement is extremely common (Fig. 15–9). The clinical appearance is commonly diagnostic, but biopsy can establish the diagnosis in equivocal cases. The lesions are generally asymptomatic, and no treatment is required.

Genital Drug Eruptions

FIXED DRUG ERUPTIONS

Fixed drug eruption typically presents as a single, oval erythematous patch, plaque, or bullae that resolves with hyperpigmentation. On the glans penis, bullous lesions typically progress rapidly to erosions (Fig. 15–10). The lesions recur at the same site after rechallenge with the offending agent. Penile fixed drug eruption generally involves the glans and prepuce.[9,10] The most commonly implicated drugs are phenolphthalein, sulfonamides, tetracyclines, barbiturates, salicylates, and penicillins.

PENILE ULCERATION

Penile ulcerations are also described after administration of the antiviral foscarnet, which is thought to act as an irritant in the urine. Foscarnet-induced ulcers occur as tender periurethral

Figure 15–10

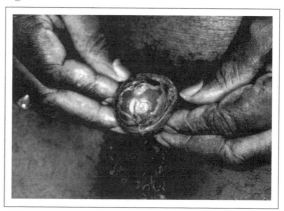

Fixed drug eruption. (See also color plates.) (Courtesy of Wilford Hall Medical Center teaching file.)

ulcerations most commonly in uncircumcised men.[11] They resolve after foscarnet therapy is discontinued. Meticulous hygiene helps to prevent ulceration.[12]

PENILE NECROSIS

Coumarin-induced necrosis of the penis may be seen 3 to 10 days after starting coumarin in patients with a relative protein C deficiency. When the penis is involved it is often associated with priapism. Coumarin has been safely readministered at small doses while overlapping with heparin anticoagulation.[13]

Contact Dermatitis

Contact dermatitis of the glans may result from spermicides, topical medications, or transfer of allergens such as the Rhus oleoresin (e.g., poison ivy) to the skin when voiding. Marked edema, often without vesiculation, characterizes these reactions. Rubber additives and lubricants in condoms are also common contact allergens. Skin testing for type IV hypersensitivity can be performed by a dermatologist if the offending agent cannot be identified.

For rubber-allergic patients, polyurethane condoms (Durex Avanti) are a good alternative. Natural membrane (lamb) condoms are generally safe for latex-sensitive individuals, but they do not protect against many sexually transmitted diseases. Trojan brand condoms contain only one accelerator and no antioxidant.[14] Some individuals with delayed-type hypersensitivity to rubber will tolerate Trojan brand condoms. Silicone is a nonsensitizing lubricant found in Ramses or Trojan-plus condoms.

A history of swelling and pruritus during intercourse occurs in 10% to 24% of condom users with type I IgE-mediated latex allergy.[15,16] Immediate-type hypersensitivity to latex may progress to anaphylaxis with repeated exposure to the allergen. RAST testing for latex protein allergy is readily available. Skin testing for type I hypersensitivity may be performed by an allergist.

For latex protein-allergic patients, polyurethane and natural membrane condoms are safe alternatives.

Irritant contact dermatitis may be seen as a result of frequent washing,[17] often in individuals who fear they have been exposed to a sexually transmitted disease. Nonallergic irritation from spermicides is common. Irritant dermatitis may also occur as a result of vigorous sexual activity or inadequate lubrication.

Infections

Ulcerative Lesions

Genital ulcers have many causes (Table 15–2). Several are discussed below.

SYPHILIS

Syphilis is a common cause of genital ulcers. Syphilitic chancres are indurated and relatively

Table 15–2
Causes of Genital Ulcers

INFECTIOUS	NON-INFECTIOUS
Syphilis	Carcinoma
Herpes simplex	Trauma
Chancroid	Aphthosis
Anaerobic erosive balanitis	Fixed drug reaction
Chlamydia/Lymphogranuloma venereum	Erythema multiforme
	Pyoderma gangrenosum
Granuloma inguinale	
Pseudomonas (ecthyma gangrenosum)	Coumarin necrosis
	Hypereosinophilic syndrome
Amoebic balanitis	
Trichomonas	Kaposi's sarcoma
Tuberculosis (mycobacteria)	
Candida (immunocompromised)	
Deep fungal (Histo, Blasto, crypto, Penicillium)	

Figure 15–11

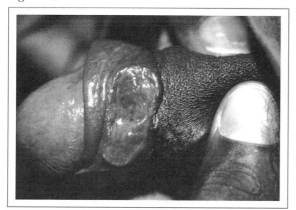

Hard syphilitic chancre. (See also color plates.)

Figure 15–12

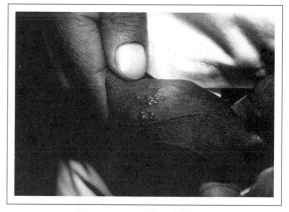

Herpes simplex. (See also color plates.)

painless (Fig. 15–11). Diagnosis at this stage is best made by darkfield examination.

HERPES SIMPLEX VIRUS

Herpes simplex virus (HSV) is another common cause of penile ulceration. Genital HSV presents with grouped vesicles, commonly on an erythematous base (Fig. 15–12). Symptoms include burning, pain, pruritus, or an associated urethritis.[18] Constitutional symptoms are more common in primary HSV.

Tzanck smears or viral culture can establish the diagnosis. ELISA tests and direct fluorescent antibody are less widely available. A Tzanck smear is a simple procedure in which the vesicle is unroofed and the base of the lesion scraped and then stained with toluidine blue or any of several commercially available Tzanck stains. Multinucleated giant cells with nuclear molding, a basophilic nuclear rim, and paler-staining central nucleus are characteristic for HSV (Fig. 15–13). Chronic ulcerative herpes (Fig. 15–14) is generally seen in immunosuppressed patients. The lesions are characterized by a thread-like pearly border. Tzanck smears can be diagnostic. Biopsies of herpetic lesions demonstrate an acantholytic blister with giant cells and characteristic nuclear cytopathic effect (Fig. 15–15). Of the laboratory methods available, viral culture is the most sensitive.[19]

Effective treatments for genital HSV include acyclovir, famciclovir, and valacyclovir. For acyclovir-resistant herpes infections, the thymidine kinase-independent agent foscarnet has been effective.[20]

CHANCROID

Chancroid, lymphogranuloma venereum, and granuloma inguinale may all affect the glans and prepuce and lead to genital ulceration. In Africa,

Figure 15–13

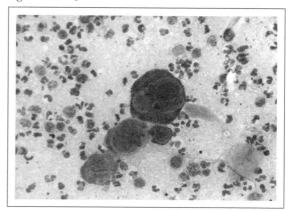

Tzanck smear. (See also color plates.)

Figure 15–14

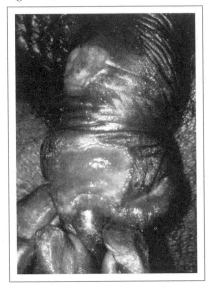

Chronic ulcerative herpes is seen in immunosuppressed patients.

Figure 15–16

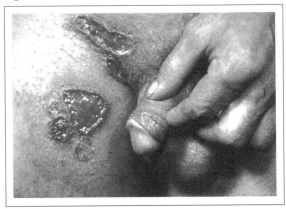

Soft chancres of chancroid. (Courtesy of Dr. Richard Vinson.)

chancroid is reported as the most common cause of genital ulcer disease. In the United States it is reported in epidemics.[21] Ulcers tend to be painful and soft (Fig. 15–16), in contrast to the hard painless chancres of syphilis. The fastidious organism may be detected by direct smear, but culture is difficult and requires a specialized cul-

ture media. Health care providers are advised to discuss culture of suspected cases of chancroid with their local health department or reference laboratory.

Treatment regimens for genital ulcers are published by the Centers for Disease Control and Prevention. Clinicians should consult current guidelines before initiating treatment. Current recommendations for chancroid include azithromycin 1 g orally in a single dose, or ceftriaxone 250 mg IM once, or ciprofloxacin 500 mg orally bid for 3 days, or erythromycin base 500 mg orally qid for 7 days.

GRANULOMA INGUINALE

Granuloma inguinale produces a large, painless ulcer with abundant friable granulation tissue (Fig. 15–17).[22] Fewer than 100 cases are reported annually in the United States.[23]

LYMPHOGRANULOMA VENEREUM

The initial papular lesion of lymphogranuloma venereum usually regresses prior to the appearance of large painful suppurative lymph nodes (buboes). Diagnosis is often made by demonstration of organisms in a biopsy speci-

Figure 15–15

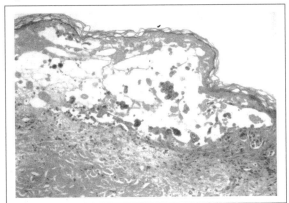

Acantholytic blister with viral cytopathic effect. (See also color plates.)

Figure 15–17

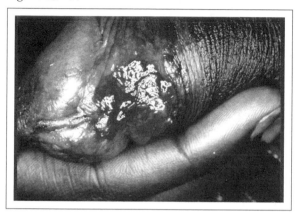

Granuloma inguinale. (See also color plates.) (Courtesy of Wilford Hall Medical Center teaching file.)

Figure 15–18

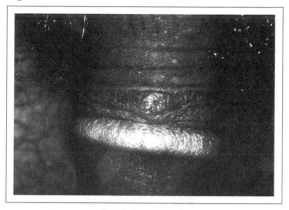

Scabies nodule. (See also color plates.)

Figure 15–19

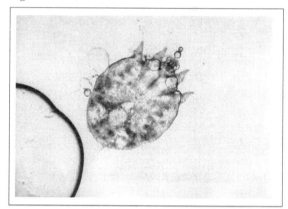

Scabies mite.

Figure 15–20

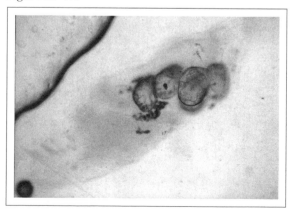

Scabies ova and feces.

men. Treatment regimens include trimethoprim-sulfamethoxasole one double strength tablet orally twice daily or doxycycline 100 mg orally bid. Treatment must be continued for at least 3 weeks or until the lesions resolve completely.

Nonulcerative Lesions

SCABIES

Scabies will often cause pruritic papules and nodules on the glans penis (Fig. 15–18). Severe nocturnal pruritus is characteristic, but may be absent in the initial 2 to 3 weeks of infestation. Identification of the *Sarcoptes scabiei* mite, eggs, or scybala (feces) confirms the diagnosis (Figs. 15–19 and 15–20). A single overnight application of 5% permethrin to the entire body is safe and effective. Immunocompromised patients may require repeated treatments or sequential treatment with permethrin, lindane, or "off label" use of oral ivermectin.[24,25]

HUMAN PAPILLOMA VIRUS

Human papilloma virus (HPV) infection may involve the distal penis in 30% to 60% of men

Figure 15–21

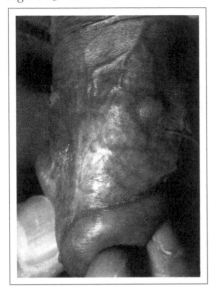

Genital wart. (See also color plates.)

(Figs. 15–21 and 15–22).[26] Many cases of genital HPV are subclinical.[27] European studies have demonstrated that men presenting with a balanoposthitis (infected glans and prepuce) may have HPV infection of the glans and prepuce.[28–30] Uncircumcised men presented with long-lasting or recurrent redness, burning, tenderness, or pruritus that was refractory to treatment with topical steroids, antifungals, or emollients. No other cause of balanoposthitis could be identified. Seventy-seven of 78 men who underwent biopsy had histologic evidence of HPV infection. Topical 5-fluorouracil has been an effective agent for the treatment of macular lesions caused by HPV.[31] Electrodessication has been used successfully to treat limited HPV balanoposthitis. Liquid nitrogen or podophyllin may also be indicated, but are limited due to pain, particularly for larger lesions. Multiple treatments are often required.

CANDIDA

Candida is responsible for up to one third of all cases of balanitis.[32,33] Patients present with glazed erythema, satellite lesions, eroded pustules, or a moist curd-like discharge (Fig. 15–23). Mild burning or pruritus is common, but pain suggests bacterial superinfection. Diabetes and antibiotics may precipitate *Candida* infections. Diagnosis is confirmed by direct smears or culture. Treatment with a topical antifungal agent or a single 150-mg dose of fluconazole results in a 90% cure rate.[34,35]

Figure 15–22

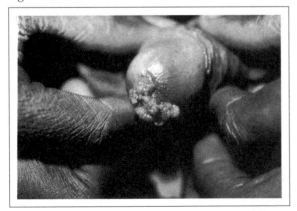

Urethral warts. (See also color plates.) (Courtesy of Wilford Hall Medical Center teaching file.)

Figure 15–23

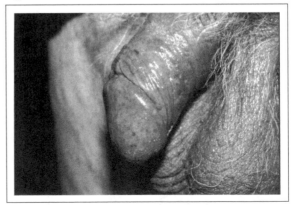

Candida balanitis. (See also color plates.)

DERMATOPHYTES

Dermatophytes commonly produce lesions on the legs and buttocks, but only rarely on the genitals.[36] Dermatophyte infections are generally treated with an topical antifungal cream applied bid. Nystatin has no effect on dermatophytes and should never be used. Clotrimazole, naftifine, and terbinafine creams are usually effective. Terbinafine has the advantage of shorter treatment duration (1 week).

BALANITIS

Bacteria commonly cause balanitis. Group B beta-hemolytic streptococci may be transmitted from the female genital tract. In prepubertal boys, group A beta-hemolytic streptococci may result from autoinoculation. As the diagnosis is generally made by culture, the choice of antibiotics for group B infections can be based on in vitro sensitivity tests, for group A streptococci generally penicillin or first-generation cephalosporins. Both types of streptococci are easily treated with an appropriate antibiotic.

Balanitis appears uncommonly in association with nongonococcal urethritis from chlamydia or mycoplasma.[37,38] Gonococcal balanoposthitis most commonly presents as an infection of a duct or sinus such as a median raphe cyst or Tyson's or Cowper's glands. Infection of the penile skin rarely causes tender ulcers, pustules, or furuncles. Gram stain and culture of the purulent discharge or urethral swabs for *Neisseria gonorrhoeae* may aid in diagnosis, although absence of urethral symptoms is common.[39]

Instead of the more common chancre (Fig. 15–11), primary syphilis may rarely present as a syphilitic balanitis (of Follman).[40] Syphilitic balanitis appears as a swollen glans covered with partially coalescent white flat papules and plaques. Numerous *Treponema pallidum* spirochetes may be demonstrated by darkfield examination.

Anaerobic erosive balanitis (AEB) results from a mixed infection of nontreponemal spirochetes and anaerobes, most commonly *Bacteroides* spp. This condition also presents as erosive and gangrenous balanitis. Most reports of AEB are in uncircumcised men who present with extensive tender erosions of the glans accompanied by a foul-smelling purulent discharge. Edema of the prepuce leading to phimosis is not uncommon. Darkfield exam demonstrates mixed spirochetes with numerous bacteria. Transmission occurs most commonly by orogenital contact. Metronidazole can produce rapid clearing of the lesions.[41] *Bacteroides* spp are also felt to play a role in *Gardnerella vaginalis*-associated balanitis.[42] Symptoms from *Gardnerella*-associated balanitis are generally mild. Patients may complain of a "fishy"-smelling preputial discharge. A venereal mode of transmission is suspected, because symptoms often began within 2 days of sexual contact.

Entamoeba histolytica may result in a severe balanitis with edema, phimosis, dysuria, and ulceration. The lesions fail to respond to antibiotic therapy.[43] The clinical picture may resemble an ulcerative carcinoma, except that patients report pain.[44] The organism may be identified by examination of the thick, creamy, blood-tinged discharge. Treatment with metronidazole and dehydroemetine has been successful.[45] In cases with limited involvement, circumcision is an alternative.[46] Such cases should be managed jointly with a specialist in infectious disease.

An erosive balanitis may occur in approximately one third of male carriers of *Trichomonas*.[47] Patients may also report an associated urethritis and adenopathy. Tinea versicolor is another rare cause of balanitis.[48] Genital cases of tinea versicolor generally respond to topical clotrimazole.

INTERTRIGO

Intertrigo presents with erythematous, tender denuded areas of skin in intertriginous areas. It commonly affects the inguinal creases (Fig. 15–24). *Candida,* gram-negative bacteria, and diphtheroids may be involved in the pathogenesis. Treatment with an anticandidal agent alone

Figure 15–24

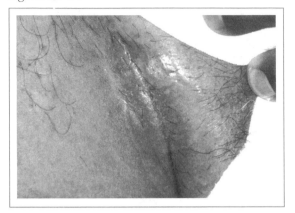

Intertrigo. (See also color plates.)

often yields disappointing results. A topical anti-candidal cream such as nystatin, miconazole, or clotrimazole applied bid, together with a mild or mid-potency steroid (such as desonide), can be helpful. Colorless Castellani's paint applied daily can also be helpful.

PUBIC HAIR INFECTION

White piedra is a common fungal infection that affects pubic hair. The fungus causes yellow-white gelatinous casts, which surround the hair shafts (Fig. 15–25). Response to topical anti-

Figure 15–25

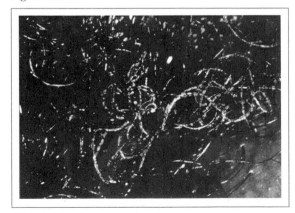

White piedra. (See also color plates.)

fungal agents is variable and recurrence is common.

SCLEROSING LYMPHANGITIS

Sclerosing lymphangitis of the penis presents as a circumferential cord or ulceration behind the corona of the penis (Fig. 15–26). The lesions frequently follow prolonged or repeated sexual intercourse, and may be associated with other sexually transmitted diseases. A full evaluation is warranted, to include physical examination, serologic testing for syphilis and AIDS, and urethral swabs for gonorrhea and chlamydia.

MOLLUSCUM CONTAGIOSUM

Molluscum contagiosum presents with umbilicated papules that may occur anywhere on genital skin. Individual lesions can be quite large, and grouped lesions may occur (Fig. 15–27). A crush preparation of the contents of the molluscum stained with toluidine blue or any Tzanck stain

Figure 15–26

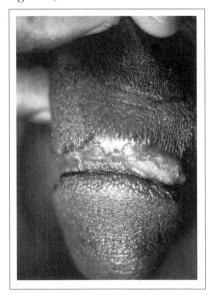

Sclerosing lymphangitis. (See also color plates.) (Courtesy of Wilford Hall Medical Center teaching file.)

Figure 15–27

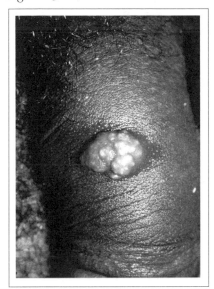

Molluscum contagiosum. (See also color plates.)

demonstrates diagnostic inclusion bodies (Fig. 15–28). Treatment may require curettage or cryotherapy. No single topical agent is consistently effective. Normal Tyson's glands occur adjacent to the frenulum (Fig. 15–29) and appear similar to the lesions of molluscum, resulting in occasional diagnostic errors.

Figure 15–28

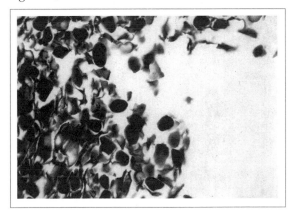

Molluscum bodies. (See also color plates.)

Figure 15–29

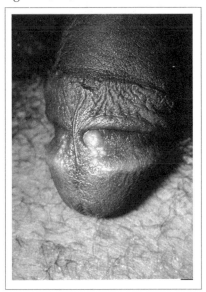

Tyson's gland. (See also color plates.)

HERPES ZOSTER

Herpes zoster may occur in the genital region. Painful dermatomal vesiculation suggests the diagnosis (Fig. 15–30). As genital lesions of zoster are generally quite painful, many clinicians treat with famciclovir 500 mg tid for 7 days or acyclovir 800 mg 5 times daily for 7 to 10 days. Immunosuppressed patients may present with herpes simplex infections in multiple dermatomes. These may be treated with acyclovir 400 mg tid or famciclovir 250 mg tid for 7 to 10 days.

NECROTIZING FASCIITIS OF THE GENITALIA

Necrotizing fasciitis of the genitalia was originally described by Fournier. Most cases have a urologic or colorectal source of infection.[49] The process begins as an area of cellulitis that progresses to an extremely painful blue-brown ecchymotic discoloration.[50] In adults, mixed gram-negative and anaerobic bacteria, especially *Bacteroides*, are isolated most frequently.[51] Two

Figure 15–30

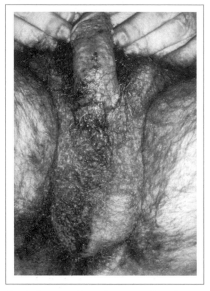

Genital zoster. (See also color plates.)

Figure 15–31

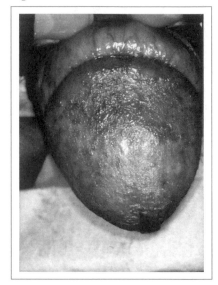

Bowen's disease. (See also color plates.)

thirds of all childhood cases occur in boys less than 3 months of age, and streptococcal and staphylococcal species are the most common isolates.[52] Both groups require urgent broad-spectrum antibiotics and surgical debridement.

Neoplasia

Erythroplasia of Queyrat and Bowen's Disease

Erythroplasia of Queyrat and Bowen's disease both represent squamous-cell carcinoma in situ involving the glans penis, foreskin, or both.[53] Typical lesions are red, slightly raised plaques (Fig. 15–31). The texture of erythroplasia of Queyrat is classically smooth and velvety, but portions of the lesion may be scaly or rough and distinction between erythroplasia of Queyrat

and Bowen's disease may be somewhat arbitrary. Lesions may be pruritic or painful. Patients may present because of bleeding or difficulty in retracting the foreskin. Recent evidence suggests that infection with human papilloma virus is the cause of most genital cancers, although the pathogenesis may also involve chronic irritation, inflammation, and trauma.[54,55] Management may include circumcision, topical 5-fluorouracil, Mohs micrographic surgery, and electrosurgery.[56,57]

Penile Carcinoma

Penile carcinoma is uncommon in the United States. Most cases are squamous-cell carcinoma and, as noted, are probably papilloma virus–induced. Lesions may present as papillary tumors, giant condylomata, or ulcerations (Fig. 15–32). Verrucous carcinoma or Buschke–Lowenstein tumor is a low-grade squamous-cell carcinoma. Verrucous carcinoma is closely linked to human

Figure 15–32

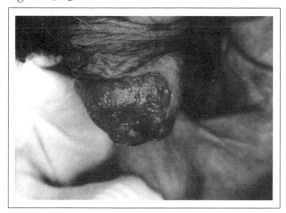

Invasive squamous-cell carcinoma. (See also color plates.)

papillomavirus infection.[58,59] Penile squamous-cell carcinoma may also arise in lesions of chronic lichen planus. Lack of circumcision may represent a risk factor for penile carcinoma.[60]

Squamous-cell carcinomas are generally treated with complete excision. Wide local excision may be appropriate for some tumors. Tissue-conserving techniques, such as Mohs micrographic surgery, can be helpful. Radiation therapy may be appropriate for some penile squamous-cell carcinomas, but is not recommended for verrucous carcinoma.[61]

Trauma

The most common traumatic injuries to the genitalia are burns, crush injury, and penetrating trauma. Penile frostbite occurs in joggers and alpine hikers.[62] Minor self-inflicted injuries, such as zipper entrapment, are relatively common. Children may experience penile tourniquet syndrome as a result of hair wrapped around the penis. The resulting penile strangulation can be dramatic.[63,64]

Scrotal Lesions

Candida

Candida readily involves scrotal skin. Please see the earlier discussion.

Tinea

Although candidiasis readily involves scrotal skin, symptomatic dermatophyte infection of scrotal skin is quite uncommon. Asymptomatic carriage of dermatophytes on scrotal skin is quite common, and topical antifungal agents should be applied to scrotal skin when tinea cruris is treated.[65]

Angiokeratomas

Angiokeratomas of Fordyce appear as numerous 1 to 4-mm red to purple lesions on the scrotum (Fig. 15–33). They are usually asymptomatic, but may cause scrotal bleeding.[66] Similar lesions may occur on the labia majora (Fig. 15–34). The lesions never involve the penile shaft and suprapu-

Figure 15–33

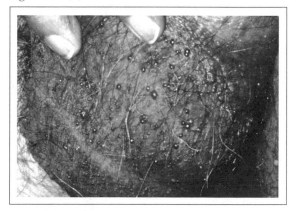

Fordyce angiokeratomas. (See also color plates.)

Figure 15–34

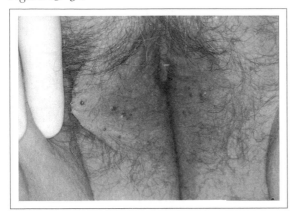

Vulvar angiokeratomas. (See also color plates.)

bic or sacral areas. If angiokeratomas are seen in these locations, a diagnosis of Fabry's disease should be considered. Patient's with Fabry's disease may report lancinating pains and may have significant renal disease.

Pyogenic Granuloma

Pyogenic granulomas present as eruptive friable, easily bleeding papules (Fig. 15–35). They may occur on the scrotum following minor trauma or with no apparent preceding trauma. Multiple pyogenic granulomas may erupt around the site where a single lesion has been treated. Currettage with electrodessication, silver nitrate cautery, or simple excision is curative.

Paget's Disease

Extramammary Paget's disease commonly affects the skin of the scrotum (Fig. 15–36). The skin of the penis and suprapubic region may also be affected (Fig. 15–37). The lesions may occur as an epidermotropic extension of an underlying urologic or gastrointestinal malignancy. Primary cutaneous extramammary Paget's disease may eventually give rise to an invasive adenocarcinoma. Surgical treatment is difficult, as the lesions are commonly multifocal and may extend far beyond the apparent clinical margin.[67]

Squamous-Cell Carcinoma

Scrotal squamous-cell carcinoma may be related to exposure to tar or soot. English chimney sweeps during the last century had a high inci-

Figure 15–35

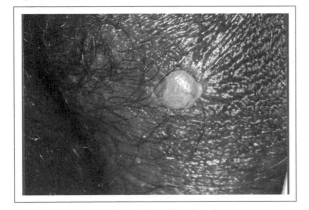

Pyogenic granuloma. (See also color plates.)

Figure 15–36

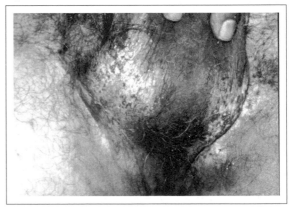

Extramammary Paget's disease. (See also color plates.)

Figure 15–37

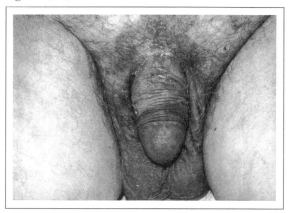

Extramammary Paget's disease. (See also color plates.)

Figure 15–38

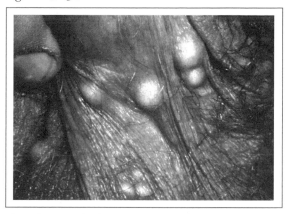

Idiopathic scrotal calcinosis.

dence of scrotal carcinoma. Today, psoriasis patients may develop scrotal carcinoma if their genitalia are not shielded during ultraviolet therapy.[68] To date, only limited data implicate the medical use of coal tar as a risk factor for scrotal carcinoma.[69,70]

As noted, Buschke–Lowenstein tumors of the penis or scrotum are well differentiated squamous-cell carcinomas associated with human papilloma virus infection.[71] The lesions are best treated with local resection. Radiation therapy should be avoided, as it has been associated with high-grade transformation of the tumor.[72]

Elephantiasis of the Male Genitalia

Idiopathic genital elephantiasis commonly affects the scrotum and prepuce out of proportion to the rest of the genitalia. Many cases may be the result of subclinical streptococcal infection.[73] Management is difficult, but some patients respond well to excision and grafting.[74]

Idiopathic Calcinosis of the Scrotum

Idiopathic scrotal calcinosis is quite common. The lesions appear as yellow or white subcutaneous

nodules (Fig. 15–38). Patients often present when the skin overlying the lesions begins to break down revealing white chalky material. The lesions are thought to arise as a result of calcification of benign cysts.[75,76] The lesions may require no specific therapy. When therapy is deemed appropriate, surgical excision is the best approach.

Note: The authors are full-time federal employees. This work is in the public domain. The views expressed are those of the authors, and are not to be construed as official or as reflecting those of the Department of Defense, the Army Medical Department, or the U.S. Air Force.

References

1. English JC, Laws RA, Keough GC, et al: Dermatoses of the glans penis and prepuce. *J Am Acad Dermatol* 37:1–24, 1997.
2. Wallace HJ: Lichen sclerosus et atrophicus. *Trans St John's Hosp Dermatol Soc* 57:930, 1971.
3. Meffert JJ, Davis BM, Grimwood RE: Lichen sclerosus. *J Am Acad Dermatol* 32:393–416, 1995.
4. Mikat DM, Ackerman HR, Mikat KW: Balanitis xerotica obliterans: A report of an 11-year-old and review of the literature. *Pediatrics* 52:25–28, 1973.
5. Meyrick Thomas RH, Ridley CM, Black MM: Clinical features and therapy of lichen sclerosus

et atrophicus affecting males. *Clin Exp Dermatol* 12:126–128, 1987.

6. Bainbridge DR, Whitaker RH, Shepheard BGF: Balanitis xerotica obliterans and urinary obstruction. *Br J Urol* 43:487–491, 1971.

7. Staff WG: Uretheral involvement in balanitis xerotica obliterans. *Br J Urol* 47:234–239, 1970.

8. Drut RM, Gomex MA, Drut R, et al: Human papillomavirus is present in some cases of childhood penile lichen sclerosis: An in situ hybridization and SP-PCR study. *Pediatr Dermatol* 15:85–90, 1998.

9. Sehgal VH, Gangarani OP: Genital fixed drug eruptions. *Genitourin Med* 62:56–58, 1986.

10. Sehgal VH, Gangarani OP: Fixed drug eruption: Current concepts. *Int J Dermatol* 26:67–74, 1987.

11. Moyle G, Barton SE, Balestrini A: Penile ulcerations with foscarnet. *Lancet* 335:547–548, 1990. Letter.

12. Lernested JO, Chonas AC: Penile ulcerations with foscarnet. *Lancet* 335:548, 1990. Letter.

13. Barkley C, Badalament RA, Metz EN: Coumarin necrosis of the penis. *J Urol* 141:946–948, 1989.

14. Fischer AA: Condom dermatitis in either partner. *Cutis* 39:281–285, 1987.

15. Turjanmaa K, Reunala T: Condoms as a source of latex allergens and contact urticaria. *Contact Dermatitis* 20:360–364, 1989.

16. Wrangsjo K, Wahlberg JE, Axelsson IGK: IgE-mediated allergy to natural rubber in 30 patients with contact urticaria. *Contact Dermatitis* 19:264–271, 1988.

17. Birley HDL, Walker MM, Luzzi GA, et al: Clinical features and management of recurrent balanitis: Association with atopy and genital washing. *Genitourin Med* 69:400–403, 1993.

18. Smith MA, Singer C: Sexually transmitted viruses other than HIV and papillomavirus. *Urol Clin North Am* 19:47–61, 1992.

19. Moseley RC, Carey L, Benjamin D, et al: Comparison of viral isolation, direct immunofluorescent and indirect immunoperoxidase techniques for detection of genital herpes simplex virus infection. *J Clin Microbiol* 13:913–918, 1981.

20. Lavoie SR, Kaplowitz LG: Management of genital herpes infections. *Semin Dermatol* 13:248–255, 1994.

21. McCarley ME, Cruz PD Jr, Sontheimer RD: Chancroid: Clinical variants and other findings from an epidemic in Dallas County, 1986–1987. *J Am Acad Dermatol* 19:330–337, 1988.

22. Rosen T, Tschen JA, Ramsdel W, et al: Granuloma inguinale. *J Am Acad Dermatol* 11:433–437, 1984.

23. Buntin DM: The 1993 sexually transmitted disease treatment guidelines. *Semin Dermatol* 13:269–274, 1994.

24. Meinking TL, Taplin D, Hermide JL, et al: The treatment of scabies with ivermectin. *N Engl J Med* 333:26–30, 1995.

25. Funkhouser ME, Omohundro C, Ross A, et al: Management of scabies in patients with human immunodeficiency virus disease. *Arch Dermatol* 129:911–913, 1993.

26. Cook LS, Koutsky LA, Holmes KK: Clinical presentation of genital warts among circumcised and uncircumcised heterosexual men attending an urban STD clinic. *Genitourin Med* 69:262–264, 1993.

27. Schneider A, Kirchmayr R, de Villiers EM, et al: Subclinical human papillomavirus infection in male sexual partners of female carriers. *J Urol* 140:1431–1434, 1988.

28. Arumainayagam JT, Sumathiapapa AHT, Smallman LA, et al: Flat condylomata of the penis presenting as patch balanoposthitis. *Genitourin Med* 66:251–253, 1990.

29. Birley HDL, Luzzi GA, Walker MM, et al: The association of human papillomavirus infection with balanoposthitis: A description of five cases with proposals for treatment. *Int J STD AIDS* 5:139–141, 1994.

30. Wikstrom A, von Krogh G, Hedblad HA, et al: Papillomavirus-associated balanoposthitis. *Genitourin Med* 70:175–181, 1994.

31. Krebs HB: Treatment of genital condylomata with topical 5-fluorouracil. *Dermatol Clin* 9:333–341, 1992.

32. Dockerty WG, Sonnex C: Candidal balano-pothitis: A study of diagnostic methods. *Genitourin Med* 71:407–409, 1995.

33. Abdullah AN, Drake SM, Wade Aah, et al: Balanitis (balanoposthitis) in patients attending a department of genitourinary medicine. *Int J STD AIDS* 3:128–129, 1992.

34. Warner E, Strashin E: Benefits and risks of circumcision. *Can Med Assoc J* 125:967–976, 1981.

35. Stary A, Goeltz-Szoets J, Ziegler C, et al: Comparison of the efficacy and safety of oral fluconazole and topical clotrimazole in patients with candida balanitis. *Genitourin Med* 72:98–102, 1996.

36. Dekio S, Sidoi J: Tinea of the glans penis. *Dermatologica* 178:112–124, 1989.

37. Bhangara RK, Thin RNT: Subpreputial carriage of aerobic microorganisms and balanitis. *Br J Venereal Dis* 59:131–133, 1993.

38. Siboulet A, Catalint F, Deubel M: Balanitis et mycoplasma. *Bull Soc Fr Dermatol Syphiligr* 82: 419–422, 1975.

39. Rosen T: Unusual presentations of gonorrhea. *J Am Acad Dermatol* 6:369–372, 1982.

40. Lejman K, Starzycki Z: Syphilitic balanitis of Folloman developing after the appearance of the primary chancre: A case report. *Br J Venereal Dis* 51:138–140, 1975.

41. Cree GE, Willis AT, Phillips KD, et al: Anaerobic balanoposthitis. *Br Med J* 284:859–860, 1983.

42. Kinghorn GR, Jones BM, Cowdhry FH, et al: Balanoposthitis associated with *Gardnerella vaginalis*. *Br J Venereal Dis* 58:127–129, 1982.

43. Rodrique RB: Amebic balanitis. *JAMA* 239:109, 1978.

44. Thomas JA, Anthony AJ: Amoebiasis of the penis. *Br J Urol* 48:269–273, 1976.

45. Moldwin RM: Sexually transmitted protozoal infections. *Urol Clin North Am* 19:93–101, 1992.

46. Cooke RA, Rodrique RB: Amoebis balanitis. *Med J Aust* 1:114–116, 1964.

47. Michalowski R: Balano-posthitis A trichomonas: Apropos de 16 observations. *Ann Dermatol Venereol* 108:731–738, 1981.

48. Nia AK, Smith EL: Pityriasis versicolor of the glans penis. *Br J Venereal Dis* 55:230, 1979.

49. Spirnak JP, Resnick MI, Hampel N, Persky L: Fournier's gangrene: Report of 20 patients. *J Urol* 131:289–291, 1984.

50. Kearney GP, Carling PC: Fournier's gangrene: An approach to its management. *J Urol* 130:695–698, 1983.

51. Finegold FM: *Anaerobic Bacteria in Human Disease*. New York, Academic Press, 1977, pp 411–481.

52. Adams JR, Mata JA, Venable DD, et al: Fournier's gangrene in children. *Urology* 35:439–341, 1990.

53. Mikhail GR: Cancers, precancers, and pseudocancers on the male genitalia: A review of clinical appearances, histopathology and management. *J Dermatol Surg Oncol* 6:1027–1035, 1980.

54. Cupp MR, Malek RS, Goellner JR, et al: The detection of human papillomavirus deoxyribonucleic acid in intrepithelial, in situ, verrucous and invasive carcinoma of the penis. *J Urol* 154:-1024–1029, 1995.

55. Sarkar FH, Miles BJ, Plieth DH, et al: Detection of human papillomavirus in squamous neoplasm of the penis. *J Urol* 147:389–392, 1992.

56. Bernstein G, Forgaard DM, Miller JE: Carcinoma in situ of the glans penis and distal urethra. *J Dermatol Surg Oncol* 12:450–455, 1986.

57. Gribetz ME, Fine EM: Neoplastic lesions of the penile gland and periglandular regions. *Clin Dermatol* 5:77–86, 1987.

58. Boshart M, zur Hausen H: Human papillomaviruses in Buschke–Lowenstein tumors: Physical state of the DNA and identification of a tandem duplication in the noncoding region of a human papillomavirus 6 subtype. *J Virol* 58:963–966, 1986.

59. Lehn H, Ernst TM, Sauer G: Transcript of episomal papillomavirus DNA in human condylomata accuminata and B-L tumors. *J Gen Virol* 65:2003–2010, 1984.

60. Maden C, Sherman KJ, Beckman AM, et al: History of circumcision, medical conditions, and sexual activity and the risk of penile cancer. *J Natl Cancer Inst* 85.19–24, 1993.

61. Schwartz RA: Verrucous carcinoma of the skin and mucosa. *J Am Acad Dermatol* 32:1–21, 1995.

62. Hershkowitz M: Penile frostbite, an unforseen hazard of jogging. *N Engl J Med* 296:1/8, 1977.

63. Farah R, Cerny JC: Penis tourniquet syndrome and penile amputation. *Urology* 2:310–311, 1973.

64. Singh B, Kim H, Wax SH: Strangulation of the glans penis by hair. *Urology* 9:170–172, 1978.

65. Chakrabarti A, Sharma SC, Talwar P: Isolation of dermatophytes from clinically normal sites in patients with tinea cruris. *Mycopathologia* 120: 139–141, 1992.

66. Hoekx L, Wyndaele JJ: Angiokeratoma: A cause of scrotal bleeding. *Acta Urol Belg* 66:27–28, 1988.

67. Knottenbelt A, Nicolai JP: Ziekte van Paget van het scrotum. *Ned Tijdschr Geneeskd* 138:914–916, 1994.

68. Taniguchi S, Furukawa M, Kutsuna H, et al: Squamous cell carcinoma of the scrotum. *Dermatology* 193:253–254, 1996.

69. Van Schooten FJ, Godschalk R: Coal tar therapy. Is it carcinogenic? *Drug Saf* 15:374–377, 1996.

70. Andrews PE, Farrow GM, Oesterling JE: Squamous cell carcinoma of the scrotum: Long-term follow-up of 14 patients. *J Urol* 146:1299–1304, 1991.

71. Kabiri H, Albouzidi A, Rachid K, et al: Tumeur de Buschke Loewenstein scrotale degeneree. *Prog Urol* 6:439–442, 1996.

72. Micali G, Innocenzi D, Nasca MR, et al: Squamous cell cacinoma of the penis. *J Am Acad Dermatol* 35:432–451, 1996.

73. Geyer H, Geyer A, Schubert J: Erysipel und elephantiasis des Skrotums. Operative und medikamentose therapie. *Urologe A* 34:59–61, 1995.

74. Ollapallil JJ, Watters DA: Surgical management of elephantisis of male genitalia. *Br J Urol* 76:213–215, 1995.

75. Michl UH, Gross AJ, Loy V: Idiopathic calcinosis of the scrotum—a specific entity of the scrotal skin. Case report. *Scand J Urol Nephrol* 28:213–217, 1994.

76. Song DH, Lee KW, Kang WH: Idiopathic calcinosis of the scrtoum: Histopatholgic observations of fifty-one nodules. *J Am Acad Dermatol* 19:1095–1101, 1988.

Margaret S. Pearle

Chapter 16

Urinary Calculi

How Common Are Urinary Stones?

Urinary tract stones (nephrolithiasis) are common, affecting nearly 5% to 10% of the population at some time during their lifetime.[1] If no prophylactic measures are initiated to prevent stone recurrence, 20% to 50% of stone patients will experience repeat stone events within 5 years.[2] Even stones that are diagnosed incidentally pose a risk; patients with asymptomatic stones have a 50% chance of becoming symptomatic within 5 years of diagnosis.[3] Not surprisingly, nephrolithiasis incurs substantial personal and financial cost to the population. The total annual cost of evaluation and treatment of nephrolithiasis in the United States is in the range of $2 billion.[4]

Surgical management of urinary tract stones has undergone a quiet revolution over the past 20 years. The development of new technology to treat stones noninvasively or with minimal invasion has nearly eliminated open stone surgery and has substantially reduced morbidity and convalescence time. The cornerstone of stone management, however, remains prevention, and new diagnostic and treatment algorithms have kept pace with surgical advances such that with institution of a medical prophylactic program, most stone recurrences can be prevented.

In many cases, primary care and emergency clinicians comprise the initial health care contact made by patients experiencing an acute stone event. Accordingly, a thorough understanding by the primary care clinician of the natural history, pathophysiology, and treatment of nephrolithiasis is mandatory.

The prevalence of nephrolithiasis is estimated at 2% to 3% in North American adults.[1] Although the peak incidence of stone disease occurs in the 3rd to 5th decade of life, many patients experience their first stone event in their late teens or early 20s.[5] Males are affected more commonly than females by a ratio of 2 or 3 to 1, and Caucasians have a higher incidence of stone disease compared to African Americans. The gender bias toward males observed in the Caucasian population is reversed in the African American population.[6–8]

Typical Presentation of an Acute Stone Event

When a urinary calculus is in transit from the kidney to the bladder, it may partially or completely obstruct the outflow of urine from the kidney, resulting in a constellation of symptoms known as renal colic. Typically, renal colic is characterized by the abrupt onset of pain originating in the flank and radiating around to the lower abdomen, groin, or testicle (labia). The occurrence of pain in the groin area is attributed to the close proximity with which the blood vessels and autonomic nerve fibers supplying the kidney and testicle (ovary), respectively, originate. The pain generally occurs in paroxysms that last a few minutes or more at a time. Because the celiac axis innervates the kidneys as well as the stomach and small intestine, renal colic is frequently associated with nausea and vomiting, often confusing the diagnosis with gastrointestinal diseases, such as acute appendicitis, perforated ulcer, colitis, or diverticulitis.

The location of the pain may reflect the location of the obstructing stone. Stones close to the kidney in the proximal ureter cause flank pain; stones in the ureter overlying the bony pelvis may cause pain in the lower abdomen; and stones in the distal ureter near the bladder often predominantly cause irritative bladder symptoms such as urinary frequency and urgency.

Patients with renal colic are often identifiable even before a history is obtained. Unlike the patient with peritonitis who lies motionless in bed to avoid any movement of his abdomen, patients with renal colic characteristically writhe in pain or pace the floor in an attempt to gain relief.

Key History

When a patient presents to the emergency room or clinician's office with symptoms attributable to a ureteral calculus, the goal is to establish a diagnosis and relieve the pain and/or obstruction. To that end, a careful history, thorough physical examination, selective laboratory tests, and radiographic imaging studies must be obtained.

A complete history regarding the onset, duration, location, and nature of the pain is critical in establishing the diagnosis of a renal or ureteral calculus. Sharp paroxysmal pain in the flank that wakes the patient from sleep is typical of renal colic. Nausea and vomiting, usually in association with pain, is a frequent accompanying occurrence. Associated fever and chills are uncommon, occurring more typically with acute pyelonephritis; however, obstructive pyelonephritis may occur in association with a ureteral stone, and prompt diagnosis of this potentially life-threatening complication of a ureteral stone is critical. Gross hematuria in the presence of renal colic is highly suggestive of urinary tract stones. However, the absence of gross hematuria does not exclude the diagnosis of a stone.

A complete medical and surgical history is essential for establishing the diagnosis and managing the patient with an acute stone event. A personal or family history of stone disease or underlying medical risk factors associated with stone formation, such as gastrointestinal disease (chronic diarrhea, intestinal resection), gout, bone disease, or chronic urinary tract infections should raise the suspicion of a urinary tract stone as a source of the pain. Medical illness may also influence the choice of imaging modality, such as avoidance of intravenous contrast in a diabetic patient at risk for nephrotoxicity. Likewise, a patient with a known solitary kidney requires urgent decompression of the collecting system to prevent renal damage if obstruction is identified. Lastly, a history of previous surgical intervention for stone disease should be elicited, as it may affect urinary tract anatomy and ultimately impact management.

Physical Examination

An elevated pulse and blood pressure are nonspecific signs that often accompany pain, but temperature is important in determining the presence of infection. Occasionally noninfected stones are associated with a low-grade fever (<100°F); however, temperatures above 100°F should raise suspicion of an obstructive pyelonephritis.

Physical examination is often remarkable only for tenderness overlying the site of stone impaction, either in the flank or anterior abdomen. The absence of peritoneal signs such as rebound or percussion tenderness should rule out an acute abdomen. Gastrointestinal diseases rarely present primarily with flank pain; rather, tenderness is usually localized to the abdominal quadrant containing the diseased organ. Examination of the testes and ovaries should be performed to determine if the pain can be reproduced with palpation, which would suggest a gonadal rather than renal etiology.

Ancillary Tests

Laboratory Studies

The minimum laboratory evaluation of the patient with a suspected renal or ureteral calculus includes a complete blood count, serum electrolyte levels, blood urea nitrogen, creatinine level, and a urinalysis. Although a mild leukocytosis (10,000 to 15,000/mm^2) is common in patients presenting with renal colic due to demargination of white blood cells in response to stress, a white blood count greater than $15,000/mm^2$ should alert the clinician to the possibility of pyelonephritis.

Serum blood urea nitrogen and creatinine provide a rough estimate of overall renal function and hydration status; an elevated creatinine level may suggest the presence of bilateral ureteral obstruction or unilateral obstruction in a patient with a functionally solitary kidney or baseline renal insufficiency. In addition, an assessment of renal function is mandatory to prevent potential nephrotoxicity if administration of intravenous contrast for radiographic imaging is considered.

Serum electrolytes should be checked to identify metabolic abnormalities such as acidosis, alkalosis, or hypokalemia. If a stone is ultimately identified, serum calcium, phosphorus, and uric acid should be measured to elucidate underlying metabolic risk factors; however, for economic reasons, these tests may be delayed until a diagnosis of stone disease is firmly established.

The urinalysis constitutes an important part of the laboratory assessment of the patient with acute renal colic. The presence of red blood cells in the urine may suggest the diagnosis of urinary tract stones, but their absence does not rule it out. In 10% to 25% of patients with an acute stone event, no red blood cells are identified in the urine; in some cases the absence of red blood cells is due to complete urinary obstruction on the affected side. Mild pyuria may be present in the urine of a patient with a stone but usually represents inflammation rather than infection. Significant pyuria, however, particularly when associated with fever and/or leukocytosis, may indicate the presence of a urinary tract infection, and a culture should be sent.

Additional urine parameters such as pH and the presence of crystals may contribute to the overall evaluation of the stone patient, although they are less crucial for diagnosis and management of the acute stone event. Urine pH greater than 7 suggests the presence of urea-splitting organisms and should raise suspicion of a struvite stone. At a urine pH below 5.5, uric acid precipitates and may form uric acid stones. Identification of crystals in the urine, such as hexagonal cystine crystals, may

be diagnostic, but pyramidal calcium oxalate crystals are common and less specific.

Imaging Studies

The cornerstone of the diagnosis of urinary tract stones is radiographic imaging. Radiographic studies should determine the size, number, and location of urinary tract stones, and they may suggest a likely composition.

PLAIN FILM RADIOGRAPH/ KIDNEY-URETER-BLADDER

Radiopaque stones comprise upwards of 90% of urinary tract stones, and consequently a plain abdominal radiograph of the kidneys, ureters, and bladder (KUB) provides a rapid screen for diagnosing a urinary calculus. Stones vary in radiodensity according to their composition (Table 16–1). Size also plays a role in the ability to identify a calculus on KUB. Oblique views increase the sensitivity of KUB for identifying urinary calculi by projecting a calculus away from a bony structure, altering the relation of the stone to overlying bowel gas, or changing the dimension of the stone penetrated by the x-ray beam. Likewise, plain nephrotomograms facilitate visualization of small stones or stones obscured by overlying stool or bowel gas.

Table 16–1

Radiodensity of Various Stone Compositions

STONE COMPOSITION	RADIODENSITY
Calcium hydrogen phosphate dihydrate (brushite)	Very opaque
Calcium oxalate monohydrate	Very opaque
Calcium phosphate (apatite)	Very opaque
Calcium oxalate dihydrate	Moderately opaque
Magnesium ammonium phosphate (struvite)	Moderately opaque
Cystine	Faint to moderately opaque
Uric acid	Radiolucent

Not all calcifications identified on KUB represent urinary tract calculi. Extraurinary calcifications may mimic urinary tract stones and must be distinguished from them with the aid of oblique or lateral views that project these calcifications away from the expected location of the kidneys or path of the ureters. Gallstones, which are characteristically multifaceted, lie in the right upper quadrant and project anterior to the kidney on a right posterior oblique view. Vascular calcifications are usually linear and lie in the expected location of major blood vessels (aorta, iliac arteries). Renal artery aneurysms can be mistaken for renal calculi because of their location within the kidney, although unlike calculi, they generally contain a lucent center. Pelvic phleboliths (calcified thrombi in pelvic veins) are typically round or oval and contain a lucent center. Although some phleboliths are easily distinguishable from ureteral or bladder calculi by their location, most require opacification of the urinary tract to discern them as discrete from the ureters.

INTRAVENOUS UROGRAM

Historically, the intravenous urogram (IVU, also called intravenous pyelogram) has been the mainstay in the diagnosis of renal and ureteral calculi. A scout film obtained prior to the administration of intravenous contrast may suggest the presence of a likely candidate for a urinary tract stone (Fig. 16–1A). Once the collecting system is opacified, the stone can be unequivocally determined to lie within the urinary tract (Fig. 16–1B). The presence, size, and location of urinary tract stones can be assessed with an IVU, as can abnormalities in urinary tract anatomy (horseshoe kidney, solitary kidney, medullary sponge kidney) and the presence and degree of obstruction either from the stone or due to underlying urinary tract anomalies. In addition, sequelae from urinary tract obstruction, such as loss of renal parenchyma from long-standing obstruction or extravasation of contrast due to forniceal rupture, may be identified. Radiolucent stones are invisible on initial KUB and IVU, but

their presence on IVU can be inferred by the presence of urinary tract obstruction and a filling defect, representing the lucent stone, in the opacified urinary tract.

The sensitivity of the IVU in diagnosing a stone and assessing its location and degree of associated obstruction depends on the quality of the study and the tenacity of the radiographer. Monitoring the study as it progresses allows the radiographer to adjust the timing of the films and the position of the patient, thereby increasing the amount of useful information obtained from the study. The judicious use of oblique views, prone positioning, delayed images, and fluoroscopy may contribute to the successful diagnosis of a difficult-to-visualize or highly obstructing stone.

ULTRASOUND

Renal sonography provides an alternative to the IVU for patients with a contrast allergy or renal insufficiency in whom the use of intravenous contrast is contraindicated, but it suffers from a number of limitations that hinder its use in the acute setting. Although sonography is highly sensitive for detecting stones larger than 5 mm in the kidney and for identifying hydronephrosis, small stones and stones in the ureter are easily missed. Distal ureteral stones, however, may often be visualized though the window of a fluid-filled bladder. An obese body habitus and increased bowel gas may preclude the identification of some stones by sonography.

RETROGRADE PYELOGRAM

Retrograde pyelography is rarely used in the acute setting for the diagnosis of urinary tract stones. However, in the patient with obstruction demonstrated by sonography in whom surgical intervention is indicated to decompress the urinary tract, retrograde pyelography may clearly define a filling defect in the ureter or kidney and show a discrepancy in the caliber of the ureter above and below the defect.

Figure 16–1

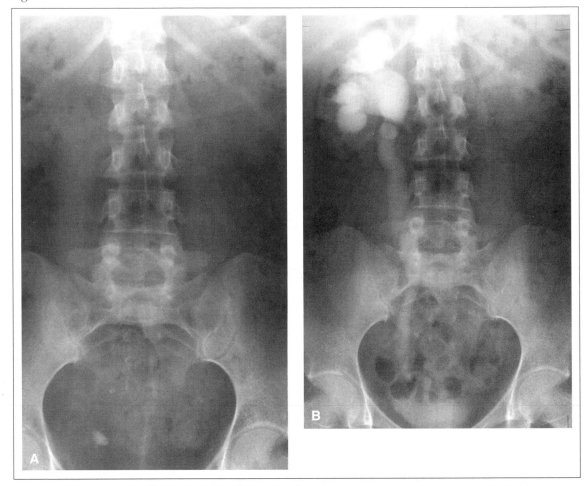

A. Large calcification in right hemipelvis. Note additional smaller calcifications scattered throughout pelvis. **B.** After administration of intravenous contrast, opacification of a markedly dilated right kidney and ureter to the level of a large distal ureteral calculus is evident.

HELICAL (SPIRAL) CT

The current imaging study of choice for the evaluation of *acute flank pain* is unenhanced, thin-cut (5-mm) helical CT.[9] With this modality, images are acquired in a helical configuration during a single breath hold, thereby eliminating respiratory motion artifact and allowing three-dimensional reconstruction of the entire urinary tract (Fig. 16–2). Helical CT has been shown to be more sensitive than IVU for detecting ureteral stones. Even

in the absence of a distinct stone, secondary signs of obstruction, such as perinephric stranding or circumferential soft-tissue attenuation, can confirm the diagnosis of a ureteral stone with a high degree of accuracy.[10] CT has the advantage of being rapid (less than a minute), highly sensitive, and readily available, and precludes the need for intravenous contrast in most cases. Although cost still favors IVU in terms of the radiographic study itself, the rapidity of diagnosis using CT and the potential for shortening time in the emergency

Figure 16–2

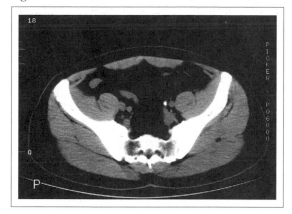

Noncontrast, helical CT showing a left middle ureteral calculus.

room may compensate for the greater cost of the study.[11]

Although CT is the preferred imaging study for the diagnosis of acute flank pain, the need for a contrast study, particularly in IVU, is not eliminated. In the patient requiring subsequent surgical intervention, radiographic visualization of the collecting system and ureter is necessary to determine the optimal form of treatment and to rule out associated anatomic anomalies that may preclude certain forms of treatment. However, an IVU may be performed electively at a later date under more favorable conditions, without the need to utilize costly emergency room time.

Algorithm for Acute Stone Event

When a patient presents to the emergency room or a doctor's office with symptoms suggestive of renal colic, the goal is to establish a diagnosis, relieve pain and/or obstruction, identify stone characteristics and anatomic features that impact management, select conservative management versus surgical treatment, and ultimately proceed with treatment if indicated. Fig. 16–3 presents an algorithm for management of the acute stone event when a patient presents with complaints suggestive of renal colic.

Management

Treatment of the Acute Stone Event

ANALGESIA

Once the diagnosis of a stone is made, attention is directed toward providing prompt pain relief. Narcotic analgesics, such as morphine sulfate or meperidine, have traditionally provided excellent pain control. A trend favoring the use of intravenous nonsteroidal analgesics such as ketorolac has recently emerged; however, reports of renal failure, particularly in patients with impaired renal function or dehydration, suggest that these agents be used judiciously if at all. Inhibition of platelet aggregation common to all nonsteroidal medications may predispose to bleeding; as such, use of these medications in patients who may require urgent or timely surgical intervention should be avoided if possible.

The use of agents aimed at reducing ureteral peristalsis and presumably renal colic and facilitating stone passage has been met with varying success. Intranasal desmopressin,[12] aminophylline, indomethacin,[13] nifedipine,[14,15] and methylprednisolone[14] have all been used to treat renal colic and facilitate stone passage, but their use has not reached widespread acceptance.

DECOMPRESSION

Subsequent management of the patient with acute renal colic depends on his or her response to analgesics, ability to maintain oral intake, and the presence of infection. A stone causing any degree of obstruction that is associated with clinical

Figure 16–3

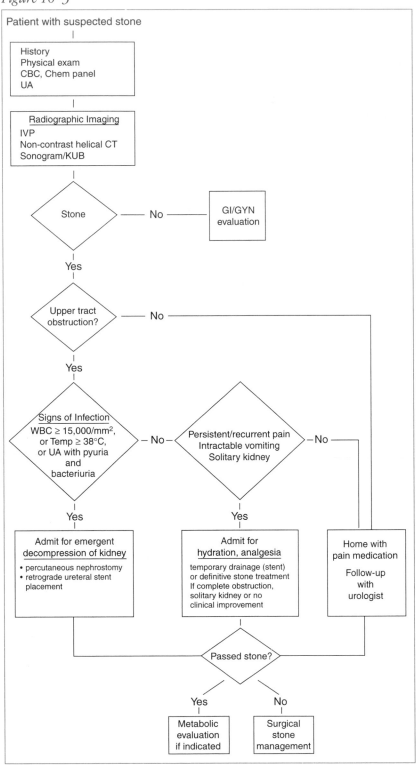

Algorithm for management of an acute stone event.

Plate 1 (Figure 15-1)

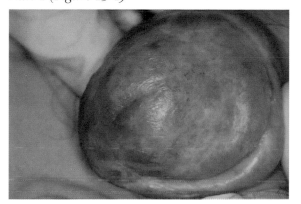

Lichen sclerosus.

Plate 2 (Figure 15-2)

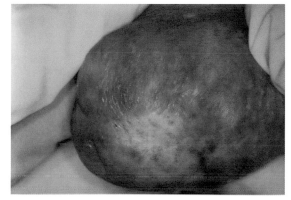

Deformity of the glans secondary to lichen sclerosus.

Plate 3 (Figure 15-4)

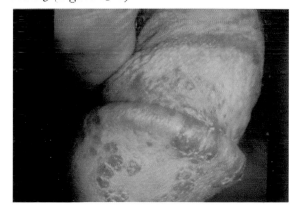

Penile psoriasis.

Plate 4 (Figure 15-5)

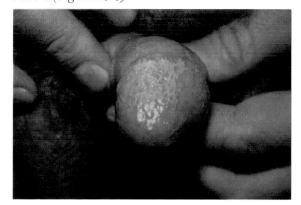

Lichen planus in an uncircumcised male.

Plate 29 (Figure 15-34)

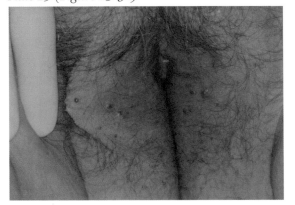

Vulvar angiokeratomas.

Plate 30 (Figure 15-35)

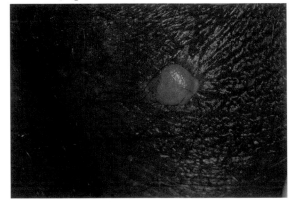

Pyogenic granuloma.

Plate 31 (Figure 15-36)

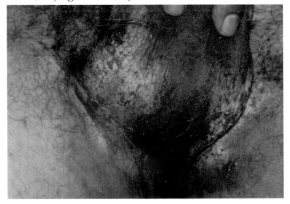

Extramammary Paget's disease.

Plate 32 (Figure 15-37)

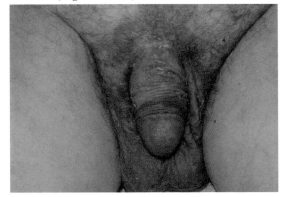

Extramammary Paget's disease.

signs of infection, such as fever, leukocytosis, or pyuria/bacteriuria, mandates urgent decompression of the collecting system because of the risk of pyonephrosis. The optimal choice of drainage, whether placement of a percutaneous nephrostomy tube or retrograde ureteral catheterization, is controversial. Percutaneous drainage offers the advantage of a larger, external drainage tube that can be monitored for output and irrigated in the event of obstruction. Alternatively, internal drainage with a ureteral stent is less cumbersome for the patient.

A prospective, randomized trial comparing the two methods of renal drainage showed no advantage of one modality over the other in terms of length of time to clinical improvement, but percutaneous nephrostomy was less costly.[16] Whichever method of drainage is chosen, it should be performed without delay. Broad-spectrum antimicrobial agents should be initiated promptly after obtaining a voided urine specimen for culture. A specimen of urine from the obstructed kidney should be sent at the time of decompression as well. Placement of a Foley catheter facilitates optimal urinary drainage, particularly in the case of a ureteral stent.

With the exception of urgent stent placement, immediate definitive surgical intervention is rarely necessary. However, timely surgical intervention is indicated in the patient in whom the stone is unlikely to pass spontaneously (diameter >6 mm), who experiences recurrent renal colic or has persistent high-grade obstruction (>1 week), or in whom occupational requirements mandate prompt treatment (e.g., airline pilots).

HOSPITALIZATION

The need for hospitalization in a patient with renal colic without signs of infection depends on the ability to achieve adequate pain relief with oral narcotic analgesics and to retain fluids without vomiting. Patients requiring continued intravenous narcotics and fluids or those with a solitary kidney (in whom urgent decompression of the collecting system is required) should be admitted to the hospital for pain control, intravenous fluids, and antiemetics.

OBSERVATION

Most ureteral calculi will pass spontaneously without the need for surgical intervention, and thus conservative management is indicated in select patients. The probability of spontaneous passage depends on stone size, the location of the stone at the time of diagnosis, and urinary tract anatomy. Small stones, regardless of their position in the urinary tract, are likely to pass spontaneously; on the other hand large stones (>6 mm) rarely pass spontaneously. Stones in the distal ureter are more likely to pass than proximally located stones. A literature review estimated rates of spontaneous passage at 12%, 22%, and 45% for stones in the proximal, middle, and distal ureter, respectively.[17] The presence of obstruction distal to the stone, such as a ureteral stricture, precludes the possibility of spontaneous passage and mandates surgical intervention.

Surgical Treatment

Determination of the optimal surgical therapy for a renal or ureteral calculus depends on the size, location, and composition of the stone and the anatomy of the collecting system and ureter. For renal stones, indications for treatment include large size, persistent pain, location in the renal pelvis where the potential for obstruction is high, and associated infection or loss of renal function. Treatment of asymptomatic calyceal stones is controversial; safe and efficacious minimally invasive surgical treatments have led some to believe that all stones should be treated prophylactically because of the likelihood of future problems. Patients with asymptomatic stones that are managed with observation and medical therapy should be treated surgically if the stone grows while on medical prophylaxis. Branched, staghorn calculi should always be managed surgically because of the potential for loss of renal function and the risk of life-threatening infection if left untreated. Formal assessment of renal function with a radionuclide renal study may be indicated in cases of marginal renal function due to long-standing obstruction. A differential function of the stone-bearing kidney of less than 20% suggests that nephrectomy rather than stone removal may be appropriate.

Options for surgical management of urinary tract stones include noninvasive, minimally invasive, and open surgical approaches. Open surgery is reserved for complex stones with extensive anatomic abnormalities requiring collecting system reconstruction, or for stones that have failed all less invasive approaches. However, more than 99% of stones can be managed with minimally invasive means including shock-wave lithotripsy (SWL), ureteroscopy, percutaneous nephrostolithotomy (PCNL), and in rare cases, laparoscopic uretero- or pyelolithotomy.

SHOCK-WAVE LITHOTRIPSY

The application of shock waves to urinary tract stones to effect fragmentation is based on acoustical physics. Stone fragments created by repeated firing of shock waves focused on the primary target stone pass spontaneously in the urine over time. Since the introduction of the technology in 1980,[18] shock-wave lithotripsy (SWL) has become the treatment of choice for most renal and ureteral calculi. Most patients undergoing SWL are treated as outpatients and return to work within 1 to 2 days. Complications associated with SWL are few and are usually related to problems with passage of stone fragments or due to direct injury to the kidney. Gross hematuria is common for a few days after lithotripsy; however, clinically significant hemorrhage occurs in less than 1% of cases.[19] There is controversy regarding long-term sequelae of SWL such as hypertension, but to date no compelling evidence has clearly established a link between SWL and hypertension.

Success rates for SWL approach 70% overall but depend on stone size, location, and composition.[20] Stone-free rates vary inversely with stone size and generally drop off substantially for stones greater than 2 cm in diameter. Likewise, complication rates and the need for ancillary procedures, such as ureteral stent placement or percutaneous nephrostomy, increase with stone size.

Incomplete stone fragmentation or fragmentation of a large stone burden may result in the accumulation of stone fragments in the ureter (steinstrasse). Although many steinstrasse resolve spontaneously, others require drainage with a percutaneous nephrostomy tube and subsequent endoscopic stone fragmentation or repeat SWL to clear stone fragments.

Stone location influences outcomes as well; higher success rates are achieved with renal pelvic stones than with calyceal stones.[21] The lower-pole calyces represent a unique anatomic location in the kidney for SWL; the dependent position of the lower-pole calyces hinders clearance of stone fragments. A meta-analysis in which stone-free rates for SWL and PCNL were stratified by stone size revealed an overall stone-free rate of only 59% for SWL compared to 91% for PCNL.[22] A prospective, randomized trial comparing SWL to PCNL for management of lower-pole stones validated the meta-analysis results and showed an even more pronounced discrepancy in outcomes favoring PCNL over SWL.[23] Consequently, SWL is reserved for only small (≤1 cm) lower-pole stones.

Stone composition influences SWL success. Hard stones, such as calcium oxalate monohydrate, fragment less efficiently than soft stones such calcium oxalate dihydrate.[24] Cystine stones are relatively resistant to shock waves, and consequently endoscopic removal with the use of intracorporeal lithotripsy is recommended.[25]

Stones in all locations in the ureter may be successfully treated with SWL. Modifications in patient positioning may be necessary to facilitate stone targeting and allow unimpeded transmission of the shock waves to the stone without encountering bone. The need to place a ureteral stent to bypass the stone is controversial, but at least for proximal ureteral stones has been shown to be unnecessary.[26–28]

Although SWL has revolutionized the surgical management of stone disease, the limitations of the technology are only now being defined. SWL is most successful for renal and ureteral calculi less than 2.5 cm and 1.5 cm, respectively, that have no associated distal anatomic obstruction. Cystine stones, large or complex stones, and lower-pole stones larger than 1 cm are best managed endoscopically. Obese patients pose a special problem for SWL; weight limitations on the gantry or table, difficulty visualizing the stone, and inability to position the stone at the shock wave focal point may preclude successful shockwave treatment, and for these patients endoscopic stone management is often required.

PERCUTANEOUS NEPHROSTOLITHOTOMY

For large or complex stones, or for stones associated with distal obstruction such as stones in a kidney with congenital ureteropelvic junction obstruction, an antegrade endoscopic approach is indicated. Percutaneous nephrostolithotomy (PCNL) involves percutaneous passage of an endoscope directly into the collecting system of the kidney through a small incision in the flank. Small stones may be retrieved intact; larger stones are fragmented using a variety of intracorporeal lithotripsy devices, and the fragments are aspirated or grasped and removed, leaving no fragments to pass spontaneously.

PCNL is performed under general anesthesia, and usually involves a 2 to 4-day hospital stay. The most common complication associated with PCNL is bleeding; the average decrease in hemoglobin is 1.2 to 2.8 g/dL.[29] In less than 1% of cases, pseudoaneurysm formation necessitates arterial embolism or rarely open exploration. Access-related injuries to adjacent structures most commonly involve the pleural space, increasing the risk of hydrothorax. Less commonly, injury to the colon, spleen, liver, or duodenum occurs, but can usually be managed conservatively. Unlike SWL, stone-free rates for PCNL are independent of stone size or location. Stone-free rates of 70% to 100% are typical.[20] PCNL can be performed in conjunction with endoscopic reconstructive procedures in the kidney such as endoscopic incision

of congenital ureteropelvic junction narrowing, ureteral stricture, or calyceal diverticulum.

The American Urological Association Nephrolithiasis Clinical Guidelines Panel pronounced PCNL, with the addition of SWL and repeat PCNL as needed, as optimal first-line treatment for staghorn calculi (Fig. 16–4).[30] In some cases, multiple percutaneous accesses into the kidney are required in order to access and remove all the stone. The use of SWL to clear residual fragments remote from the nephrostomy tract has been advocated as an adjunct to PCNL; however, a trend toward repeat endoscopic procedures to definitively remove residual fragments has decreased the use of SWL in this setting.

URETEROSCOPY

Ureteral and some renal calculi may be treated by a retrograde endoscopic approach using a

Figure 16–4

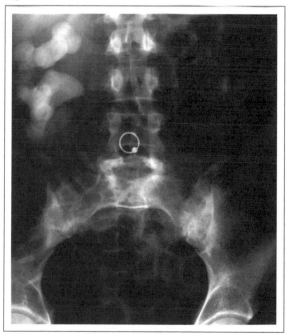

Massive complete right staghorn calculus and faintly opacified left staghorn calculus.

small-caliber semirigid or actively deflectable flexible ureteroscope (Fig. 16–5). With current technology, virtually the entire urinary tract may be accessed with a ureteroscope. A variety of intracorporeal lithotripsy devices with small-caliber, flexible probes are available for stone fragmentation through the ureteroscope (laser, electrohydraulic, or pneumatic lithotripsy devices). Likewise, multipronged graspers and baskets are available to retrieve intact stones or fragments from the ureter. After complete stone fragmentation, the ureteroscope is withdrawn from the ureter. Ureteroscopy is usually performed as an outpatient procedure. Complications of ureteroscopy are few, and include ureteral perforation and late ureteral stricture formation, both of which occur with a frequency of less than 2%.

LAPAROSCOPIC STONE REMOVAL

Laparoscopic stone removal is an alternative to open surgery as a "salvage" procedure in the rare event that endoscopic procedures fail. The safety and feasibility of laparoscopic ureterolithotomy

Figure 16–5

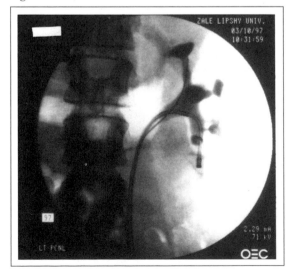

Small-diameter, actively deflectable, flexible ureteroscope advanced onto a stone in a lower pole calyx.

and pyelolithotomy have been demonstrated in anecdotal reports in the literature.[31,32]

Medical Evaluation and Management

Despite advances in endoscopic technology that have reduced the morbidity and increased the safety of endoscopic stone removal, the role of a medical prophylactic program remains undiminished. The natural history of stone disease is unchanged by surgical therapy; indeed, the risk of stone recurrence after SWL is greater for patients not treated with medical therapy compared to those undergoing targeted medical treatment.[33]

PATIENT SELECTION

One of the controversies regarding medical management of stone disease surrounds patient selection. High-risk patients such as those with recurrent, active stone disease, or first-time stone formers with a family history of stones, medical risk factors, or nephrocalcinosis clearly warrant evaluation for medical treatment. However, the need for evaluation and treatment of first-time stone formers without obvious risk factors is debatable. A favorable response to simple conservative measures such as increased fluid intake and dietary moderation supports a selective approach to first-time stone formers.[34,35] However, a 50% rate of recurrence for first-time stone formers within 5 years of the first stone event is compelling evidence for evaluation of all patients after their first stone episode.[5,36] Indeed, the profile of metabolic abnormalities of first-time stone formers is no different than that of recurrent stone formers.[37]

EVALUATION

HISTORY A variety of medical conditions are associated with an increased risk of stone formation, and these disorders should be elicited. Chronic diarrheal syndrome due to gastrointestinal disease or surgery (intestinal resection, intestinal bypass, Crohn's disease, ulcerative colitis, pancreatic insufficiency, sprue) may be associated with uric acid or calcium oxalate stones as a result of dehydration, metabolic acidosis, and hyperoxaluria. Likewise, gout may be associated with uric acid or calcium oxalate stone formation on the basis of hyperuricosuria and/or low urine pH. Both hyperthyroidism and hyperparathyroidism are associated with hypercalciuria. In the presence of brain tumors or peptic ulcer disease, hyperparathyroidism may be a manifestation of multiple endocrine neoplasia syndrome. Recurrent urinary tract infections with urease-producing organisms such as *Proteus, Klebsiella,* or *Pseudomonas* cause an alkaline urine environment conducive to struvite stone formation.

MEDICATION HISTORY   The use of stone-provoking medications should be elicited from the history. Calcium supplements or vitamin D, commonly prescribed for prevention of osteoporosis, may cause hypercalciuria. Acetazolamide, a carbonic anhydrase inhibitor, causes metabolic acidosis and consequently hypocitraturia, low urine pH, and hypercalciuria. Large doses of vitamin C (more than 1 g daily), which is metabolized to oxalate, may cause hyperoxaluria.

DIETARY HISTORY   A dietary history should quantify fluid intake and identify environmental risk factors for stone formation such as dehydration, salt abuse, a high-calcium or oxalate diet, or overindulgence in animal protein.

SIMPLIFIED EVALUATION   The choice of a simplified versus detailed metabolic evaluation depends on the risk category and motivation of the patient. Identification of a positive family history of stones or medical conditions predisposing to stone formation should prompt a detailed metabolic evaluation. On the other hand, for first-time stone formers without obvious risk factors, a simplified evaluation may suffice. However, an extensive outpatient evaluation identifies metabolic abnormalities in 90% to 95% of patients compared with only 68% or 75% of patients evaluated with 1 or 2, 24-hour urine collections, respectively.[38,39]

A simplified evaluation includes a medical and dietary history, serum chemistries, urinalysis, a plain abdominal radiograph, a stone analysis, and a single 24-hour urine collection. The serum chemistry profile may identify systemic abnormalities such as hypercalcemia due to hyperparathyroidism, hyperurisemia associated with gout or hyperchloremia, hypokalemia and low serum bicarbonate associated with distal renal tubular acidosis. Microscopic analysis of the urine may reveal crystals indicative of the underlying disorder, such as hexagonal cystine crystals in cystinuria. Pyuria and bacteriuria suggest urinary tract infection that may be associated with struvite stones. Extremes of urine pH may reveal a propensity for struvite stones (pH >7.5) or uric acid or calcium oxalate stones (pH<5.5). In some cases, knowledge of the stone composition provides a diagnosis of the primary metabolic derangement; cystine stones reflect cystinuria, uric acid stones occur only in an acid urine, and struvite stones indicate infection with urea-splitting bacteria.

A standardized battery of biochemical assays and physicochemical measurements can be applied to a single 24-hour urine collection to identify risk factors for stone disease using a variety of available kits that facilitate urine collection and analysis. The collected urine is stored in a container with an appropriate preservative, and a well-mixed aliquot of the preserved urine is sent in a specimen container to a central laboratory for measurement of urinary biochemical parameters. Metabolic (calcium, oxalate, uric acid, citrate, and pH) and environmental (total volume, sodium, sulfate, phosphorus, and magnesium) risk factors as well as physicochemical risk factors (urinary saturation of stone-forming salts) are analyzed and graphically displayed.

EXTENSIVE EVALUATION   The extensive ambulatory evaluation includes 2, 24-hour urine collections with the patient on his or her usual diet and fluid intake followed by a single 24-hour urine collection after a week-long diet restricted in sodium (100 mEq/day), calcium (400 mg/day), and oxalate (limited intake of dark green leafy vegetables such as spinach and broccoli, nuts, brewed tea, and chocolate). The restricted diet facilitates identification of hypercalciuria and enables distinction of hypercalciuria subtypes. Additionally, environmental risk factors may be identified by comparison of urinary biochemical parameters from a random and restricted diet.

A fasting and calcium load test is performed by collecting a 2-hour urine specimen after an overnight fast, followed by a 4-hour urine sample after ingestion of 1 g calcium in a liquid synthetic diet. A urinary calcium/creatinine ratio measured after both the fast and the load can distinguish the various etiologies of hypercalciuria.

The 24-hour urine collections are analyzed for total volume, pH (by pH electrode), creatinine, sodium, potassium, calcium, magnesium, phosphorus, citrate, uric acid, oxalate, and sulfate. The adequacy of the urine collection is assessed by measuring urine creatinine with respect to body weight; the average daily creatinine level for women is 17.2 mg/kg and for men is 22.1 mg/kg. Serum chemistries are obtained after the random urine collections and after a week of dietary restriction and include calcium, phosphorus, magnesium, sodium, potassium, bicarbonate, creatinine, chloride, uric acid, and alkaline phosphatase. Thyroid function tests and lipid profiles are optional. Blood is measured for serum immunoreactive PTH after the overnight fast. Urine is evaluated microscopically and a qualitative cystine determination is made. Bone mineral densities measured at the spine, hip, and forearm assess bone loss prior to consideration of calcium restriction.

Diagnosis

Diagnostic criteria for the primary causes of stone disease are summarized in Table 16–2.

HYPERCALCIURIA   Hypercalciuria is the end result of a variety of pathophysiologic disorders. Absorptive hypercalciuria (AH), the most common form of hypercalciuria, is due to intestinal overabsorption of calcium with consequent hypercalciuria and suppression of parathyroid function. AH is clas-

sified as type I or type II based on the response to a low-calcium diet; hypercalciuria persists despite dietary restriction in type I but not type II. Both forms are characterized by normal serum calcium and phosphorus, normal or suppressed serum immunoreactive PTH, normal or slightly high fasting urinary calcium (<0.11 mg/100 mL glomerular filtration), and increased urinary calcium (>0.2 mg/mg creatinine) after an oral calcium load.[40]

Renal hypercalciuria (RH) is due to impaired renal tubular calcium reabsorption, leading to calcium loss and secondary hyperparathyroidism. Normocalcemia, elevated PTH, and high fasting urinary calcium characterize RH.

Primary hyperparathyroidism, the most common form of resorptive hypercalciuria, is a relatively rare cause of hypercalciuria. Excessive secretion of PTH from a parathyroid adenoma leads to bone resorption and increased renal synthesis of 1,25-$(OH)_2$D, which in turn enhances intestinal absorption of calcium; the net effect is an elevated serum and urine calcium. Primary hyperparathyroidism is recognized by hypercalcemia, hypophosphatemia, inappropriately high serum PTH, and hypercalciuria.

HYPERURICOSURIA   Hyperuricosuria, defined as urinary uric acid greater than 600 mg/day, predisposes to calcium oxalate or uric acid stone formation as a result of supersaturation of the urine with respect to monosodium urate or uric acid.[41] The most common cause of hyperuricosuria is a purine-rich diet. At a pH below 5.5, the undissociated form of uric acid predominates, leading to uric acid stone formation, while at a pH above 5.5, sodium urate formation promotes calcium oxalate stone formation through heterologous nucleation.

HYPOCITRATURIA   Citrate inhibits calcium stone formation by complexing with calcium, thereby reducing urinary saturation of calcium oxalate and calcium phosphate. Citrate also directly inhibits calcium oxalate and calcium phosphate crystal growth.[42]

Table 16–2

Diagnostic Criteria for Primary Causes of Calcium Stone Formation

	SERUM			URINE					
	CALCIUM	PHOSPHORUS	PTH	RESTRICTED DIET CALCIUM	FASTING CALCIUM[a]	POST-LOAD CALCIUM[b]	URIC ACID	OXALATE	CITRATE
Absorptive hypercalciuria I	nl	nl	nl	↑	nl/↑	↑	nl	nl	nl
Absorptive hypercalciuria II	nl	nl	nl	nl	nl	↑	nl	nl	nl
Renal hypercalciuria	nl	nl	↑	↑	↑	↑	nl	nl	nl
Hyperparathyroidism	↑	↓	↑	↑	↑	↑	nl	nl	nl
Hyperuricosuric calcium	nl	nl	nl	nl	nl	nl	↑	nl	nl
Hypocitraturic calcium	nl	nl	nl	nl	nl	nl	nl	nl	↓
Renal tubular acidosis	nl	nl	nl	nl/↑	↑	nl	nl	nl	↓
Enteric hyperoxaluria	nl	nl	nl/↑	nl	nl	nl	nl	↑	↓
Gouty diathesis	nl	nl	nl	nl	nl	nl	nl/↑	nl	nl

[a] Fasting urinary calcium is obtained after an overnight fast.

[b] Post-load urinary calcium is obtained 4 hours after ingestion of a 1-g oral calcium load.

Hypocitraturia (citrate <320 mg/day) may represent an isolated abnormality, but more commonly it occurs in association with a variety of disorders that have as a common endpoint, acidosis. Acidosis enhances citrate reabsorption while alkalosis promotes citrate excretion. Distal renal tubular acidosis (RTA) is characterized by a high urinary pH (>6.8), high serum chloride, and low serum potassium and bicarbonate. RTA is confirmed by demonstrating an inability of the urine to acidify in response to an ammonium chloride load. Chronic diarrheal states produce hypocitraturia by inducing systemic acidosis as a result of intestinal alkali loss in stool. Thiazide-induced hypocitraturia is associated with hypokalemia and intracellular acidosis.

HYPEROXALURIA Hyperoxaluria (oxalate >40 mg/day) may be due to high substrate availability (vitamin C), increased oxalate production due to enzymatic derangements in the biosynthetic pathway of glyoxalate (primary oxalosis), or increased intestinal absorption (enteric hyperoxaluria). The most common etiology is enteric hyperoxaluria, which is associated with inflammatory small bowel disease or intestinal bypass surgery or resection. The mechanism of increased oxalate absorption is twofold. First, poorly absorbed bile salts and fatty acids may increase colonic mucosal permeability to oxalate.[43] Second, intestinal fat malabsorption enhances complexation of fatty acids with divalent cations (calcium, magnesium) in the intestinal lumen, thereby reducing binding with oxalate and increasing the pool of free oxalate available for absorption.[44] Intestinal disease is also associated with other abnormalities predisposing to stone formation, such as dehydration, acidosis, and hypocitraturia.

GOUTY DIATHESIS Gouty diathesis describes a stone-forming propensity characterized by low urinary pH (<5.5) of unclear etiology, which may or may not be associated with gouty arthritis. At a urine pH <5.5, the undissociated form of uric acid predominates and predisposes to both uric acid and calcium oxalate stone formation.

CYSTINURIA Cystinuria is an inherited transport disorder that results in excessive urinary excretion of dibasic amino acids (cystine, ornithine, lysine, and argenine). Cystine stone formation is a consequence of the low solubility of cystine in urine (250 mg/L), which is determined by pH and the presence of urinary electrolytes and macromolecules.[45]

INFECTION STONES The formation of magnesium ammonium phosphate, or struvite stones, is due to chronic infection with urea-splitting organisms (*Proteus, Pseudomonas, Klebsiella*). Urease catalyzes the hydrolysis of urea, leading to ammonium production and alkaline urine, which favors precipitation of magnesium, ammonium, and phosphate.

Algorithm for Metabolic Evaluation

An algorithm for metabolic evaluation is shown in Figs. 16–6 and 16–7. Note that dehydration may be a factor for all stone compositions. Further, the risk factors are not mutually exclusive, and a stone-forming patient may have several risk factors.

Treatment

Table 16-3 summarizes the treatment regimens for metabolic abnormalities.

CONSERVATIVE THERAPY

Conservative dietary therapy entails increased fluid intake and dietary modification. Increased fluid intake (most importantly water) increases urinary output and lowers urinary saturation of stone-forming salts.[34,46] Conservative therapy alone is often effective in reducing the incidence of stone recurrence, but should always accompany directed medical therapy for patients in whom specific metabolic abnormalities are identified. A high fluid intake to ensure a daily urine output of over 2 L is recommended for all forms of nephrolithiasis. Moderate dietary calcium restriction (400 to 600 mg daily) is recommended only

Figure 16–6

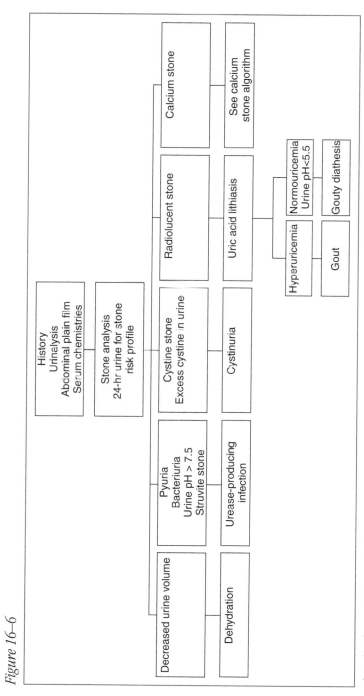

Algorithm for metabolic evaluation.

Figure 16–7

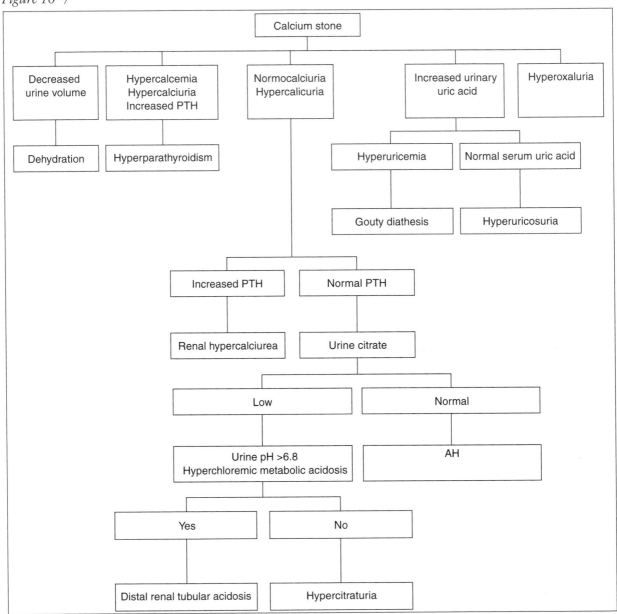

Algorithm for calcium stone metabolic evaluation.

Table 16–3

Selective Medical Treatment Regimens Based on Underlying Metabolic Abnormalities

INDICATION	TREATMENT	PHYSIOLOGIC ACTION	PHYSICOCHEMICAL ACTION
Absorptive hypercalciuria I	Thiazides	↓Urinary calcium (transient effect)	↓Urinary saturation of calcium salts
	Potassium citrate	↓Urinary citrate ↑Urinary citrate	↑Inhibitor activity ↓Urinary saturation of calcium salts
	Sodium cellulose phosphate	↓Urinary calcium ↓Intestinal calcium absorption ↓Urinary calcium	↓Urinary saturation of calcium salts
Absorptive hypercalciuria II	Low-calcium diet	↓Intestinal calcium absorption ↓Urinary calcium	↓Urinary saturation of calcium salts
Renal hypercalciuria	Thiazides	↓Urinary calcium (sustained effect) ↓Intestinal calcium absorption (indirect effect)	↓Urinary saturation of calcium salts
Hyperuricosuric calcium nephrolithiasis	Allopurinol Potassium citrate	↓Urinary uric acid ↑Urinary citrate	↓Urate-induced crystallization of calcium salts ↓Urinary saturation of calcium salts ↓Urate-induced crystallization of calcium salts
Hypocitraturic calcium nephrolithiasis	Potassium citrate	↑Urinary citrate ↑Urinary pH	↑Inhibitor activity ↓Urinary saturation of calcium salts
Enteric hyperoxaluria	Low-oxalate diet Potassium citrate	↓Urinary oxalate ↑Urinary citrate	↓Urinary saturation of calcium oxalate ↑Inhibitor activity
	Calcium citrate	↑Urinary citrate ↓Urinary oxalate	↓Urinary saturation of calcium oxalate ↑Inhibitor activity ↓Urinary saturation of calcium oxalate
	Magnesium gluconate	↑Urinary magnesium	↓Urinary saturation of calcium oxalate
Gouty diathesis	Potassium citrate	↑Urinary citrate ↑Urinary pH	↓Urinary saturation of calcium oxalate ↓Urinary saturation of uric acid ↓Undissociated uric acid
Cystinuria	D-penicillamine or α-mercaptopropionylglycine	Forms mixed disulfide bond with cystine ↓Urinary cystine	↓Urinary saturation of cystine
Infection stones	Acetohydroxamic acid	↓Activity of urease ↑Urinary pH ↓Urinary ammonium	↓Urinary saturation of struvite

for AH patients with normal bone density. Salt abuse is associated with hypercalciuria and hypocitraturia and leads to increased of saturation monosodium urate. Consequently, moderate salt restriction (100 mEq daily) is advisable.

A diet high in animal protein provides an acid ash and purine load, which increases the risk of hyperuricosuria, hypocitraturia, and low urine pH. Mild restriction of animal proteins may be beneficial in patients with uric acid or calcium oxalate stones. Lastly, restriction of oxalate-rich foods, particularly for patients with enteric hyperoxaluria, may reduce urinary oxalate. Foods containing high levels of oxalate include brewed tea, chocolate, nuts, and dark green leafy vegetables such as spinach and broccoli.

HYPERCALCIURIA

The mechanism responsible for intestinal hyperabsorption of calcium is unknown; consequently, treatment of AH is aimed at increasing renal calcium reabsorption. Thiazide diuretics have no effect on intestinal calcium absorption, but act directly at the distal renal tubule to stimulate calcium reabsorption. In addition, thiazides act indirectly at the proximal tubule to enhance calcium reabsorption there as well. Although thiazides have a sustained hypocalciuric effect in patients with RH, the effect in patients with AH is lost after 18 to 24 months of treatment.[47]

A variety of thiazide diuretics are available for use in AH, including trichlormethiazide (4 mg/day) or hydrochlorothiazide (25 to 50 mg/day). A nonthiazide diuretic, indapamide (2.5 to 5 mg/day), has a similar mechanism of action.[48] To counteract thiazide-induced hypokalemia and hypocitraturia, supplementation with potassium citrate (10 to 20 mEq twice daily) is recommended. For patients in whom the hypocalciuric action of thiazides is lost, a brief (6 months) drug holiday and substitution with an alternative form of therapy is recommended before resuming the thiazide.

Sodium cellulose phosphate (10 to 15 g/day with meals) is a nonabsorbable ion-exchange resin that binds intraluminal intestinal calcium, thereby reducing calcium availability for absorption. Sodium cellulose phosphate may induce hypomagnesemia by complexing intestinal magnesium. Likewise, complexation with calcium and other divalent cations in the intestine may promote hyperoxaluria by increasing oxalate availability. A word of caution: sodium cellulose phosphate may lead to a negative calcium balance by stimulating parathyroid function. Accordingly, use of the drug should be limited to patients with severe AH and *normal* bone density.

AH patients who normalize urinary calcium in response to a low-calcium diet (AH-II) may be treated with mild dietary calcium restriction (400 to 600 mg/day) if they have normal bone density. However, in patients with evidence of bone loss, a liberalized dairy intake and initiation of a thiazide diuretic may be prudent.

The treatment of primary hyperparathyroidism is surgical; parathyroidectomy results in normalization of urinary and serum calcium and a subsequent reduction in stone formation.[49] In some cases, estrogen administration in postmenopausal women may counteract the effect of primary hyperparathyroidism and obviate the need for surgery.[50]

HYPERURICOSURIA

Allopurinol (300 mg/day) is a xanthine oxidase inhibitor that prevents the conversion of hypoxanthine to xanthine and ultimately to uric acid. Relatively few side effects are associated with allopurinol administration; however, the occurrence of a skin rash should prompt immediate discontinuation of the drug because of the risk of progression to Stevens–Johnson syndrome. Elevation of liver enzymes may occur, but is usually reversible upon discontinuation of the drug.

HYPOCITRATURIA

Hypocitraturia is treated with potassium citrate at a starting dose of 40 to 60 mEq daily in divided doses. Administration of potassium citrate delivers an alkali load that enhances urinary citrate excretion and increases renal calcium reabsorption.[51] In patients unable to tolerate potassium citrate, sodium citrate or sodium bicarbonate provide an alternative therapy; however, the sodium-induced increase in urinary calcium and monosodium urate may counteract the beneficial effect of the increased inhibitory activity.

HYPEROXALURIA

In patients with enteric hyperoxaluria due to intestinal disease, calcium supplementation may be beneficial. Direct binding of oxalate by calcium reduces the availability of oxalate for absorption. As such, calcium should be administered with meals to optimize oxalate binding. Careful monitoring of urinary calcium is advised in order to identify hypercalciuria, which is usually rare in these patients, who often have markedly low baseline urinary calcium.

Potassium citrate therapy corrects hypocitraturia and low urinary pH that often accompanies intestinal malabsorption. Likewise, magnesium supplementation may correct hypomagnesiuria; however, magnesium may exacerbate diarrhea, attenuating any beneficial effect.

Pyridoxine (vitamin B₆) supplementation reduces the production of oxalate by enhancing conversion of glyoxalate to glycine, reducing the substrate available for conversion to oxalate. Although pyridoxine administration may be beneficial for primary hyperoxaluria, it plays a limited role in enteric hyperoxaluria because most of the urinary oxalate derives from dietary oxalate and only a small proportion originates from the metabolic pathway.

GOUTY DIATHESIS

The low urine pH characteristic of gouty diathesis responds well to potassium citrate (30 to 60 mEq daily in 2 or 3 divided doses). The rise in urinary pH favors the dissociated form of uric acid and prevents uric acid stone formation. Calcium oxalate stone formation is prevented as well by citrate-induced inhibition of calcium oxalate crystallization and the decrease in calcium oxalate saturation due to complexation with calcium.

CYSTINURIA

The goal of therapy for cystinuria is to increase cystine solubility and reduce the risk of cystine stone formation. High fluid intake is critical in maintaining a cystine concentration below the solubility limit; however, the solubility of cystine varies according to pH. Alkali therapy is aimed at producing a urine pH between 6.5 and 7.0; at higher urine pH, the risk of calcium phosphate stone formation increases. Potassium citrate (30 to 60 mEq/day in divided doses) effectively alkalinizes the urine to a modest degree.

When fluid and alkali therapy are inadequate in controlling cystine stone formation, the addition of a chelating agent such as D-penicillamine or tiopronin (α-mercaptopropionylglycine) will reduce cystine excretion. The free sulphydryl group of these agents undergoes a thiol–sulphydryl exchange with cystine, producing a more soluble complex. Tiopronin (800 to 2000 mg/day in 3 or 4 divided doses) is better tolerated than D-penicillamine, but is itself associated with side effects such as pancytopenia and nephrotic syndrome.

INFECTION STONES

The mainstay of therapy for infection stones is surgical removal of the stones and eradication of urea-splitting organisms. In limited cases, sterilization of the urine after SWL for patients with residual fragments is possible with the use of long-term antibiotics.[52] The use of acetohydroxamic acid, a urease inhibitor, prevents formation of struvite stones, but its use if limited due to frequent side effects.

Education

Although surgical advances in the management of stone disease receive attention in the lay press, medical breakthroughs in stone prophylaxis receive little attention. Clinicians are often uncomfortable with the evaluation and medical management of stone disease and fail to make an effort to identify underlying metabolic derangements responsible for stone formation and to initiate medical treatment. All patients should be informed of the option of medical evaluation and management, and at the very least should undergo a limited evaluation for systemic causes of stone disease and be advised of conservative dietary measurements.

Errors

One of the most serious errors in the management of stone disease is failure to diagnose and promptly treat a stone associated with obstructive pyelonephritis. When a patient with known stone disease is diagnosed with acute pyelonephritis, an imaging study should be obtained to identify an obstructing stone as the potential source of infection, even in the absence of classic signs of an acute stone. Likewise, imaging should be performed in a patient without known stone disease diagnosed with acute pyelonephritis, if he or she fails to respond appropriately to antibiotics.

Unfortunately, consultation with a urologist often occurs only after the patient becomes seriously ill during admission to the hospital for presumed uncomplicated pyelonephritis, and treatment of obstructive pyelonephritis is substantially delayed. If an obstructing stone is identified, prompt decompression of the collecting system with a percutaneous nephrostomy tube or ureteral stent is mandatory to relieve the obstruction and prevent progression to sepsis.

Controversies

SURGICAL MANAGEMENT

One of the current controversies in the surgical management of stones involves the optimal therapy for distal ureteral stones. Both SWL and ureteroscopy are highly efficacious and associated with few complications. Proponents of SWL cite the noninvasive nature of the procedure, the need for minimal anesthesia, and the rapid convales-

cence. Advocates of ureteroscopy argue that the procedure is nearly 100% effective and is associated with less uncertainty of fragment passage compared to SWL. Currently two prospective, randomized trials are underway to compare the efficacy and patient satisfaction for the two treatment modalities in patients with distal ureteral stones.

Technological advances in ureteroscope design and instrumentation have enabled access and treatment of stones in virtually all locations in the kidney and ureter. Consequently, some authors have advocated the use of endoscopy over shock-wave lithotripsy for all upper urinary tract stones. Ongoing studies comparing efficacy and morbidity of the two modalities will help direct practitioners in their choice of surgical treatment.

MEDICAL THERAPY

The need for medical evaluation and management of stone-forming patients is controversial. Ready access to noninvasive and minimally invasive surgical modalities has led some to disparage the role of medical therapy. However, Parks and Coe estimated that a medical preventative program would result in cost savings of $3226 per patient/year compared with patients not treated medically.[4] Moreover, a meta-analysis of randomized, controlled clinical trials evaluating the efficacy of drug treatment for the prevention of stone recurrence confirmed the benefit of treatment in lowering the incidence of stone recurrence and validated the use of medical therapy for stone metaphylaxis.[53]

Emerging Concepts

Surgical treatment of stone disease has progressed at a rapid pace over the last two decades. Currently, over 85% of stones can be treated noninvasively. However, an increasing trend toward endoscopic management of renal and ureteral calculi as a result of improved technology, along with relatively few improvements in shock-wave lithotripsy technology, may in some ways represent a technologic step backward toward greater invasiveness.

Our focus for the future should be on prevention of stone recurrence. Clinical trials evaluating the efficacy of new drugs for stone prevention are often poorly designed and nonuniform, making comparison between drug treatments problematic. Guidelines for standardization of trial design and primary outcomes should facilitate evaluation of new drugs and encourage future drug development.

References

1. Johnson CM, Wilson DM, O'Fallon WM, et al: Renal stone epidemiology: A 25 year study in Rochester, Minnesota. *Kidney Int* 16:624–631, 1979.

2. Marshall V, White RH, Chaput de Saintonage M, et al: The natural history of renal and ureteric calculi. *Br J Urol* 47:117–124, 1975.

3. Glowacki LS, Beecroft ML, Cook RJ, et al: The natural history of asymptomatic urolithiasis. *J Urol* 147:319–321, 1992.

4. Parks JH, Coe FL: The financial effects of kidney stone prevention. *Kidney Int* 50:1706–1712, 1996.

5. Blacklock NJ: The pattern of urolithiasis in the Royal Navy. In Hodgkinson A, Nordin BEC (eds): *Renal Stone Research Symposium*. London, Churchill, 1969, p 33.

6. Sarmina I, Spirmak JP, Resnick MI: Urinary lithiasis in the black population: An epidemiological study and review of the literature. *J Urol* 138:14–17, 1987.

7. Michaels IK, Nakagawa Y, Miura N, et al: Racial variation in gender frequency of calcium urolithiasis. *J Urol* 152:2228–2232, 1994.

8. Rous SN: A review of 171 consecutive patients with urinary lithiasis. *J Urol* 126:376–379, 1981.

9. Dalrymple NC, Verga M, Anderson KR, et al: The value of unenhanced helical computerized tomography in the management of acute flank pain. *J Urol* 159:735–740, 1998.

10. Smith RC, Verga M, Dalrymple N, et al: Acute ureteral obstruction: Value of secondary signs of helical unenhanced CT. *AJR* 167:1109–1113, 1996.

11. Chen MY, Sagoria RJ: Can noncontrast helical computed tomography replace intravenous urography for evaluation of patients with acute urinary tract colic? *J Emerg Med* 17:299–303, 1999.

12. El-Sherif AE, Salem M, Yahia H, et al: Treatment of renal colic by desmopressin intranasal spray and diclofenac sodium. *J Urol* 153:1395–1398, 1995.

13. Flannigan GM, Clifford RPC, Carver RA, et al: Indomethacin; an alternative to pethidine in ureteral colic. *Br J Urol* 55:6–9, 1983.

14. Borghi L, Meschi T, Amato F, et al: Nifedipine and methylprednisolone in facilitating ureteral stone passage: A randomized, double-blind placebo-controlled study. *J Urol* 152:1095–1098, 1994.

15. Caravati EM, Runge JW, Bossart PJ, et al: Nifedipine for the relief of renal colic: A double-blind, placebo-controlled clinical trial. *Ann Emerg Med* 18:352–354, 1989.

16. Pearle MS, Pierce HL, Miller GL, et al: Optimal method of urgent decompression of the collecting system for obstruction and infection due to ureteral calculi. *J Urol* 160:1260–1264, 1998.

17. Hübner WA, Irby P, Stoller ML: Natural history and current concepts for the treatment of small ureteral calculi. *Eur Urol* 24:172–176, 1993.

18. Chaussy C, Brendel W, Schmiedt E: Extracorporeally induced destruction of kidney stone by shock waves. *Lancet* 2:1265–1268, 1980.

19. Knapp PM, Kulb TB, Lingeman KE, et al: Extracorporeal shock wave lithotripsy-induced perirenal hematomas. *J Urol* 139:700–703, 1988.

20. Pearle MS, Clayman RV: Outcomes and selection of surgical therapies of stones in the kidney and ureter. In: *Kidney Stones: Medical and Surgical Management*. Philadelphia, Lippincott-Raven, 1996, pp 709–755.

21. Politis G, Griffith D: ESWL: Stone-free rates based upon stone size and location. *World J Surg* 5:255–258, 1987.

22. Lingeman JE, Siegel YI, Steele B, et al: Management of lower pole nephrolithiasis: A critical analysis. *J Urol* 151:663–667, 1994.

23. Lingeman JE, Lower Pole Study Group: Prospective randomized trial of extracorporeal shock wave lithotripsy and percutaneous nephrostolithotomy for lower pole nephrolithiasis: Initial long-term follow up. *J Endourol* 11:S95, 1997.

24. Dretler SP: Stone fragility—a new therapeutic distinction. *J Urol* 139:1124–1127, 1988.

25. Hockley NM, Lingeman JE, Hutchinson CL: Relative efficacy of extracorporeal shock wave lithotripsy and percutaneous nephrostolithotomy

in the management of cystine calculi. *J Endourol* 3:273–285, 1989.

26. Albala DM, Clayman RV, Meretyk S: Extracorporeal shock wave lithotripsy for proximal ureteral calculi: To stint or not to stint? *J Endourol* 5:277–281, 1991.

27. Hendrikx AJM, Bierkens AAF, Oosterhof GON, DeBruyne FMJ: Treatment of proximal and mid ureteral calculi: A randomized trial of in situ and pushback extracorporeal lithotripsy. *J Endourol* 4:353–364, 1990.

28. Danuser H, Ackermann DK, Marth DC, et al: Extracorporeal shock wave lithotripsy in situ or after push-up for upper ureteral calculi: A prospective randomized trial. *J Urol* 150:824–826, 1993.

29. Segura JW, Patterson DE, LeRoy AJ, et al: Percutaneous removal of kidney stones: Review of 1,000 cases. *J Urol* 134:1077–1081, 1985.

30. Segura JW, Preminger GM, Assimos DG, et al: Nephrolithiasis clinical guidelines panel summary report on the management of staghorn calculi. *J Urol* 151:1648–1651, 1994.

31. Micali S, Moore RG, Averch TD, et al: The role of laparoscopy in the treatment of renal and ureteral calculi. *J Urol* 157:463–466, 1997.

32. Gaur DD: Retroperitoneal endoscopic ureterolithotomy: Our experience in 12 patients. *J Endourol* 7, 1993.

33. Fine JK, Pak CYC, Preminger GM: Effect of medical management and residual fragments on recurrent stone formation following shock wave lithotripsy. *J Urol* 153:27–33, 1995.

34. Borghi L, Meschi T, Amato F, et al: Urinary volume, water and recurrence in idiopathic calcium nephrolithiasis: A 5-year randomized prospective study. *J Urol* 155:839–843, 1996.

35. Hosking DH, Erickson SB, Van den Berg CJ, et al: The stone clinic effect in patients with idiopathic calcium urolithiasis. *J Urol* 130:1115–1118, 1983.

36. Williams RC: Long-term survey of 538 patients with upper urinary tract stones. *Br J Urol* 35:416, 1963.

37. Pak CYC: Should patients with single renal stone occurrence undergo diagnostic evaluation? *J Urol* 127:855–858, 1982.

38. Pak CY: Medical management of nephrolithiasis in Dallas: Update 1987. *J Urol* 140:461–467, 1988. Review.

39. Yagisawa T, Chandhoke PS, Fan J: Comparison of comprehensive and limited metabolic evaluations in the treatment of patients with recurrent calcium urolithiasis. *J Urol* 161:1449–1452, 1999.

40. Pak CYC, Britton F, Peterson R, et al: Ambulatory evaluation of nephrolithiasis: Classification, clinical presentation and diagnostic criteria. *Am J Med* 60:19–30, 1980.

41. Pak CYC, Waters O, Arnold L, et al: Mechanism for calcium nephrolithiasis among patients with hyperuricosuria: Supersaturation of urine with respect to monosodium urate. *J Clin Invest* 59:426–431, 1977.

42. Smith LH, Meyer JL: Growth of calcium oxalate crystals. II. Inhibition by natural urinary crystal growth inhibitors. *Invest Urol* 13:36–39, 1975.

43. Dobbins JW, Binder H: Effect of bile salts and fatty acids on the colonic absorption of oxalate. *Gastroenterology* 70:1096–1100, 1976.

44. Earnest DL, Williams HE, Admirand WH: A physicochemical basis for treatment of enteric hyperoxaluria. *Trans Assoc Am Clinicians* 88:224–234, 1975.

45. Pak CYC, Fuller CJ: Assessment of cystine solubility in urine and of heterogeneous nucleation between cystine and calcium salts. *Invest Urol* 129:1066–1070, 1983.

46. Pak CYC, Sakhaee K, Crowther C, Brinkley L: Evidence justifying a high fluid intake in treatment of nephrolithiasis. *Ann Intern Med* 93:36–39, 1980.

47. Preminger GM, Pak CYC: Eventual attenuation of hypocalciuric response to hydrochlorothiazide in absorptive hypercalciuria. *J Urol* 137:1104–1109, 1987.

48. Borghi L, Meshi T, Guerra A, Novarini A: Randomized prospective study of a nonthiazide diuretic, indapamide, in preventing calcium stone recurrences. *J Cardiovasc Pharmacol* 22:S78–S86, 1993.

49. Kaplan RA, Snyder WH, Stewart A, Pak CYC: Metabolic effects of parathyroidectomy on asymptomatic primary hyperparathyroidism. *J Clin Endocrinol Metab* 42:415–426, 1976.

50. Selby PL, Peacock M: Ethinyl estradiol and norethindrone in the treament of primary hyperparathyroidism in postmenopausal women. *N Engl J Med* 314:1481–1485, 1986.

51. Nicar MJ, Hsu MC: Urinary response to oral potassium citrate therapy for urolithiasis in a private practice setting. *Clin Ther* 8:219–225, 1986.

52. Michaels EK, Fowler JEJ: Extracorporeal shock wave lithotripsy for struvite renal calculi: Prospective study with extended followup. *J Urol* 146:728–732, 1991.

53. Pearle MS, Roehrborn CG, Pak CYC: Meta-analysis of randomized trials for medical prevention of calcium oxalate nephrolithiasis. *J Endourol*, in press.

Edmund S. Sabanegh

Impotence

How Common Is Erectile Dysfunction?

A National Institutes of Health (NIH) consensus panel standardized the definition of erectile dysfunction, or impotence (as it was formerly known), as "the inability to achieve or maintain an erection sufficient for satisfactory sexual performance."[1] Between 20 and 30 million men in the United States experience some degree of erectile dysfunction. The prevalence of erectile dysfunction increases with age, rising from 22% at age 40 up to 50% by age 70.[2]

The diagnosis and treatment of erectile dysfunction have undergone a marked metamorphosis over the past 20 years. Early treatment options were limited to penile implants and a variety of relatively ineffective oral therapies. Social stigma of the diagnosis, and a public perception that erectile dysfunction was a normal sequela of aging, led to underreporting of the disease. Advances in our understanding of the physiology of erection, marked media interest, and the development of more effective, less invasive therapies have resulted in an outpouring of patient interest in the problem.

Large population-based studies have revealed that erectile dysfunction does not have to be a natural consequence of aging but may be a result of other diseases or conditions that are amenable to treatment.[2] It is against this backdrop that the primary care clinician and the specialist alike must approach this diagnosis. This chapter is intended to provide a framework for a systematic, goal-directed approach to this common problem.

Physiology of Erection

Erections represent the end-result of a complex interplay between neuronal, hormonal, vascular, and smooth-muscle factors. Visual stimuli, desire, and perception are integrated at the level of the central nervous system resulting in autonomic outflow to the penis to stimulate an erection. Sensory stimuli from the penis are important to maintain an erection via a spinal reflex from the pudendal nerve.

The penis is composed of three erectile bodies—the paired corpora cavernosa and the corpus spongiosum, which surrounds the urethra. Each erectile cylinder consists of a central mass of trabecular smooth muscle within which is embedded an intercommunicating system of endothelial-lined vascular spaces, called lacunar spaces or sinusoids. The corporal bodies are individually surrounded by a dense collagenous sheath called the tunica albuginea. During arousal, parasympathetic outflow from the central nervous system initiates an erection by relaxing the trabecular smooth muscle of the corpora cavernosa and dilating the helicine arteries of the penis. Increased arterial inflow (5 to 10-fold from flaccid state) into the lacunar spaces results in an increase in the diameter of the central erectile tissue within the relatively rigid tunica albuginea. The resulting increase in intracorporal pressure obstructs venous drainage, further elevating intracorporal pressure to near arterial pressures, and resulting in a rigid erection.

A variety of neurotransmitters have been implicated in the smooth-muscle relaxation that initiates erection. Originally, acetylcholine was felt to be solely responsible, but more recent studies suggest that noncholinergic, nonadrenergic agents including nitric oxide and vasointestinal peptide are more important. Nitric oxide released from the endothelial cells induces trabecular smooth-muscle relaxation via stimulation of guanylate cyclase and production of cyclic guanosine monophosphate (cGMP). Cyclic GMP is an important intracellular messenger and is metabolized to GMP by the phosphodiesterase enzyme. These pathways, and our emerging understanding of the effects of neurotransmitters on the penis, have allowed the development of effective pharmacologic therapies for erectile dysfunction.

Principal Diagnoses

Erectile dysfunction can result from any disease process that affects the nervous, endocrinologic, vascular, or smooth-muscle systems. Risk factors for erectile dysfunction are summarized in Table 17–1. Erectile dysfunction may occur from one or more of three common mechanisms: failure to initiate, failure to fill (arteriogenic), or failure to store (veno-occlusive).

Failure to initiate an erection is typically the result of central nervous system pathology such as psychogenic causes or endocrinologic dysfunction such as hypogonadism. In addition, it may result from peripheral nervous diseases such as spinal radiculopathies, surgical trauma, or multiple sclerosis, in which penile innervation is impaired.

Erectile dysfunction from failure to fill is due to inadequate arterial blood delivery to the lacunar spaces. The underlying arterial insufficiency may be secondary to atherosclerotic or traumatic etiologies. Risk factors for atherosclerotic disease are well known to include smoking, advanced age, diabetes mellitus, known coronary artery or peripheral vascular disease, hypertension, and hypercholesterolemia. Traumatic penile arterial injuries occur most commonly as a result of a straddle injury such as a fall onto a bicycle crossbar or top tube, or from a motor vehicle accident with pelvic fractures.

Inability to occlude venous outflow during erection results in a "failure to store" type of erectile dysfunction. This is secondary to inadequate intracorporal smooth-muscle function and is associated with atherosclerosis, prior priapism with resulting intracorporal ischemia, and trauma.

Typical Presentation

Failure to initiate erection due to psychogenic causes typically presents as an acute onset of erectile dysfunction. Patients may describe significant antecedent stressors, marital or spousal issues, or situational dynamics impacting their sex life. This diagnosis may be easily suspected if a patient notes normal erections with one partner but not with another partner. A sudden onset of erectile dysfunction also is seen in spinal cord injury, pelvic or perineal surgery, or pelvic trauma.

Failure to initiate erection due to hypogonadism, or failure to fill, typically presents as a gradual and progressive problem, because the erectile dysfunction mirrors the severity and duration of the underlying medical problem (e.g., hypertension, hypercholesterolemia). Patients typically note a gradual decline in penile rigidity over time regardless of partner. Stressors may exacerbate erectile dysfunction, and secondary marital discord may result.

Failure to store typically presents as a gradually progressive onset of a failure to maintain a

Table 17–1

Risk Factors for Erectile Dysfunction

Failure to Initiate (Neurologic)
Psychiatric disease (depression, anxiety)
Endocrinopathy (hypogonadism)
Spinal radiculopathies/spinal cord injury
Pelvic or perineal surgery
Alcohol or other substance abuse

Failure to Fill (Arteriogenic)
Advanced age
Hypertension
Smoking
Coronary artery or peripheral vascular disease
Diabetes mellitus
Hypercholesterolemia/hyperlipidemia
Trauma to pelvis

Failure to Store (Veno-occlusive)
Atherosclerosis
Trauma
History of priapism (ischemia)

rigid penile erection, even though the initial rigidity is normal. With advancing severity, the duration of erection may be limited so that initial penile rigidity is impaired. Further, failure to initiate and failure to store may coexist.

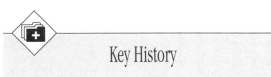

Key History

The appropriate evaluation of the patient with erectile dysfunction should include a comprehensive but focused medical and sexual history, physical examination, and basic laboratory tests. The clinician must be sensitive to the patient's underlying concerns in discussing this intensely personal issue, but must not shy away from the need to obtain detailed information to allow a complete assessment.

The patient's sexual and medical history are the most important components of the clinical evaluation for erectile dysfunction. Sexual history should include an assessment of the onset of dysfunction (acute or gradual) and the frequency, duration, and quality of erections. Historical information about the acuteness of onset and level of libido may provide clues to the etiology of erectile dysfunction (Table 17–2). Acute onset may be the result of a new medication or psychogenic factors. Acute onset in conjunction with pelvic surgery or trauma should raise suspicion for a vascular or nerve injury. If the patient's erectile dysfunction is more gradual and is accompanied by a simultaneous decrease in libido, the diagnosis of a hypogonadal state should be considered.

Table 17–2
Clues from History

PRESENTATION	SUSPECT
Acute onset	Psychogenic, medications
Acute onset + trauma/surgery	Nerve or vascular injury
Gradual onset, decreased libido	Hypogonadal state

A variety of erectile function questionnaires have been developed and may facilitate an objective assessment of sexual function. One such questionnaire, the EF index, is shown in Table 17–3.[3] Overall scores on this index range from 1 to 25. Scores of 20 or higher indicate normal erectile function while scores of 10 or less describe moderate to severe erectile dysfunction.

A brief medical history should be obtained with specific emphasis on medical, surgical, and psychiatric factors that may affect sexual function (Table 17–4).

Physical Examination

Overall

Although usually confirmatory of the diagnosis suggested from the medical history, the physical exam will occasionally yield unsuspected findings such as lumbosacral radiculopathy or signs of systemic or endocrinologic disease. Thus, physical examination should include an assessment of the male secondary sexual characteristics in addition to a focused evaluation of the vascular, neurologic, and genitourinary systems (Table 17–5).

Observation of normal male hair, body fat, and muscle patterns suggests adequate virilization and androgen levels. A breast exam should be performed to rule out gynecomastia, which could be suggestive of an underlying endocrinopathy due to elevated prolactin or estrogen levels. Patients with prolactinomas, while uncommon, will occasionally have decreased libido and erectile dysfunction as the presenting complaint. In addition, hyperprolactinemia can be caused by liver disease and medications such as phenothiazines. Hyperestrogenemia is usually secondary to obesity with enhanced peripheral aromatization of testosterone to estradiol in adipose tissue. Both prolactin and estrogen act centrally to inhibit GnRH release with a resulting decrease in testosterone levels, producing a "failure to initiate" pattern of erectile dysfunction.

Table 17–3

EF Index "Over the Past Six Months"[3]

		Very low 1	Low 2	Moderate 3	High 4	Very high 5
1. How do you rate your confidence that you could get and keep an erection?		Very low 1	Low 2	Moderate 3	High 4	Very high 5
2. When you had erections with sexual stimulation, how often were your erections hard enough for penetration?	No sexual activity 0	Almost never/never 1	A few times 2	Sometimes 3	Most times 4	Almost always/always 5
3. During sexual intercourse, how often were you able to maintain your erection after you had penetrated (entered) your partner?	Did not attempt intercourse 0	Almost never/never 1	A few times 2	Sometimes 3	Most times 4	Almost always/always 5
4. During sexual intercourse, how difficult was it to maintain your erection to completion of intercourse?	Did not attempt intercourse 0	Extremely difficult 1	Very difficult 2	Difficult 3	Slightly difficult 4	Not difficult 5
5. When you attempted sexual intercourse, how often was it satisfactory for you?	Did not attempt intercourse 0	Almost never/never 1	A few times 2	Sometimes 3	Most times 4	Almost always/always 5

A thyroid exam should also be performed to screen for goiter or other pathology that could result in hypothyroidism, another unusual cause of erectile dysfunction.

Genitourinary

The genitourinary exam should include a thorough assessment of testicular and penile anatomy. Decreased testicular size or a change in consistency may suggest a hypogonadal etiology for erectile function. The lower limits of normal length and width for a mature testis are approximately 4 and 2.5 cm, respectively. When the testes are damaged before puberty, they are small and firm; with postpubertal damage, they are usually soft and small.

A complete examination of the penis will provide important clues to the etiology of the dysfunction. Careful palpation of the corpora cavernosa may reveal firm superficial plaques on the surface of the tunica, so-called Peyronie's plaques. These may cause curvature of the penis during erection, making intercourse uncomfortable or impossible. Fibrotic or nodular corpora may suggest ischemia or prior intracavernosal therapy.

Neurologic

A focused neurologic exam should include an assessment of penile sensation. During the rectal and prostate examinations, anal sphincter tone and the bulbocavernosus reflex can be evaluated, reflecting sacral root function. Absence of a bulbocavernosal reflex does not in and of itself indicate neurologic dysfunction because it may be absent in up to 30% of neurologically normal men. More sophisticated neurologic testing, including dorsal nerve conduction latency, evoked potential measurements, and penile biothesiometry, has been developed but is seldom indicated in the routine workup of erectile dysfunction.

Table 17–4
Medical History

Chronic disease
    Anemia
    Diabetes mellitus
    Renal failure
Cardiovascular risk factors
    Hypertension
    Known coronary artery or peripheral vascular disease
    Hypercholesterolemia
Endocrinologic disease
    Hypothyroidism
    Hypogonadism
    Hyperprolactinemia
Neurologic disease
    Disk disease
    Multiple sclerosis
Psychiatric disease
    Depression
    Anxiety disorder
Surgical history
    Pelvic surgery (prostatectomy)
    Laminectomy
Trauma (e.g., pelvis, penis)
Medications
    Antihypertensives
    Antidepressants
    H_2 receptor blockers
    Antihyperlipidemics
Habits
    Smoking
    Alcohol
    Recreational drugs (e.g., marijuana, cocaine)

Table 17–5
Physical Exam

EXAMINATION	PATHOLOGY
Overall appearance (loss of virilization)	Hypogonadism
Body habitus	
Hair pattern	
Genitourinary	
Testis—decreased size	Hypogonadism
Penis	
Curvature	Peyronie's disease
Plaques or fibrosis	Prior ischemia, priapism, intracavernosal therapy
Neurologic	
Sensation/bulbocavernosal reflex	Radiculopathy, diabetes mellitus
Vascular	Arterial insufficiency
Peripheral pulses	
Other	
Breast (e.g., gynecomastia)	Hyperprolactinemia, hyperestrogenemia
Thyroid	Hypothyroidism

Ancillary Testing

Laboratory Evaluation

Laboratory testing has a role in select patients with erectile dysfunction (Table 17–6). Testing should be tailored to the individual patient to avoid the expense of a battery of unnecessary lab work. A general metabolic survey with serum electrolytes, fasting blood glucose, complete blood count (CBC), and lipid profiles should be obtained on all patients if not performed in the past year or if clinically indicated (e.g., suspicion of new-onset diabetes). A serum thyroid panel may also be considered if clinically warranted.

Routine endocrine screening of impotent men with serum testosterone and prolactin assays re-

Vascular

The vascular system can be evaluated by palpating the lower extremity pulses. In the setting of a high clinical suspicion of arterial injury, such as in a young man with acute onset of erectile dysfunction after pelvic trauma, more advanced vascular testing is indicated. Such testing is described later in the chapter.

Table 17–6

Indications for Laboratory Tests

LABORATORY VALUE	INDICATIONS TO OBTAIN
General metabolic survey (CBC, electrolytes, lipid profile, blood glucose)	Not tested within 12 months, or clinical suspicion of abnormality
Serum total testosterone (AM)	Small testis or decreased libido
Serum prolactin	Low serum testosterone or decreased libido
Thyroid function test	Clinical suspicion of hyperthyroidism or hypothyroidism

mains controversial. The broad-screening viewpoint would support an initial assessment of serum testosterone, either total or free, in the setting of decreased libido, testicular atrophy, or clinical suspicion of hypogonadism.[4–6] Some authors argue for routine screening in all men, but this strategy may not represent a cost-effective approach to the problem given the low incidence of detected endocrinopathies in the absence of clinical signs and symptoms of hypogonadism.[7] Serum testosterone measurements should be performed on morning specimens because of the diurnal secretion pattern. If the initial measurement is low, a repeat level should be determined, because up to 40% of follow-up assays will be normal.

Serum prolactin measurement is indicated in the subset of patients with low serum testosterone levels, decreased libido, or gynecomastia. Ideally, serum prolactin levels should be drawn in the morning, after a 20-minute rest to eliminate stress-induced hyperprolactinemia. In addition, any drug that may increase prolactin levels, such as phenothiazines, should be discontinued for at least 24 hours prior to prolactin determination. Men with hyperprolactinemia will require pituitary imaging with an MRI of the sella turcica to rule out a prolactinoma.

Additional Testing

Specialized testing is rarely indicated in the average patient with erectile dysfunction, although it may be helpful in two categories of patients: those in whom the diagnosis of psychogenic etiology is being considered and those with risk factors for penile artery injury, such as a history of pelvic trauma. These tests are considered with the caveat that they may significantly increase the cost of the evaluation without altering the treatment.

Nocturnal penile tumescence (NPT) testing assesses the degree of erectile dysfunction during sleep and is helpful in distinguishing between organic and psychogenic dysfunction. A variety of devices have been developed from the simplest—the snap-gauge, which is a ring with several bands that is placed around the penis at bedtime and will reveal broken bands if a nocturnal erection has occurred—to the more sophisticated Rigiscan device, which makes repetitive measurements of rigidity from the base and tip of the penis. Lack of test standardization limits the results of these studies, but documentation of nocturnal erections with these tests suggests a psychogenic diagnosis.

More advanced vascular testing should be considered in the rare patient with the acute onset of erectile dysfunction after pelvic trauma. Color duplex Doppler ultrasound of the cavernosal arteries before and after intracavernosal injection of a smooth-muscle relaxant-vasodilator (such as prostaglandin E_1) will help determine the adequacy of arterial inflow. Pelvic angiography is indicated in the setting of an abnormal ultrasound and will allow precise anatomic localization of an arterial injury. More invasive tests, such as dynamic infusion cavernosometry and cavernosography, which involve intracavernosal irrigation with pressure measurements and fluoroscopy, were promoted for vascular screening over a decade ago, but with advances in ultrasound imaging, such tests have now been largely relegated to a historic role in the vascular workup.

Algorithm for Ancillary Tests

An algorithm for integrating the ancillary tests is shown in Fig. 17–1. Note that many impotent patients will not require any specialized tests.

Treatment

The treatment for erectile dysfunction must be goal oriented based on the expectations of the patient and his partner for a satisfactory sexual experience. After excluding any reversible causes of erectile dysfunction (see the next section), therapy should follow a stepwise progression from first to third-line treatments. First-line treatment is characterized as the least invasive with the lowest risk profile and the broadest utility to a majority of patients. Second and third-line therapies have progressive increases in both invasiveness and treatment morbidity. Levels of treatment are summarized in Fig. 17–2. Specific contraindications for first-line therapies are reviewed in Table 17–7. Side effects from various therapies are summarized in Table 17–8.

Identification of Reversible Causes

Up to 25% of cases of erectile dysfunction have been attributed to prescription and nonprescription medications as well as illicit drug use. Certain classes of drugs are more commonly associated with reversible dysfunction (Table 17–9). This listing is not intended to be all inclusive, as there have been anecdotal reports of dysfunction associated with thousands of medications. Although it may be difficult to alter a patient's medications, depending on the clinical condition being treated, often a switch to another treatment agent will minimize the side effects. For example, antihypertensive agents are among the most frequently implicated drugs contributing to erectile dysfunction. Thiazide diuretics and beta-blockers seem to have the most profound negative effects on erection as compared to calcium channel blockers and angiotensin-converting enzyme inhibitors. Alpha-adrenergic blockers and angiotensin-converting enzyme inhibitors are probably the least likely to cause dysfunction.

In addition to medications, high-risk lifestyle factors such as lack of exercise, cigarette smoking, excessive alcohol consumption, or recreational drug use appear to play significant roles in the onset of erectile dysfunction. The potential for resolution with lifestyle modification remains to be proven.

First-Line Therapy

ORAL AGENTS

SILDENAFIL   Since approval by the FDA in 1998, sildenafil (Viagra) has enjoyed widespread popularity as an oral therapy for erectile dysfunction. The drug is a potent, selective inhibitor of type V phosphodiesterase, resulting in persistent high levels of cyclic GMP. Cyclic GMP causes smooth-muscle relaxation and increased blood flow, resulting in penile engorgement. Sildenafil has proven to be effective in 69% to 93% of patients, with excellent efficacy across a spectrum of diagnoses including psychogenic, organic, and mixed erectile dysfunction.[8–10]

Sildenafil is administered as an "on-demand" (prn) medication in doses of 25, 50, or 100 mg, to be used no more than once daily. Onset of action is within 20 to 60 minutes of ingestion and requires sexual stimulation to be effective.

Reported side effects include headaches (16%), flushing (10%), dyspepsia (7%), and nasal congestion (4%). In addition, 2% to 3% of patients will report transient vision disturbances such as a blue tint to the vision, increased light sensitivity, or blurred vision. Sildenafil use is *contraindicated* in patients on any nitrate therapy. Concurrent nitrate and sildenafil use has been associated with cardiac-related deaths.

Figure 17-1

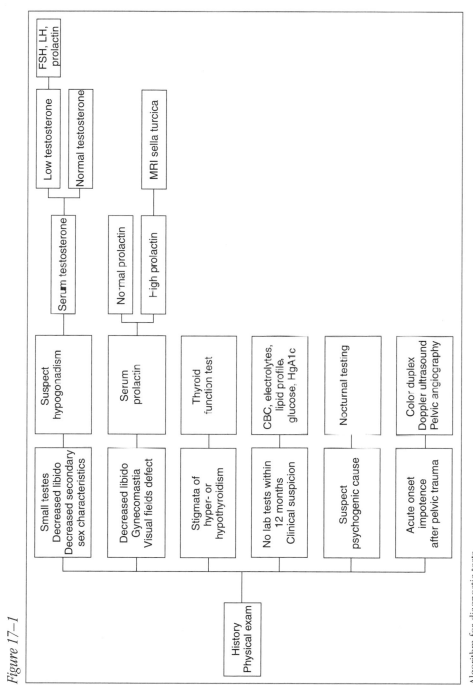

Algorithm for diagnostic tests.

Figure 17–2

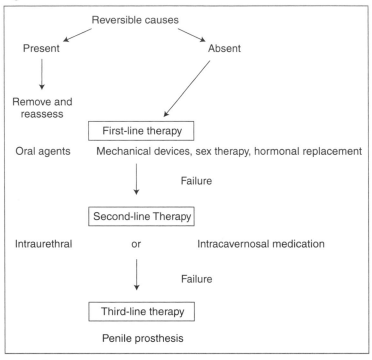

Levels of treatment.

YOHIMBINE Yohimbine (Yocon) is an alpha$_2$-adrenergic receptor antagonist derived from the bark of the Central African Yohimbine tree. It has been used in some form for the treatment of erectile dysfunction for over 100 years. The mecha-nism of action remains unclear, but it is postulated to act centrally via blockade of the presynaptic alpha$_2$ receptors, leading to increased levels of norepinephrine, facilitating arousal. Outcome analysis has been limited by poor study designs, although a recent review of placebo-controlled trials reported positive responses in 34% to 73% of treated patients versus 9% to 28% for placebo.[11]

A number of dosing regimens have been utilized but the most common is 5.4 mg orally three times a day. Beneficial effects usually require several weeks of use. Adverse effects have occurred in 10% to 30% of men and are generally mild, including anxiety, headache, mild increases in blood pressure, and gastrointestinal disturbance.

Table 17–7

Contraindications for First Line Therapy

THERAPY	CONTRAINDICATIONS (ABSOLUTE—A, OR RELATIVE—R)
Medication	
Sildenafil	Nitrate use (A)
Yohimbine	Hypertension (R)
Vacuum erectile devices	Anticoagulation (R)
	Coagulation disorders (R)
Endocrinologic therapy	Known prostate cancer or symptomatic BPH (A)
	Coronary artery disease (R)
	Hyperlipidemia (R)

VACUUM CONSTRICTION DEVICES

Vacuum constriction devices represent a safe, noninvasive, and simple therapy for erectile dys-

Table 17–8

Side Effects of Various Therapies

	SIDE EFFECTS
First-Line Therapy	
Sildenafil (Viagra)	Headaches
	Flushing
	Dyspepsia
	Nasal congestion
	Visual disturbance
Yohimbine (Yocon)	Anxiety
	Headache
	Hypertension
	Gastrointestinal disturbance
Vacuum constriction device	Penile pain
	Ecchymosis
	Retarded ejaculation
Androgen replacement	Accelerated BPH or prostate cancer
	Polycythemia
	Sleep apnea
Second-Line Therapy	
Intracorporal injection	Priapism
	Penile fibrosis
	Pain/hematoma
Intraurethral alprostadil agent	Penile pain
	Hypotension
	Priapism
Third-Line Therapy	
Penile prosthesis	Mechanical failure
	Infection
	Erosion

function. These devices utilize a lubricated air-tight tube placed over the penis to create negative external pressure, which increases arterial inflow to the penis (Fig. 17–3). After an erection is achieved, a flexible constriction band is placed around the base of the penis to reduce venous outflow. The band must be removed within 30 to 60 minutes of placement.

Initial satisfaction rates with vacuum devices range from 67% to 93%.[12,13] There is a significant rate of patient dropout with this therapy, largely

Table 17–9

Drugs Commonly Associated With Erectile Dysfunction

Antiandrogens	Histamine receptor blockers (Cimetidine)
Antiarrhythmics	Narcotics
Antidepressants	Recreational drugs (alcohol, marijuana,
Antihypertensives	cocaine, heroin)
Antipsychotics	Tranquilizers

due to the lack of spontaneity inherent with usage and discomfort from the constricting band. The adverse effects include penile pain, ecchymosis, and retarded ejaculation. Special care must be taken with paraplegics and other sensory-compromised men to ensure the constricting band is not excessively tight or inadvertently left in place for too long, as this has been associated with severe complications including penile skin necrosis. Anticoagulant use or coagulation disorders represent relative contraindications to use, although there appears to be minimal risk if used carefully.

SEXUAL THERAPY

Sexual and behavioral therapy may be helpful for the occasional patient with psychogenic erectile dysfunction. Therapy is directed at reducing psychosocial stressors that precipitated the sexual dysfunction. Couples counseling is indicated for those in whom marital discord is identified as a significant contributing factor. Clinical depression may first manifest as erectile dysfunction. Standard depression therapy including medical management and psychotherapy may result in resolution of sexual dysfunction. Similarly, patients with major psychosocial stressors may respond to instruction in relaxation and stress reduction techniques.

Success rates for sexual counseling remain difficult to quantify due to the wide variety of therapies utilized and the lack of long-term follow-up. In general, sex therapy as a solo treatment appears to have fairly low long-term efficacy with high patient dropout rates.[14] Therapy in conjunction with other treatments such as oral erectile agents may result in improved success.

Figure 17–3

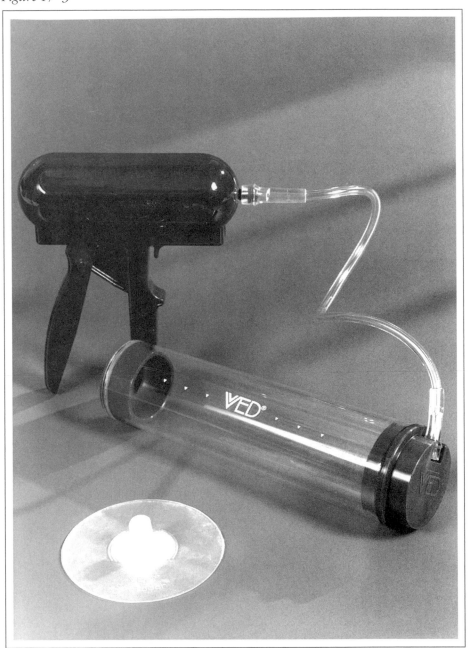

Vacuum constriction device. (Courtesy of Mission Pharmaceutical.)

HORMONE REPLACEMENT

Androgen replacement therapy may be effective in improving erectile dysfunction in the occasional patient with either primary (testicular failure) or secondary (hypogonadotropic hypogonadism) hypogonadism. A trial of therapy is indicated for men with low serum testosterone levels and poor libido. Due to potential health risks, androgen therapy is *not* indicated for patients with normal baseline androgen levels.

Testosterone replacement may be provided either by parenteral (intramuscular) or transdermal delivery systems. Oral testosterone therapies are to be avoided due to poor efficacy and the potential for serious hepatotoxicity. The two most commonly utilized parenteral formulations are testosterone cypionate and enanthate. They are administered via intramuscular injection in doses of 200 to 300 mg every 2 to 6 weeks. Dose and dosing intervals are adjusted based on clinical response and serum testosterone levels.

Transdermal testosterone formulations offer the advantage of more closely mimicking physiologic delivery and avoiding the requirement for parenteral injections. Transdermal agents are available as Testoderm, which must be applied to shaved scrotal skin, and Androderm, which can be applied to any skin surface. Currently, patches must be replaced on a daily basis, although more extended delivery systems are under development. Transdermal patches are substantially more expensive than parenteral formulations.

Patients receiving androgen replacement therapy should be carefully counseled regarding the significant potential health risks from this therapy. Although use has not been conclusively linked to the de novo development of prostate cancer, it is well known to accelerate the growth of existing prostate cancer or benign prostatic hypertrophy (BPH).[15] All men over age 40 receiving therapy require a baseline serum prostate-specific antigen (PSA) level and digital rectal exam followed by at least yearly exams thereafter. Testosterone should *not* be administered to patients with a known history of prostate cancer or symptomatic BPH. It should be employed with caution in patients with significant coronary artery disease or hyperlipidemia due to the potential for inducing alterations in serum lipid profiles. The hematocrit level should be checked several months after starting therapy, because a rare patient will develop polycythemia. Testosterone replacement has also been associated with the development or worsening of sleep apnea.

Second-Line Therapy

INTRACAVERNOSAL MEDICATION

Intracavernosal self-injection remains an excellent therapeutic option in selected patients. Candidates should have good manual dexterity and a history of good compliance with medical therapies, as efficacy and side effects are exquisitely dose dependent. Physicians who prescribe intracavernosal and intraurethral medications must be adept in the recognition and therapy of serious side effects, such as priapism (described later).

The three most commonly utilized agents are alprostadil (prostaglandin E_1, Caverject), phentolamine (Regitine), and papaverine. They have been used alone or in various combinations with success rates ranging from 61% to 95%.[16,17] Alprostadil is the most commonly used monotherapy and has received FDA approval for treatment of erectile dysfunction. Initial alprostadil dose ranges from 5 to 20 μg with the lower range reserved for men with psychogenic impotence or neuropathic etiologies, such as spinal cord injury. The majority of older patients with organic dysfunction will require 15 to 20 μg to achieve a satisfactory response. Dosages are titrated to achieve an erection lasting 30 to 60 minutes. Once a proper dose is identified, patients are instructed in the proper sterile technique for self-administration including intracavernosal injection into the superolateral aspect of the proximal shaft of the penis while avoiding the subcutaneous veins. Direct pressure should be applied to the needle site after the injection to prevent hematoma formation. Men should be instructed to inject no more than once per day and no more than three times per week.

Complications of intracavernosal injection therapy include prolonged erection or priapism, penile fibrosis, and penile pain. Although there is no standard definition for priapism, most authors believe intervention is necessary for erections lasting longer than 4 hours. Rates of priapism are related to drug dose and agents utilized, ranging from 2% with alprostadil to 4% with papaverine.[16,17] Timely recognition and therapy for prolonged erection can prevent penile ischemia, which can render the penis incapable of erections regardless of the therapy utilized. Intracorporal treatments for priapism are summarized in Table 17–10.[18] All the treatments involve vasoactive substances, so vital signs should be closely monitored during administration. If priapism fails to respond to medical therapy, surgical shunting may become necessary.

Penile fibrosis appears related to trauma to the corpora from repeated needle injections and chemical injury from the specific agent utilized, with about a 4% incidence in patients treated with papaverine-based therapy and less than 1% incidence with alprostadil. Risk of penile fibrosis can be minimized by using smaller needles, varying the site of injection, decreasing the frequency of usage, and utilizing proper injection technique.

Penile pain is commonly observed after injection and appears to be a major contributing factor to the high dropout rate with injection therapy. Pain is highest with alprostadil monotherapy, but

Table 17–10

Intracorporal Treatments for Priapism

Intracorporal aspiration of 1–20 mL of blood with 10 mL of saline irrigation

Vasoactive agents (use *only* one)—may repeat q 5 minutes

Phenylephrine 200–500 µg

Epinephrine 10–20 µg

Ephedrine 50–100 µg

Norepinephrine 10–20 µg

may be reduced by alkalinizing the agent with sodium bicarbonate.

INTRAURETHRAL THERAPY

The excellent systemic absorption via the urethra forms the basis of intraurethral delivery of vasoactive substances to treat erectile dysfunction. Alprostadil (MUSE) is the only FDA-approved drug for intraurethral use, with doses ranging from 125 to 1000 µg. The drug is formulated into a small suppository that is delivered into the urethral meatus after urination, using a plastic applicator. Onset of erection occurs within 10 minutes of administration.

Despite initial reports of outstanding success and high in-clinic erection rates during drug titration, subsequent results have been disappointing, with less than 50% of patients able to have intercourse using this technique.[19] The majority of patients will require doses of 500 µg or higher.

Side effects have been minor, although up to one third of patients will have significant penile pain. Priapism has been reported but is relatively rare as compared to intracavernosal alprostadil use. Hypotension has also been reported in 3% to 4% of men.

Third-Line Therapy

Third-line therapy involves surgical implantation of a penile prosthesis and is generally reserved for patients who have failed first and second-line treatment regimens. This should be utilized as a last resort, because the erectile tissue is irreversibly damaged during implantation, preventing future response to other therapy should the prosthesis fail for any reason.

There are two main types of prosthesis. The first variety is malleable or semirigid at all times. It is simple to implant with rare mechanical breakdowns, but suffers from relatively poor concealability of the erection. The second variety of implant is inflatable and involves a complex system of penile cylinders, hydraulic reservoir, and intrascrotal pump. This system has a higher mechanical failure rate although this has markedly improved in recent years with technologic advances. Inflatable prostheses yield a more natural appearance than the malleable or semirigid prostheses. All varieties of prosthesis are susceptible to erosion or infection, complications that can necessitate removal. Despite the invasive nature of this therapy, it retains relatively high patient and partner satisfaction rates.[20]

Indications for Referral

Most patients with erectile dysfunction can be managed in the primary care setting with a goal-directed regimen as outlined. However, several categories of patient may benefit from referral to a urologist (Table 17–11). Patients who have failed first or second-line therapy may benefit from referral. Although second-line therapy can be offered in the primary care environment, the physician should be comfortable managing the complications of these therapies, because good outcomes require prompt recognition and treatment.

Patients, especially younger men, with a history of perineal or genital trauma and the acute onset of erectile dysfunction should receive a urologic referral for more specialized vascular testing. Arterial revascularization can successfully restore potency in a subset of patients with traumatic arterial injury. In addition, men with significant penile curvature or Peyronie's disease may benefit

Table 17–11
Indications for Urologic Referral

Failure of first- or second-line therapy
Suspicion of anatomic abnormality
Arterial injury (perineal trauma with acute onset of dysfunction)
Peyronie's disease (penile curvature)

from penile straightening procedures by a urologist. Occasionally, additional subspecialty help may be needed with an endocrinologist for the management of complicated endocrinopathies or with a psychiatrist or psychologist for the management of refractory depression or psychosexual disorders.

Emerging Concepts

Over the next decade, a phlethora of noninvasive treatments will emerge with an increasing emphasis on oral and topical administration. Growing understanding of smooth-muscle factors and their implications for erectile function may eventually allow genetic testing and therapy for high-risk patients.

Note: The author is a full-time federal employee. This work is in the public domain. The views expressed are those of the author, and are not to be construed as official or as reflecting those of the Department of Defense, the Army Medical Department or the U.S. Air Force.

References

1. NIH Consensus Development Panel on Impotence: Impotence. *JAMA* 270:83, 1993.
2. Feldman HA, Goldstein I, Hatzichristou DG, et al: Impotence and its medical and psychosocial correlates: Results of the Massachusetts male aging study. *J Urol* 151:54, 1994.
3. Rosen R, Goldstein I, Padma-Nathan H: *The Process of Care Model for the Evaluation and Treatment of Erectile Dysfunction.* New Brunswick, NJ, The University of Medicine and Dentistry of New Jersey Robert Wood Johnson Medical School, 1998.
4. Johnson AR, Jarow JP: Is routine endocrine testing of impotent men necessary? *J Urol* 147:1542, 1992.
5. Buvat J, Lemaire A: Endocrine screening in 1,022 men with erectile dysfunction: Clinical significance and cost-effective strategy. *J Urol* 158:1764, 1997.

6. Citron JT, Ettinger B, Rubinoff H, et al: Prevalence of hypothalamic-pituitary imaging abnormalities in impotent men with secondary hypogonadism. *J Urol* 155:529, 1996.

7. Govier FE, McClure D, Kramer-Levien D: Endocrine screening for sexual dysfunction using free testosterone determinations. *J Urol* 156:405, 1996.

8. Buvat J, Gingell C, Jardin A, et al: Sildenafil (Viagra), an oral treatment for erectile dysfunction: A 1-year, open-label, extension study. *J Urol* 157:204, 1997.

9. Christiansen E, Hodges M, Hollingshead M, et al: Sildenafil (Viagra), a new oral treatment for erectile dysfunction (ED): Results of a 16 open dose escalation study. *Int J Impot Res* 8:147, 1996.

10. Eardley I, Morgan R, Dinsmore W, et al: Oral administration of sildenafil, improves penile erections in patients with male erectile dysfunction (med). A double-blind, placebo controlled study with patients and partner outpatient diary as efficacy end points. *Eur Urol* 158:573, 1996.

11. Ernst E, Pittler MH: Yohimbine for erectile dysfunction: A systematic review and meta-analysis of randomized clinical trials. *J Urol* 159:433, 1998.

12. Cookson MS, Nadig PW: Long-term results with vacuum constriction device. *J Urol* 149:290, 1993.

13. Baltaci S, Aydos K, Kosar A, et al: Treating erectile dysfunction with a vacuum tumescence device: A retrospective analysis of acceptance and satisfaction. *B J Urol* 76:757, 1995.

14. Tiefer L, Schuetz-Mueller D: Psychological issues in diagnosis and treatment of erectile disorders. *Urol Clin North Am* 22:767, 1995.

15. Svetec DA, Canby ED, Thompson IM, et al: The effect of parenteral testosterone replacement of prostate specific antigen in hypogonadal men with erectile dysfunction. *J Urol* 158:1775, 1997.

16. Fallon B: Intracavernous injection therapy for male erectile dysfunction. *Urol Clin North Am* 22:833, 1995.

17. Manning M, Junemann KP: Pharmacotherapy of erectile dyfunction. In Hellstrom WJG (ed): *Male Infertility and Sexual Dysfunction.* New York, Springer, 1997, p. 440.

18. Lee M, Cannon B, Sharifi R: Chart for preparation of dilutions of α-adrenergic agonists for intracavernous use in treatment of priapism. *J Urol* 153:1182, 1995.

19. Padma-Nathan H, Hellstrom WJG, Kaiser FE, et al: Treatment of men with erectile dysfunction with transurethral alprostadil. *N Engl J Med* 336:1, 1997.

20. Lewis RW: Long-term results of penile prosthetic implants. *Urol Clin North Am* 22:847, 1995.

James H. Gilbaugh III

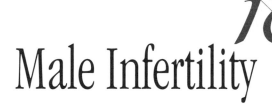

Male Infertility

How Common Is Male Infertility?

Roughly 15% of American couples are subfertile as defined by the inability to initiate a pregnancy after 1 year of unprotected intercourse. This represents over 2 million couples, and the incidence seems to be increasing. In approximately half of these couples, there is a significant male factor. Most of these couples will initially present to a family physician for evaluation.

Traditionally, the female was evaluated first, with male factor evaluation being performed if the female factor testing was normal. A better strategy involves first evaluating the male, because this is less expensive and may avoid potentially invasive testing of the female.

This chapter will serve to review male reproductive physiology, methods used in the diagnosis of possible male factor subfertility, and medical and surgical approaches to treatment. In Chapter 18B, male sterilization will be addressed with attention to technical aspects and controversies surrounding possible secondary health problems.

Principal Diagnoses

The most important cause of male infertility is varicocele, since this condition is easily corrected and a good pregnancy rate may be expected. Other diagnoses to consider are genital tract obstruction, hypogonadotropic hypogonadism, hyperprolactinemia, antisperm antibodies, genital tract infection, anejaculation, and retrograde ejaculation.

Review of Male Reproductive Physiology

Hypothalamic–Pituitary–Gonadal Axis

The male hypothalamic–pituitary–gonadal axis is responsible for production of androgens as well as spermatogenesis. The decapeptide gonadotropin-releasing hormone (GnRH) is synthesized in and released by the hypothalamus, and transported to the pituitary gland via the portal venous system. GnRH secretion occurs in a pulsatile fashion. Release of GnRH results in secretion of luteinizing hormone (LH) and follicle-stimulating hormone (FSH) from the anterior pituitary gland. LH and FSH are released into the circulation. LH acts on a specific receptor in testicular Leydig cells to stimulate testosterone production. FSH acts primarily on a receptor in the Sertoli cells and is felt to be involved in the initiation of spermatogenesis.

A complex feedback inhibition mechanism is present to control release of LH and FSH. Testosterone and estrogen as well as nonsteroidal mediators such as activin and inhibin are involved in this feedback control mechanism to regulate androgen levels and sperm production. Ongoing research continues to provide new insight into the complex mechanisms involved in male reproductive physiology.

Spermatogenesis

Spermatogenesis is the process by which the precursor germ cells progress through a number of stages of maturation, ultimately culminating in the formation of mature spermatozoa. The precursor germ cells, termed spermatogonia, are present from birth but are quiescent until puberty. Beginning at puberty, some of the spermatogonia give rise to more spermatogonia (stem cell replacement) while others ultimately undergo maturation to spermatozoa. During spermatogenesis, the germ cells migrate from the basement membrane to the lumen of the seminiferous tubule. Spermatogonia undergo mitotic division to become primary spermatocytes. The diploid primary spermatocyte then undergoes meiotic division, resulting in two haploid secondary spermatocytes, and these in turn mature to become spermatids and ultimately mature spermatozoa. The entire maturation process from spermatogonia to mature sperm takes approximately 74 days.

Sperm Transport

Following production, mature sperm are transported via the lumen of the seminiferous tubules to the rete testis, which coalesces to become the efferent ducts of the testis. Sperm are then transported through the efferent ducts to the epididymis. The epididymis is a coiled tubular structure approximately 4 meters in length encased in a connective tissue sheath and surrounding the posterior aspect of the testis. Anatomically, the epididymis is divided into the caput (head), corpus (body), and cauda (tail) and it is here that sperm are felt to gain motility and the ability to fertilize ova.

Ejaculation

Sperm are transported from the epididymis to the prostate during ejaculation, where they mix with fluid from the prostate and seminal vesicles. The ejaculatory event is comprised of seminal emission and ejaculation proper. Seminal emission refers to the deposition of sperm into the prostatic urethra by muscular contraction of the vasa deferentia and seminal vesicles mediated by the sympathetic nervous system.

Ejaculation is the forceful expulsion of semen out of the urethra. This occurs secondary to the rhythmic contraction of periurethral and pelvic floor muscles, mediated by the parasympathetic nervous system, in conjunction with closure of the bladder neck, which is sympathetically stimulated.

Key History

Medical History

The evaluation of the potentially subfertile male begins with a careful history and physical examination. The duration of subfertility should be determined and whether any pregnancies have been achieved in the present relationship. Any pregnancies or attempts at pregnancies in previous relationships should also be ascertained, as well as any previous fertility evaluation or treatment. Frequency and timing of intercourse are discussed to determine the couple's level of understanding with respect to reproductive physiology. The wife's age, regularity and character of menstrual cycle, and gynecologic history should be obtained, which can be facilitated by having the patient's wife present during the initial interview.

A detailed medical history should be taken with emphasis on factors that may influence fertility. Any history of cryptorchidism (undescended testes) or pediatric inguinal surgery should be elicited. Cryptorchidism of one or both testes has been associated with decreased spermatogenesis. Often, a patient will have undergone orchiopexy in conjunction with inguinal herniorrhaphy during infancy but will be unaware of this surgery. A history of other pediatric genitourinary surgeries or problems such as hypospadias, bladder neck reconstruction, or testicular torsion should be noted, as well as the age of onset of puberty.

A history of any urinary tract infections or sexually transmitted diseases should be noted, as these can be associated with genital ductal obstruction. Mumps orchitis was formerly a significant cause of testicular atrophy but is fortunately rare today in reproductive-age-range males due to childhood immunizations. Any significant previous trauma to the genitalia may impact fertility by causing atrophy of the testes, obstruction of the epididymis, or immunologic causes due to anti-sperm antibody production with the breakdown of the blood–testis barrier.

Any type of systemic illness that results in elevated body temperatures may impair spermatogenesis. These effects may not be reflected in the semen analysis immediately and may result in diminished semen parameters for 3 to 4 months following the illness due to the length of spermatogenesis and transit of sperm through the ductal system. For this reason, any abnormal semen analysis results associated with a history of recent febrile illness should be repeated over the ensuing 3 to 4 months to eliminate this confounding factor as a cause of the abnormalities.

Certain diseases can be associated with male subfertility. Neurologic disorders such as multiple sclerosis or spinal cord injury may cause impairment of ejaculation. A number of prescription medications can affect spermatogenesis. Sulfasalazine, used in the treatment of inflammatory bowel disease, will frequently cause severe oligo-asthenospermia. Cessation of the drug will often lead to restoration of normal seminal parameters, but unfortunately this will typically result in worsening of the underlying bowel disease. Other drugs commonly associated with diminished fertility include cimetidine, nitrofurantoin, spironolactone, colchicine, and allopurinol. Recent studies have suggested a possible impairment of sperm fertilizing ability with use of calcium channel blockers.

A history of cancer is of obvious importance, as chemotherapy and radiation therapy used in the treatment of any type of cancer may be gonadotoxic, and the damage to the seminiferous epithelium is often irreversible. Interestingly, men with certain forms of cancer such as lymphoma in sites distant to the testes will often have impaired semen parameters prior to any form of treatment.

Social History

A careful social history should be obtained to determine any exposure to toxic chemicals, heat, or radiation in the patient's work environment or hobbies. Prolonged direct exposure to toxins such as pesticides, herbicides, or organic solvents may reduce sperm counts or cause azoospermia. Exposure to ambient temperatures over 100°F for extensive periods of time, as may be seen in some workplaces or with use of hot tubs, saunas, or heated waterbeds, may result in reduced semen parameters.

Whether cigarette smoking may have a causal role in male subfertility has been controversial but some studies have shown reduced spermatogenesis with use of more than 20 cigarettes per day. Alcohol abuse may lead to diminished spermatogenesis by either direct toxic or hormonal effects, although mild to moderate use has not been shown to adversely affect fertility. Recreational drugs such as marijuana have been associated with decreases in sperm count, motility, and morphology. The effects are often reversible with discontinuation of the drugs.

The use of anabolic steroids can significantly impair spermatogenesis. Anabolic steroid use has unfortunately been on the rise lately, in particular among high school and college athletes. These drugs interfere with the hypothalamic–pituitary–gonadal axis and can lead to irreversible sterility even with only short-term use. Some physicians have used androgens either orally or parenterally in the treatment of male infertility in an attempt to enhance sperm production, with worsening of seminal parameters or azoospermia resulting.

Lastly, a careful review of systems should be obtained. The patient should be asked about any chronic respiratory problems, anosmia, headaches, or visual field defects to eliminate the rare possibility of Kartagener's syndrome (situs inversus, bronchiectasis, sinusitis, and immotile cilia), Kallman's syndrome (agenesis of olfactory lobes causing anosmia, and hypogonadal hypogonadism) or pituitary tumor.

Physical Examination

The physical examination of the potentially sub-fertile male should be thorough. Initially, the patient is examined with respect to secondary sexual characteristics. Attention is directed to the presence or absence of gynecomastia, which could be indicative of hyperprolactinemia or a hyperestrogenic state. The abdomen should be palpated for the presence of any masses or scars. Often an individual will have undergone herniorrhaphy or orchiopexy during infancy without being told of this by his parents.

The penis is examined and the location of the meatus is noted. Hypospadias can be associated with mechanical problems related to improper deposition of semen in the vaginal vault. There is also conjecture that this congenital abnormality may be associated with diminished semen quality as a result of a partial androgen insensitivity state.

The scrotal contents should be examined with the patient standing. The testes are evaluated with respect to size, location, and consistency. The length and width can be measured and recorded. Diminished testicular size is often associated with concomitant decrease in semen parameters. Testes of very soft consistency can also be indicative of impaired function. The presence or absence of a vas deferens on each side should be noted. The spermatic cords are palpated between the thumb and forefinger for the presence of varicoceles.

Varicoceles are defined as dilated veins of the pampiniform plexus and are the most common treatable cause of male infertility. Varicoceles are graded on a scale of 1 to 3. Grade 1 varicoceles are palpable as an impulse only when the patient performs a Valsalva maneuver. Grade 2 varicoceles are palpable both with and without Valsalva, and grade 3 varicoceles are visible through the scrotum as well as palpable without Valsalva. It is important to examine the patient after he has been standing for at least 10 minutes and in a warm room to accurately identify varicoceles.

A digital exam of the prostate is important to exclude the possibility of prostatitis. Prostate massage can be performed and the expressed prostatic fluid examined microscopically for the presence of inflammatory cells. The prostate may sometimes feel boggy in the presence of a large ejaculatory duct cyst or obstruction but this diagnosis is usually made with transrectal ultrasound.

Ancillary Tests

Semen Analysis

The laboratory evaluation of the subfertile male begins with the semen analysis. The specimen is usually collected by masturbation in a clean, wide-mouthed container after an abstinence period of 2 to 5 days. Special nonspermicidal condoms are available for use with coitus as an alternative. The specimen should be kept at approximately body temperature and delivered to the lab within 1 to 2 hours of collection. At least two or three specimens should be obtained over a 1 to 2-month time interval in the initial evaluation. If significant discrepancy is noted between the samples, then additional specimens are obtained as necessary.

The semen analysis is performed in the laboratory according to standardized techniques. Initially, the semen volume is measured and viscosity and color are recorded. Sperm density is quantified manually using a hemocytometer or counting chamber. Although computer assisted semen analysis (CASA) has been widely used as a research tool, manual examination by an experienced technician is the accepted standard in clinical practice.

If no sperm are noted on the counting chamber, the specimen is subjected to centrifugation and the pellet is examined for the presence of small numbers of sperm.

Assessment of sperm motility is then performed. The term "motility" refers to the percentage of sperm that are moving, while forward progression is a quantitative assessment of the quality of sperm movement in a forward direction. Forward progression is typically graded on a scale of 0 (no movement) to 4.0 (excellent, straight movement in a forward direction).

Sperm morphology is determined based on any of a number of classification schemes. Typically, sperm are classified as normal (oval) or into a number of abnormal categories (head defects, tail defects, tapering forms, immature) with percentages of each type listed. The normal range for morphology depends on the classification system used.

The presence and quantity of round cells are noted. It is difficult to differentiate seminal white blood cells from immature sperm cells without the use of special immunohistochemical stains. Sperm agglutination can be indicative of the presence of antisperm antibodies, and several different types of tests are available to evaluate this possibility. Special stains and other tests are available to evaluate the viability of sperm when none of the sperm are motile.

Although no "fertile–infertile" cut-off point can be determined for semen parameters, the probability of male fertility decreases with decreasing semen parameters. The average sperm density is approximately 70 million per mL, but studies have shown fecundity rates do not significantly decrease until sperm density is below 20 million per mL. Generally accepted "limits of adequacy" for the various semen parameters have been defined and are summarized in Table 18A–1. A glossary of commonly used terms related to classification of semen analysis abnormalities is shown in Table 18A–2.

Postcoital test

More sophisticated tests of sperm function are available although their place in the clinical evaluation of male infertility remains controversial. The postcoital test (PCT) measures the ability of sperm to penetrate the cervical mucus. The test is performed by examining a woman's cervical mucus several hours after intercourse during the expected time of ovulation. Although no standard exists for interpretation of the PCT, there should be several sperm with good forward progression per high-powered field on microscopic examination. An abnormal test in the presence of grossly normal semen parameters can be indicative of male or female antisperm antibodies or anatomic abnormalities.

Sperm Penetration Assay

In vitro tests of sperm–mucus interaction, which use bovine cervical mucus, are available in order to help determine whether abnormal PCT results are of male or female origin. The sperm penetration assay (SPA) or "hamster test" measures the ability of human sperm to penetrate hamster eggs

Table 18A–1

Semen Analysis: Minimal Limits of Adequacy

Volume: 1.5–5.0 mL
Sperm density: >20 million/mL
Motility: >50%
Forward progression: >2.0 (scale 0–4.0)
Normal morphology: >35% by WHO criteria
                    > 14% by strict criteria
Absence of pyospermia, agglutination, and hyperviscosity

Table 18A–2

Glossary of Semen Analysis Terms

Azoospermia: Zero sperm count
Aspermia: Absence of ejaculate
Oligospermia or oligozoospermia: Low sperm count or density
Asthenospermia or asthenozoospermia: Low sperm motility and/or forward progression
Teratozoospermia: Low percentage of morphologically normal sperm
(When more than one parameter is abnormal, the above terms may be combined, as in oligoasthenospermia—low sperm density and motility.)

processed to remove the species-specific zona pellucida. Although several studies have shown a correlation between the SPA and sperm-fertilizing ability with in vitro fertilization, the exact role of this test in the evaluation of the subfertile male remains unclear.

Endocrine Tests

Although endocrine causes of male subfertility are uncommon, accounting for no more than 3% of cases in most series, initial endocrine evaluation of the potentially subfertile male is usually undertaken. Serum FSH, LH, and testosterone levels are obtained during the first visit. If the testosterone level is low, then a repeat testosterone level is obtained in addition to a prolactin level to evaluate the possibility of hyperprolactinemia. In the obese male, a serum estradiol level should be obtained to determine whether a hyperestrogenic state may exist. Testosterone is converted to estrogen in fatty tissue by the action of the enzyme aromatase, and estrogen exerts inhibitory effects on the release of gonadotropins from the pituitary gland. Although several studies have shown the incidence of endocrine disorders to be low in men with sperm densities above 10 million, baseline gonadotropin levels may be important in assessing the potential effectiveness of empiric hormonal therapy. Tests of thyroid function have been shown to be needed only in individuals who exhibit clinical signs of hyper- or hypothyroidism.

Ultrasonography

Radiologic imaging, in particular ultrasound, has become important in the evaluation of male-factor infertility. Varicoceles are usually diagnosed by physical examination. In individuals where the physical exam for varicoceles is equivocal, usually due to the patient's body habitus, scrotal ultrasound has proven to be very helpful. The procedure is inexpensive and noninvasive and typically available in the urologist's office.

The exact ultrasound criteria to use as diagnostic of a varicocele remain controversial, although many centers regard spermatic veins greater than 2.5 mm and that increase with Valsalva or demonstrate reversal of flow as varicose. Because most studies have shown a correlation between size or grade of the varicocele and its impact on fertility, the routine use of scrotal ultrasound to detect "subclinical" varicoceles is discouraged.

In patients with low semen volumes (<1.5 mL) and azoospermia or severely decreased sperm motility, partial or complete obstruction of the ejaculatory ducts within the prostate is a diagnostic consideration. In the past, this diagnosis was made by surgical exposure of the vas deferens in conjunction with vasography. Transrectal ultrasound of the prostate and seminal vesicles has all but eliminated the need for vasography. The finding of dilated seminal vesicles in conjunction with a midline cystic structure or calcifications in the prostate is diagnostic of ejaculatory duct obstruction. Ultrasound may also be used in such individuals to perform transrectal aspiration of the dilated seminal vesicles in order to confirm the presence of sperm.

Testis Biopsy

If the initial semen analyses reveal azoospermia, then in general terms, the patient has either genital ductal obstruction or a sperm production problem. In most series, approximately one third of azoospermic patients are obstructed and two-thirds have testicular hypofunction. In the case of azoospermia, the serum FSH level is the most important prognostic test. If the serum FSH level is normal or mildly elevated, the possibility of ductal obstruction exists and the patient should next undergo diagnostic testicular biopsy. Studies have shown that if the serum FSH level is more than 2 to 3 times the upper limit of normal (typically more than 20 or 30 mIU/mL), this is evidence that the patient has an "untreatable" production problem. In these patients, testicular biopsy is unnecessary unless the couple wishes to pursue extraction of sperm from the testicle for use with advanced reproductive techniques (see "Assisted Reproductive Techniques" later in the chapter).

Testicular biopsy can be performed through an open technique in conjunction with exploration of the epididymis and spermatic cord, utilizing a small incision "window technique" or percutaneously using a Tru-Cut needle. The open techniques are usually performed in a hospital or ambulatory surgery center with general, regional, or local anesthesia. Percutaneous needle biopsy is typically performed in the urologist's office utilizing local anesthetic. Although percutaneous needle biopsy is less invasive and associated with lower costs, the quality of histology is usually not as good when compared with the open techniques. Unilateral testicular biopsy is usually performed unless there is significant testicular size discrepancy or other complicating factor such as previous inguinal surgery or history of scrotal trauma.

Microscopic examination of the testicular biopsy will reveal one of several histologic patterns: normal spermatogenesis, hypospermatogenesis, maturation arrest, or germ cell aplasia (Sertoli cell only). If normal spermatogenesis is noted in the azoospermic patient, then the presence of genital ductal obstruction is confirmed and further investigation with possible microsurgical reconstruction is undertaken. Although conditions causing nonobstructive azoospermia such as severe hypospermatogenesis or maturation arrest were formerly considered untreatable, pregnancy is now possible for many of these individuals with the use of assisted reproductive techniques.

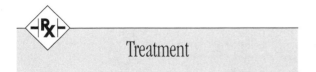

Treatment

Following the initial evaluation, and based on what is felt to be the cause or causes of the male-factor problem, different treatment options are re-

viewed with the patient and his wife. In approximately 25% of men with subfertile semen parameters, no treatable cause is identified, and these men are classified as having "idiopathic infertility." Treatment of male-factor subfertility problems can be classified as medical or surgical.

Medical therapy for male infertility can be divided into two general categories: specific therapy and empiric therapy. Specific therapy is utilized when a definable abnormality is present and treatment exists to correct it. Empiric therapy involves treatment of patients with idiopathic semen parameter abnormalities.

Specific Therapy

VARICOCELES

Varicoceles are the most common cause of male factor infertility. The incidence of varicoceles in the general population is approximately 15%. This incidence rises to 35% to 40% of subfertile men and is as high as 80% in men who have previously initiated a pregnancy (secondary infertility). The vast majority of varicoceles occur on the left side, and this left-sided predominance is felt to be due to the fact that the internal spermatic vein drains into the renal vein on the left side while the right internal spermatic vein drains into the inferior vena cava. The incidence of bilateral varicoceles depends on method of detection but is less than 10% in most series. The finding of an isolated right varicocele should alert the clinician to the possibility of vena caval obstruction secondary to tumor or thrombosis. (An isolated right varicocele thus should prompt an expedited workup for cancer, specifically, renal cell carcinoma.) Varicoceles are felt by most experts to cause testicular dysfunction by increasing the intrascrotal temperature.

Numerous studies have shown the effectiveness of varicocelectomy with respect to both improvement in semen quality (increased sperm density and motility and improved morphology) and pregnancy rates. Most studies have demonstrated improved semen quality in approximately 75% of men after varicocelectomy, with pregnancy rates as high as 40%.

Varicoceles may be corrected by a number of methods including surgical ligation by either subinguinal, inguinal, laparoscopic, or retroperitoneal approaches or by percutaneous embolization. Most male infertility specialists now favor a microscopic inguinal or subinguinal approach due to decreased recurrence rates compared to laparoscopic or retroperitoneal approaches. In the case of percutaneous embolization, costs are higher and success rates are lower than surgical ligation, although percutaneous embolization remains the modality of choice for recurrences after attempted surgical correction.

Surgical correction is typically performed in a hospital or ambulatory surgery center. Under general anesthesia or intravenous sedation, an inguinal or subinguinal incision is made and the spermatic cord is dissected out and delivered from the wound. After opening the enveloping spermatic and cremasteric fascial layers, the dilated internal spermatic veins are dissected out and double ligated with sutures using magnifying loupes or an operating microscope. The internal spermatic arteries, lymphatics, and the vas deferens along with its blood supply are preserved. Patients typically return to work in 2 to 3 days.

GENITAL TRACT OBSTRUCTION

Obstruction of the genital duct can occur at any level and is often amenable to surgical treatment. Congenital bilateral absence of the vas deferens (CBAVD) is the most common cause of obstructive azoospermia. Unfortunately, reconstruction is not possible in these cases, and treatment consists of microscopic epididymal sperm aspiration (MESA) or testicular sperm extraction (TESE) in conjunction with in vitro fertilization.

When obstruction occurs within the vas deferens or epididymis, usually due to previous vasectomy, epididymitis, or trauma, microsurgical reconstruction can be performed. The procedure is performed under a general anesthetic in a hos-

pital or ambulatory surgery center setting. Depending on the location of the obstruction, the distal vas deferens is anastomosed to either the vas deferens or the epididymal tubule proximal to the level of the obstruction using an operating microscope and microsutures of 9–0 and 10–0 nylon. With modern microsurgical techniques, success rates are excellent. In the case of vasal obstruction, microsurgical vasovasostomy results in return of sperm in the ejaculate in 80% to 90% of cases with pregnancy ensuing in 65% to 70%. When microsurgical epididymovasostomy is performed for epididymal obstruction, there is restoration of patency in 70% and pregnancy rates of 40%.

When transrectal ultrasound of the prostate reveals the presence of obstruction of the ejaculatory ducts, transurethral resection of the ejaculatory ducts (TURED) may be performed. Under a general or spinal anesthetic, a resectoscope is passed through the urethra into the prostate. Tissue is resected from the floor of the prostate until the obstructing cyst is unroofed or the dilated ejaculatory ducts are visualized. Following this procedure, there is often rapid return of sperm in the semen, with pregnancy quickly following.

HYPOGONADOTROPIC HYPOGONADISM

While hypogonadotropic hypogonadism (HH) is present in only a small percentage of patients with male-factor infertility, successful treatment is very common. Causes include congenital HH (Kallman's syndrome), idiopathic HH, or acquired HH secondary to pituitary tumors, trauma, anabolic steroid use, or pituitary failure. Treatment involves gonadotropin replacement initially with human chorionic gonadotropin (hCG) given 2000 IU intramuscularly three times per week followed by addition of human menopausal gonadotropins (hMG, a combination of FSH and LH) 75 IU three times per week intramuscularly if sperm counts have not improved after 8 to 12 weeks of hCG therapy. While on hCG and hMG, serum FSH, LH, and testosterone should be monitored at 1 month to titrate the dose. Also, a semen analysis should be rechecked at 3 months. Interestingly, pregnancy rates are very high in these couples, often with sperm densities as low as 5 million per mL.

HYPERPROLACTINEMIA

Hyperprolactinemia has been implicated as a cause of both male infertility and impotence. Prolactin exerts a negative influence on hypothalamic release of GnRH and is felt to have an inhibitory effect on the binding of LH to Leydig cells in the testis. Patients with hyperprolactinemia should undergo pituitary gland imaging with MRI or CT scan of the brain to detect pituitary adenomas. Individuals with macroadenomas generally require surgical extirpation, while those with microadenomas respond to medical treatment with bromocryptine or cabergoline. Hypothyroidism is estimated to be a cause in approximately 0.6% of male infertility cases. Patients typically have normal serum FSH and LH levels with elevated prolactin and decreased testosterone levels. Semen analyses show decreases in all parameters. Treatment with thyroxine will often restore fertility.

ANTISPERM ANTIBODIES

Antisperm antibodies can be a cause of male-factor infertility. Because production of mature spermatozoa does not commence until puberty, sperm are antigenically foreign with respect to the immune system. Events that disrupt the "blood–testis barrier" of the seminiferous tubules expose sperm surface antigens to the immune system leading to the production of antisperm antibodies. Risk factors for development of antisperm antibodies include patients with a history of epididymo-orchitis, testicular trauma or torsion, or scrotal surgery. Antisperm antibodies can affect fertility by binding to sperm tails, inhibiting motility; or by binding to sperm heads, inhibiting sperm fertilizing ability.

Treatment in the past involved use of corticosteroids in an attempt to suppress antisperm antibody production. Unfortunately, most studies have shown low-dose steroid regimens to be of no benefit and high-dose regimens to be fraught with serious complications such as avascular necrosis of the hip. Although some centers still employ moderate-dose cyclic steroid regimens, most experts now feel that assisted reproductive techniques are the best treatment for this problem.

ASSISTED REPRODUCTIVE TECHNIQUES

Assisted reproductive techniques (ART) involve the manipulation of sperm and/or eggs. The most commonly employed modalities are intrauterine insemination (IUI) and in vitro fertilization with embryo transfer (IVF-ET). Prior to using semen for any type of assisted reproduction, it is necessary to process it to remove prostaglandins, white blood cells, bacteria, and other debris. In addition, processing may enhance the quality of sperm motility.

A number of methods are available for sperm processing depending on the desired outcome. The "swim up" technique involves first washing the sperm using sperm processing medium and centrifugation, following which fresh medium is added and the most motile sperm swim into the supernatant and are extracted and used for ART. Density gradient techniques usually employ Percoll, a colloidal suspension of silica particles, or similar compounds in layers of different concentrations. Following centrifugation, the best-quality sperm may be found at the bottom of the processing tube and used for ART. Although the yield of sperm may be lower with density gradient techniques, the sperm have been shown to be of high quality with enhanced motility and improved fertilizing capacity.

IUI involves placing processed semen into the uterine cavity. The semen must be processed using one of the previously mentioned techniques, as the naturally present prostaglandins cause significant uterine irritation. Insemination is performed at the time of ovulation, typically using urinary ovulation prediction kits that measure the LH surge. The sperm are concentrated to a volume of less than 1 cc and loaded into a syringe with a plastic insemination catheter. The catheter is inserted through the cervix into the upper uterine cavity where the sperm are deposited. This procedure bypasses the barrier effect of the cervix and cervical mucus and places the sperm closer to the fallopian tubes where fertilization occurs. Most studies have shown modest increases in pregnancy rates when IUI is used in the treatment of male factor infertility. Most pregnancies occur within 3 or 4 inseminations, with few pregnancies occurring after more than 6 inseminations in most series. Success rates are low when less than 5 million motile sperm are inseminated, but pregnancies have been documented with as few as 200,000 motile sperm. Pregnancy rates may be improved with concomitant controlled ovarian hyperstimulation using clomiphene citrate or human menopausal gonadotropin.

IVF-ET involves controlled stimulation of the ovaries to initiate development of multiple follicles during the female reproductive cycle. Follicle development is followed with serial ultrasound evaluation and serum estradiol levels. When follicle size is adequate, human chorionic gonadotropin is administered to cause follicular maturation. The follicles are aspirated transvaginally with ultrasound guidance. The aspirated oocytes are then combined with processed sperm in a Petri dish. Following 48 hours incubation, the oocytes are assessed, and typically 2 to 3 embryos are transferred into the uterus using a transfer catheter. Surplus embryos may be cryopreserved. Numerous studies have revealed lower fertilization and pregnancy rates for male-factor infertility patients using conventional IVF-ET.

Because of these lower fertilization and pregnancy rates and the need for motile sperm, sperm micromanipulation techniques were developed specifically for severe male-factor infertility. Intracytoplasmic sperm injection (ICSI) involves injection of a single sperm into the cytoplasm of the oocyte using a microinjection pipette and a phase contrast microscope. Assessment of fertilization and embryo transfer is identical to conventional IVF-ET. Patients with severe oligospermia or asthenospermia, immunologic infertility, or failed conventional IVF-ET are candidates for IVF with ICSI. Patients with genital ductal obstruction not amenable to reconstruction such as CBAVD or failed vasovasostomy or epididymovasostomy may undergo MESA or TESE in conjunction with IVF with ICSI. Recently, pregnancies have been documented in patients with azoospermia and severe hypospermatogenesis on testicular biopsy—so-called nonobstructive azoospermia—using TESE and IVF with ICSI. The incidence of birth defects has not been shown to be significantly higher in children conceived using these advanced assisted reproductive techniques, but propagation of possible gene defects related to male infertility is a concern.

With sophisticated ART, there has been a trend towards ignoring potentially treatable male-factor infertility problems and proceeding directly to treatment with IVF-ET with or without ICSI when an abnormal semen analysis is discovered. This approach is suboptimal for several reasons. Studies of the cost-effectiveness of different infertility treatments have consistently shown lower costs per delivery for treatment of male-factor problems such as varicoceles when compared with proceeding directly to IVF. In addition, the tremendous expense of IVF puts this technology beyond the financial means of many couples when these services are not covered by health insurance. Furthermore, not all couples are willing to accept IVF from a moral or ethical standpoint. Lastly, studies of male infertility patients reveal serious underlying health problems such as testicular cancer in a small but measurable fraction of these patients.

INFECTION

Infection of the male reproductive tract is another treatable cause of male-factor infertility. Irritative voiding symptoms, painful ejaculation, or urethral discharge may be indicative of prostatitis or urethritis. In some asymptomatic patients, the finding of prostatic tenderness in conjunction with elevated white blood cells in the prostatic fluid or the finding of white blood cells on semen analysis (pyospermia) may indicate infection. Genital tract infections are most commonly caused by gram-negative bacilli, *Neisseria gonorrhoeae*, and

Chlamydia trachomatis. Cultures should be obtained and treatment instituted with antibiotics possessing activity against these pathogens and with good penetration into the genitourinary tract. Recommendations from the Centers for Disease Control should be consulted (see Chapter 7). Current first-line management in the United States of gonorrhea includes ceftriaxone, and of chlamydia by doxycycline or the fluoroquinolones levofloxacin and floxacin. Patients should be treated for 2 to 4 weeks and reevaluated to insure the adequacy of treatment. Persistent pyospermia after antibiotic therapy may be indicative of causes of genital tract inflammation other than infection, especially if cultures are not obtained or are negative.

DISORDERS OF EJACULATION

Disorders of ejaculation include retrograde ejaculation and anejaculation. Retrograde ejaculation, where sperm enter the bladder during ejaculation, can occur with previous bladder neck surgery, diabetes mellitus, or with some neurologic conditions. The diagnosis is made by the finding of sperm on examination of a postejaculation urine specimen. Retrograde ejaculation will sometimes respond to medical therapy with imipramine 25 mg orally twice a day or alpha-sympathomimetic agents such as pseudoephedrine 60 mg orally four times a day. Medications are taken continuously for at least 2 weeks and discontinued if there is no improvement. In cases unresponsive to medical therapy, postejaculate urine may be processed in order to extract the sperm for use with assisted reproductive techniques.

Anejaculation, the complete absence of ejaculation, may occur with spinal cord injury, multiple sclerosis, or after retroperitoneal surgery such as retroperitoneal lymph node dissection for testicular cancer. Anejaculation is treated with electroejaculation or surgical retrieval of sperm from the vas deferens or epididymis in conjunction with assisted reproductive techniques. Electroejaculation is performed using an electrical probe inserted into the rectum. An electrical generator is used to transmit low-voltage pulses via the rectal probe to the anterior rectal wall. The energy level is increased until ejaculation ensues, typically at less than 20 volts. The ejaculate is collected in a container with sperm-washing medium and the patient is catheterized to collect any retrograde ejaculate. Both specimens are then processed and used for assisted reproduction. Because electroejaculation is not currently FDA approved, this modality is only available at a limited number of centers. In areas where electroejaculation is not available, surgical extraction of sperm from the vas deferens or epididymis is the treatment of choice. Some patients with cervical spinal cord injuries will ejaculate in response to vibratory stimulation of the glans penis using a commercially available vibrator.

Empiric Therapy

Many empiric therapies have been tried over the years in the treatment of idiopathic oligoasthenospermia. Some of the most common of these treatments involve medications with a hormonal action. The antiestrogens clomiphene citrate (25 mg orally per day, with FSH and testosterone monitoring each month to titrate the dose, and a semen analysis 4 months after therapy begins) and tamoxifen have been studied in a number of controlled and uncontrolled trials in patients with normal gonadotropin levels over the past 30 years. Although several controlled studies have shown significant improvements in sperm density and/or motility as well as improved pregnancy rates, other studies have not and therefore controversy remains. Treatment with androgens given either orally or intramuscularly has not been shown to have a beneficial effect in most studies and may further suppress sperm production via feedback inhibition of the hypothalamic–pituitary–gonadal axis. A number of other medications and health supplements have been purported to improve semen parameters including kallikreins, nonsteroidal antiinflammatory agents, bromocriptine, zinc, L-carnitine, and a variety of herbs. Controlled studies demonstrating efficacy for these agents are lacking.

Recent studies have demonstrated an increase in the level of reactive oxygen species (ROS) in the seminal fluid of men with diminished semen parameters. In light of this observation, many centers have recommended antioxidant vitamin supplements to such patients. Although no controlled studies exist regarding the use of antioxidants, the low cost and minimal side effects make them an attractive adjuvant therapy. My current antioxidant regimen includes vitamin C 1000 mg orally per day, vitamin E 400 IU orally per day, and multivitamin 1 tablet orally per day.

Conclusion

The primary care clinician has an important role in the investigation of possible male-factor infertility. The male member of any couple presenting for infertility investigation should be fully evaluated to eliminate preventable causes of male infertility such as tobacco or drug use or heat exposure, rule out the possibility of a serious underlying medical condition, and treat genital tract infection if found. Patients with other correctable conditions affecting fertility should be referred to a urologist for further evaluation and treatment.

Bibliography

Carbone DJ: Male reproductive physiology and assisted reproductive technology. *AUA Update Series* 18: 162–167, 1999.

Gilbaugh JH III: Intrauterine insemination. In Lipshultz LI, Howards SS (eds): *Infertility in the Male.* St. Louis, Mosby-Year Book, 1997.

Gilbaugh JH III, Lipshultz LI: Nonsurgical treatment of male infertility: An update. *Urol Clin North Am* 21: 531–548, 1994.

Goldstein M: Surgical Management of male infertility and other scrotal disorders. In Walsh PC, Retik AB, Vaughn ED, Wein AJ (eds): *Campbell's Urology,* ed 7. Philadelphia, Saunders, 1998.

Nagler HM, Luntz RK, Martinis FG: Varicocele. In Lipshultz LI, Howards SS (eds): *Infertility in the Male.* St. Louis, Mosby-Year Book, 1997.

Sigman M, Lipshultz LI, Howards SS: Evaluation of the subfertile male. In Lipshultz LI, Howards SS (eds): *Infertility in the Male.* St. Louis, Mosby-Year Book, 1997.

James H. Gilbaugh III

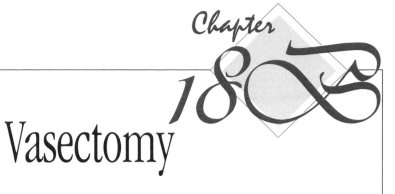

Vasectomy

How Commonly Is Vasectomy Performed?

Each year approximately half a million American men undergo surgical sterilization via vasectomy. The proper preoperative assessment and counseling, surgical technique, and controversies surrounding possible adverse health consequences will be reviewed.

Preoperative Assessment and Counseling

Individuals considering vasectomy should be interested in achieving permanent sterilization. During the initial visit, a careful medical history should be obtained to ensure that no medical contraindications to the procedure exist such as bleeding diatheses, scrotal infection, or epididymitis. Physical examination is performed with emphasis on the genitalia to assure the presence of vasa deferentia bilaterally and to rule out testicular cancer. Alternative forms of birth control should be reviewed and the physician should feel that the patient understands the potential permanency of the procedure.

The technical aspects of the vasectomy procedure should be carefully reviewed during the initial consultation. The use of anatomic diagrams is particularly helpful, as many patients are unfamiliar with male reproductive anatomy and the exact nature of the vasectomy procedure. In addition, the potential complications should be thoroughly discussed, as a number of medical malpractice cases have been successful based on a lack of proper informed consent.

The possibility of bleeding with hematoma formation (potentially requiring hospitalization to treat) should be discussed, because many of the patients are paying for the procedure out of pocket and/or do not have health insurance that would cover the costs of the subsequent treatment. As with any surgical procedure, the possibility of infection exists. This can occur in the form of a scrotal wound infection or epididymitis. Rare complications such as testicular loss should be discussed, especially if the patient has undergone previous scrotal of inguinal surgery where the testicular vasculature may have been compromised. Chronic testicular pain may ensue with the incidence being approximately 0.1% but as high as 5% in some series.

It should be emphasized to the patient that he needs to consider himself as potentially fertile until azoospermia is demonstrated on a postvasectomy semen analysis. Whether centrifuged or uncentrifuged semen specimens should be examined, and whether one or multiple azoospermic samples should be required, remains controversial. Most physicians who perform vasectomies feel that demonstrating azoospermia in one uncentrifuged semen specimen after the procedure is adequate. The possibility of spontaneous recanalization should be discussed. Historically, this has been noted to occur in approximately one out every 5000 vasectomies. Lastly, a discussion of the controversies surrounding vasectomy and a purported increased risk of problems such as prostate cancer (discussed later in the chapter) should be held. While no form of birth control except abstinence is 100% successful and risk-free, in experienced hands, vasectomy is a safe and effective means of sterilization.

Open Technique

Vasectomy is typically performed in an office setting under local anesthesia. The procedure room should be warm to encourage scrotal relaxation. The scrotum is shaved, then prepped using a warm antiseptic solution of choice. The procedure can be performed through bilateral scrotal incisions or a single incision along the median raphe of the scrotum. The vas is palpated and isolated from the remaining spermatic cord structures, following which local anesthetic is infiltrated into the scrotal skin and perivasal sheath (Fig. 18B–1).

A small vertical incision is made in the scrotal skin over the vas deferens, following which the vas is dissected out and delivered. The perivasal vessels are dissected away from the vas and a small segment is excised. The ends may be cauterized, ligated with sutures, or clipped with hemoclips depending on surgeon preference. Interposition of perivasal fascia around the testicular end of the vas using sutures is performed by some and may reduce the rate of recanalization. Hemostasis should be assured and then the incision is closed with interrupted absorbable sutures.

The patient is advised to rest and apply ice to the scrotum for 24 hours after the procedure and to avoid sex or vigorous activity such as exercise

Figure 18B–1

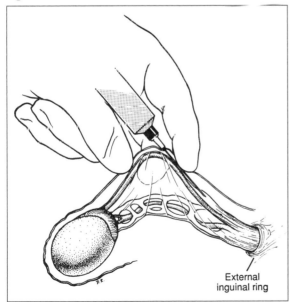

Local anesthetic is infiltrated into the scrotal skin and perivasal sheath. (Drawing courtesy of Dr. Marc Goldstein, Center for Male Reproductive Medicine and Microsurgery, Department of Urology, The New York Hospital–Weill Medical College of Cornell University.)

or heavy lifting for one week. As during the initial consultation, the patient should again be advised to consider himself as potentially fertile until postoperative azoospermia is assured.

No Scalpel Technique

A "no scalpel" vasectomy technique developed in China utilizing a special set of instruments has recently gained popularity in the United States. The initial preparation is identical to that of a conventional vasectomy. Following infiltration with local anesthetic, the vas deferens is fixed beneath the scrotal skin with a fixation clamp (Fig. 18B–2). A sharp-pointed curved dissecting clamp is used to puncture the scrotal skin, and the vas deferens is penetrated and delivered through the scrotal puncture with a twisting motion (Fig. 18B–3). The vasal vessels are dissected away from the vas and then the ends ligated or cauterized according to surgeon preference as with conventional vasectomy.

The scrotal puncture site typically does not require sutures to close. Postoperative instructions are the same as for conventional vasectomy. The "no scalpel" technique is purported to be less painful and have a lower incidence of complications such as scrotal hematoma. Several companies now manufacture "no scalpel" vasectomy instruments and have marketed them on the Internet. It is now common for patients to present specifically requesting this procedure.

Purported Health Consequences

Over the years, studies have looked at a possible association of vasectomy with a number of secondary health problems. Sperm production occurs within the testis protected from the ele-

Figure 18B–2

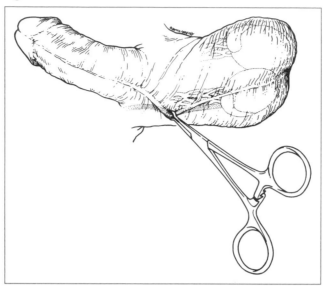

The vas deferens is fixed beneath the scrotal skin with a fixation clamp. (Drawing courtesy of Dr. Marc Goldstein, Center for Male Reproductive Medicine and Microsurgery, Department of Urology, The New York Hospital–Weill Medical College of Cornell University.)

Figure 18B–3

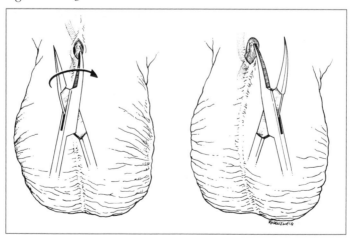

Left. A sharp-pointed curved dissecting clamp is used to puncture the scrotal skin. *Right.* The vas deferens is penetrated and delivered through the scrotal puncture with a twisting motion. (Drawing courtesy of Dr. Marc Goldstein, Center for Male Reproductive Medicine and Microsurgery, Department of Urology, The New York Hospital–Weill Medical College of Cornell University.)

ments of the immune system by the so-called blood–testis barrier provided by the Sertoli cells. Following vasectomy, the blood–testis barrier is disrupted, exposing sperm to the immune system which reacts by producing antibodies against them.

Postulating circulating immune complexes as the cause, a study published in 1978 reported an increased incidence of atherosclerosis in a small group of monkeys that had undergone vasectomy and were fed a high-cholesterol diet. This initial study provoked intense research in this area, but follow-up animal and human studies have failed to reveal any demonstrable association between vasectomy and atherosclerotic vascular disease. Studies of possible links between vasectomy and other immune complex-mediated diseases such as systemic lupus erythematosus and rheumatoid arthritis have similarly failed to reveal any association.

Several studies over the past 15 years have suggested a possible link between vasectomy and prostate cancer. A recent review of the literature and meta-analysis of existing studies have concluded that no association exists between vasectomy and prostate cancer. The current recommendation is that men who have undergone vasectomy be screened for prostate cancer based on the same guidelines as nonvasectomized men.

Bibliography

Bernal-Delgado E, Latour-Perez J, Pradas-Arnal F, et al. The association between vasectomy and prostate cancer: A systematic review of the literature. *Fertil Steril* 1998;70:191–200.

Li S, Goldstein M, Zhu J, et al. The no-scalpel vasectomy. *J Urol* 1991;145:341–344.

Schlegel PN, Goldstein M. Vasectomy. *AUA Update Series* 1994;11:98–103.

J. Bruce Redmon
Jon L. Pryor

Chapter
19

Male Menopause

Perhaps because of their unique anatomic location, the male testes have from earliest times been recognized as the source of some unique factor conferring "maleness." The Greeks and Romans used testicular preparations from goats and wolves as sexual stimulants. Brown-Séquard, the 19th century French physician and early endocrinologist, gave himself an animal testicular extract and reported improved vigor and capacity for work. In the early 20th century, men underwent monkey testicular implants with expectations of increased energy, improved cognitive function, and reversal of gray hair.

Subsequently, some physicians in the 1930s and 1940s began to speak of a male menopause, typically described as a syndrome of middle-aged men characterized by a wide variety of sexual, constitutional, and emotional complaints reminiscent of the female menopause. After the discovery of testosterone as the predominant male hormone, testosterone therapy was advocated by some as treatment for the male menopause. Clinical trials and anecdotal case reports, typically uncontrolled, suggested remarkable benefits.

Today, as the number of individuals living to older ages increases, there is increasing interest in the aging process and the changes of aging that rob us of our youth and vigor. For men, much of this interest has focused on declining testosterone levels in older men and the question of whether testosterone treatment can ameliorate, prevent, or even reverse real or perceived changes of aging. Because the term male menopause is an oxymoron (literally, menopause means "cessation of monthly"), a number of alternative names have been suggested for a male aging syndrome, linked at least in part to falling testosterone levels. These include the male climacteric, andropause, viropause, male midlife crisis, and most recently, the low testosterone syndrome. Whatever the name, a whole host of signs and symptoms have been attributed to the male menopause (Table 19–1).

We will review the scientific evidence for and against the existence of a male menopause as it may relate to age-associated changes in that most important of all testicular factors—testosterone.

Table 19–1

Suggested Signs and Symptoms of the Male Menopause

Decreased energy	Erectile dysfunction
Fatigue	Hot flashes
Decreased libido	Decreased strength and endurance
Depression, irritability	Decreased memory
Decreased enjoyment of life	Palpitations
Headache	Falling asleep after dinner

How Common Is Male Menopause?

The prevalence of male menopause varies, depending on the definition used to characterize the condition. Men aged 40 to 51 years old were asked the question, "Is there a male climacteric?" From 32% to 59% of respondents answered positively. When a subset of men were interviewed, 18% said they were climacteric. If male menopause is defined as hypogonadism, the estimates vary from 5% to 20% of older men having low total testosterone levels and as high as 50% to 60% of older men having low free testosterone levels.

Physiology

What Is a Normal Testosterone Level?

Testosterone is secreted episodically throughout the day and circulating levels vary accordingly. The variation of testosterone levels follows a circadian rhythm, highest in the early morning hours and lowest in the afternoon. As a result, laboratory reference values are quite broad, typically 300 to 1200 ng/dL. Up to 15% of normal men may have testosterone levels that dip as low as 100 ng/dL during a 24-hour period, a value that would be unquestionably hypogonadal if present on a consistent basis. Stress and illness can also transiently lower testosterone levels in a man with otherwise normal gonadal function.

To complicate things further, the vast majority of testosterone (95% or more) circulates bound to proteins, predominantly sex hormone binding globulin (SHBG) and albumin. Testosterone bound to SHBG is tightly bound and not readily dissociable, while testosterone bound to albumin and other proteins readily dissociates and is biologically active. Thus, the free fraction of testosterone (approximately 2% of the total testosterone pool) or the fraction that is not bound to SHBG (approximately 70% of the total testosterone pool) may be better indicators of the true gonadal status. Unfortunately, accurate measurement of free testosterone is difficult and various assay methods give very different results.

For practical purposes, a morning total testosterone measurement is an adequate and reliable indicator of gonadal function. An abnormal testosterone level should always be confirmed by repeat measurement. In some cases, multiple measurements extending over a several-month period may be necessary to accurately determine whether a man is truly hypogonadal. Measurement of free testosterone or non-SHBG-bound testosterone in addition to total testosterone may be helpful in situations in which levels of SHBG are either increased or decreased (Table 19–2).

Older men with definite hypogonadism (testosterone values <200 ng/dL) should have an evaluation to try and establish the cause. Men with small soft testes and elevated gonadotropins (i.e., LH and FSH) have primary testicular failure and do not need further testing in most cases. If gonadotropin levels are inappropriately normal or low, however, evaluation of overall pituitary function is appropriate, including measurement of prolactin and thyroid hormone levels, screening for hemochromatosis with a serum percent iron saturation or ferritin, and MRI of the pituitary and hypothalamus.

How aggressively to investigate older men with borderline testosterone levels in the 200 to 300 ng/dL range and normal gonadotropin levels is debatable. Laboratory screening with prolactin, thyroid levels, and iron studies is reasonable. MRI imaging is expensive and unlikely to be informative in most cases. Imaging studies can probably be reserved for men who have localized symptoms such as headache or visual problems or who have other clinical or laboratory evidence of pituitary dysfunction.

Do Testosterone Levels Decline with Age?

There is now general consensus that testosterone levels decline with age. Data from both large epidemiologic studies, such as the Massachusetts Male Aging Study, and smaller studies of well-defined groups of healthy men support this conclusion. Because SHBG levels increase with age, free testosterone levels typically show an even greater decline with age than does total testosterone. In the Massachusetts Male Aging Study, a cross-sectional study of 1700 community-dwelling men between the ages of 39 and 70, total testosterone levels declined by about 0.5% per year. SHBG increased by 1.2% per year, and both free testosterone and albumin-bound testosterone decreased by approximately 1% per year. Overall, free testosterone levels were about one-third lower in 70-year-olds compared to men aged 40. Testosterone levels were higher by about 10% to 15% in nonobese, healthy men compared to men with obesity or other chronic medical

Table 19–2

Conditions Affecting Sex Hormone Binding Globulin (SHBG) Levels

INCREASED SHBG	DECREASED SHBG
Hyperthyroidism	Hypothyroidism
Liver disease	Nephrotic syndrome
Estrogen therapy	Androgen treatment
Growth hormone deficiency	Growth hormone excess
Aging	Obesity

conditions. Nonetheless, testosterone levels declined with age in both groups at a similar rate.

Despite an age-related decline in testosterone levels, most older men still have total testosterone levels within the normal range. In the Massachusetts Male Aging Study, only 5% of men had a total serum testosterone level below 250 ng/dL. Data from the Telecom Study, a large epidemiologic study of 1400 Parisian men ages 20 to 60, revealed 5% of men with total testosterone values below 350 ng/dL. At the University of Washington, researchers over the years have recorded total testosterone levels from almost 100 healthy elderly man ages 60 to 80. Twenty percent of these men had testosterone levels below 300 ng/dL. If one looks at free or "bioavailable" testosterone levels rather than total testosterone, however, the percentage of older man with levels below the normal range for young men increases. Up to 50% to 60% of older men may have low free or bioavailable testosterone values using reference norms for young men.

What Target Tissues Are Affected By Low Testosterone Levels?

In the male, androgens play an important role in sexual and reproductive function, body composition, bone and lipid metabolism, and hematopoiesis. Young men who are severely hypogonadal, such as after complete orchiectomy, or men with severe hypogonadotropic hypogonadism, will typically have testosterone values below 100 ng/dL and will manifest corresponding signs and symptoms of testosterone deficiency. Hypogonadal young men report decreased frequency of erections and sexual events, decreased number of nocturnal erections, and decreased sexual desire and sexual fantasies. Compared to eugonadal men they report increased feelings of anger, depression, fatigue, and confusion. They have a more "female" body habitus with increased body fat, decreased muscle mass and

muscle strength, and decreased body hair. Bone density is also decreased, and they are at greater risk for osteoporosis compared to eugonadal men.

Testosterone replacement for these men reverses or significantly ameliorates virtually all of the above manifestations of androgen deficiency. Libido, number of spontaneous and nocturnal erections, and reported sexual activity increase. Treated hypogonadal men report increased levels of energy, initiative, overall sense of well-being, and improved mood. Muscle size, strength, and lean body mass increase, and fat mass may decrease. Bone density also increases.

The normally aging male is in many ways strikingly similar to the hypogonadal male (Table 19–3). The aging male experiences decreased quality of erections, a changing body habitus with increased fat mass, decreased muscle mass and strength, and decreased bone density. In the middle-aged man who is also complaining of fatigue, decreased energy, anxiety, depression, or poor memory, it is tempting to attribute these complaints to an age-related decline in testosterone. On the other hand, the majority of older men have testosterone levels well above the testosterone levels seen in hypogonadal young men, in whom most of the effects of testosterone replacement have been studied.

Table 19–3

Androgen Targets and Changes in Aging Men

TARGET	CHANGES WITH AGING
Sexual and reproductive function	Decreased libido, erectile dysfunction, increased prostate volume, increased prevalence of prostate cancer
Body composition	Decreased muscle mass and strength, increased fat mass, decreased androgen-dependent hair growth
Bone metabolism	Decreased bone density
Mood, cognitive function (?)	Decreased spatial cognition
Hematopoiesis	Decreased hemoglobin level

The question then becomes, what level of testosterone is "too low" and would benefit from testosterone supplementation in otherwise healthy older men? This question cannot be answered today, and may never be fully answered. Nonetheless, as discussed in the next section, there are some data to help guide clinicians facing this dilemma.

Pathophysiology

Aging, Testosterone, and Sexual Function

Age is the strongest risk factor for erectile dysfunction. In the Massachusetts Male Aging Study, the proportion of men who considered themselves "completely impotent" increased from 5% at age 40 to 15% by age 70. As discussed, testosterone is important for normal sexual function.

However, several studies, including the Massachusetts Male Aging Study, have failed to find a clear relationship between testosterone levels and erectile function in older men. Thus, although aging is associated with both lower testosterone levels and decreased erectile function, these appear to be independent associations. The explanation for this may lie in studies that have attempted to define a dose relationship between erectile function and testosterone.

When nocturnal erections were monitored in men with a wide range of testosterone levels from frankly hypogonadal to clearly normal, a significant falloff in the frequency and quality of nocturnal erections was seen only when the testosterone level fell below 200 ng/dL. Because most older men will have testosterone levels greater than this level, it seems unlikely that declining testosterone is a significant contributor to the age-associated decline in erectile function. Similarly, testosterone therapy appears to be of little benefit in the treatment of erectile dysfunction unless testosterone levels are severely low.

The dose relationship between sexual interest and testosterone level is not well defined. Severely hypogonadal men do report improved libido with testosterone therapy. Positive effects of testosterone therapy in men with normal testosterone levels but low sexual interest have been reported but are modest, at best. Peter Snyder and colleagues at the University of Pennsylvania School of Medicine recently studied 108 older men with mean serum testosterone levels of 370 ng/dL in a 3-year, double-blind, placebo controlled trial of transdermal testosterone therapy. In these men, testosterone therapy had no significant effect on sexual function as assessed by questionnaire responses.

In summary, epidemiologic data and limited data from long-term, controlled clinical trials do not support the notion that modest decreases in testosterone that may occur with aging are a primary determinant of declining sexual function.

Aging, Testosterone, and Body Composition

Men tend to gain weight up to around age 40, after which total body weight remains relatively stable. However, beginning in middle age, there is a decline in muscle or lean body mass and a concomitant increase in fat mass. In effect, older men begin to develop a body composition more like that of hypogonadal men.

Testosterone increases muscle protein syn thesis and muscle size and strength. This has been demonstrated both in hypogonadal young men given testosterone replacement therapy and in normal men given supraphysiologic doses of testosterone. In hypogonadal men, 10 weeks of testosterone therapy to raise the testosterone level from 72 ng/dL to a normal level of 510 ng/dL (a 7-fold increase) increased fat-free (i.e., lean body) mass by about 10% and bench press and squat strength by 20% to 45%. Normal men given very large doses of testosterone enanthate (600 mg IM every week) increased their testosterone levels from a normal baseline value of 400 ng/dL to supraphysiologic levels of 2800 ng/dL (also a 7-fold increase). After 10 weeks of treatment, fat-free mass increased by 4.5% and bench press and squat strength increased by 10% to 13%. Comparing these results suggests a law of diminishing returns may be in effect—the lower (more abnormal) the starting testosterone level, the greater the relative benefit on body composition and muscle strength.

What about older men with "low normal" or "borderline low" testosterone levels? Several studies have now addressed this question, with predictable results. When older men were given testosterone therapy to raise the testosterone level from baseline values of 300 to 350 ng/dL to treatment values of 400 to 700 ng/dL (1.5 to 2-fold increase), only minimal increases in lean body mass (approximately 2%) were seen. Effects on muscle strength were mixed. Some studies found no effect on muscle strength, while others found modest increases in some but not all measures of muscle strength or function. Body fat either remained unchanged or decreased slightly in these studies. In the longest and largest controlled trial to date, that of Snyder and colleagues already described, 3 years of testosterone therapy to raise testosterone levels from an average baseline value of 367 ng/dL to 625 ng/dL (a 1.7-fold increase) resulted in a 3% (4 lb) increase in fat-free mass and a 12% (7 lb) decrease in fat mass. Testosterone therapy had no effect on multiple measures of muscle strength or function including knee extension/flexion strength, hand grip strength, and time to climb stairs. By way of comparison, in one study of elderly nursing-home residents given resistance exercise training for 10 weeks, muscle strength increased over 100% and significant increases were seen in gait velocity and stair-climbing power!

In summary, testosterone can increase muscle size and strength in any man if given in a large enough dose. In older men with "low normal" or "slightly low" testosterone levels, the effects of raising testosterone to the mid-normal range on body composition and muscle strength are trivial to modest. Testosterone therapy may also decrease fat mass, although this has not been a consistent finding across studies. Regular exercise, including some resistance training, may be more effective.

Aging, Testosterone, and Bone Density

Testosterone regulates bone metabolism in men, although the exact mechanisms involved are not entirely established. Androgen receptors are present on osteoblasts, suggesting a role for direct anabolic action of testosterone on bone formation. Testosterone may also inhibit bone resorption, an effect probably mediated through testosterone conversion to estrogen. In any event, men, like women, achieve peak bone mass in early adulthood and then continually lose bone mass with advancing age. Hypogonadism is a cause of osteoporosis in men as well as women, and hormone replacement therapy—estrogen for women, testosterone for men—increases bone mass in hypogonadal individuals.

Do falling testosterone levels lead to decreases in bone density in older men? Will testosterone therapy for older men slow or reverse the bone loss of aging and prevent fracture? Although long-term studies will be necessary to fully answer these questions, several short-term studies have attempted to address these questions using surrogate biochemical markers of bone metabolism. In general, these studies have found no effect on most markers of bone metabolism. One study, however, did find a decrease in urinary hydroxyproline excretion, a marker of bone resorption.

In the 3-year controlled trial of Snyder and colleagues, bone density in the lumbar spine increased significantly in both the placebo (2.5%) and testosterone (4.2%) treatment groups. These increases were not significantly different between the two groups. Bone density at the hip did not change in either group. Two observations from this study are important. First, 98 of the 108 men in this study were judged at baseline to have diets somewhat deficient in calcium and vitamin D. These men were given a supplement of 500 mg of calcium and 125 units of vitamin D daily throughout the 3-year study. It is likely this calcium and vitamin D supplementation contributed to the significant increase in vertebral bone mineral density seen in the placebo group. Secondly, although overall the increase in vertebral bone mineral density with testosterone did not reach statistical significance compared to placebo, there was a clear inverse relationship between the pre-treatment testosterone level and the incremental benefit from testosterone therapy. That is, the lower the baseline testosterone level, the greater the benefit of testosterone therapy on vertebral bone mineral density. The testosterone effect appeared to be particularly significant for men with baseline testosterone levels below 300 ng/dL.

In summary, based on limited data available to date, older men with decreased vertebral bone density and testosterone levels below 300 ng/dL may benefit from testosterone therapy. Ensuring adequate intake of calcium and vitamin D is important in all men and may be as important as testosterone therapy in men with normal or only slightly low testosterone values.

Aging, Testosterone, Mood, and Cognitive Function

As noted earlier, a whole litany of psychological, emotional, constitutional, and cognitive complaints have been suggested as manifestations of a male menopause. These include fatigue, depressed mood, irritability, decreased sexual interest, and diminished overall zest for life. With the exception of decreased sexual interest, data to support a positive association between age and any of these symptoms appear to be lacking. The prevalence of depression and other symptoms typically associated with a male menopause did not vary with age in the Massachusetts Male Aging Study. Testosterone levels in depressed and non-depressed men have not shown any consistent difference.

Testosterone therapy in severely hypogonadal men is often accompanied by self-reported increases in sexual interest, mood, energy, and general sense of well-being. Similar responses have been reported anecdotally or in nonblinded, uncontrolled trials of testosterone therapy given to older men with male menopause symptoms. Few randomized controlled trials of testosterone ther-

apy in older men have prospectively assessed end-points related to cognitive function, mood, and general well-being. Published trials have sought and failed to demonstrate significant effects of testosterone therapy in the following areas: depression rating; tests of memory, recall, verbal fluency, visual and verbal memory, and fine-motor speed; and in self-assessed ratings of social functioning, pain, mental health, vitality, general health and energy, and sexual function.

The most consistent and strongest positive findings for testosterone therapy have been in the area of increased sexual interest and libido. Weak positive effects have been reported on tests of spatial cognition. In the 3-year controlled trial of Snyder and colleagues, data were collected on a variety of quality of life, general health, and sexual function parameters. Only one outcome—perception of physical function—showed a significant difference between placebo and testosterone treatment. As with other outcomes in this study, there was a significant association between the baseline testosterone level and the testosterone effect on subjects' perception of their physical function at the end of the trial. The greatest effects again appeared to occur in men with baseline testosterone levels below 300 ng/dL.

In summary, anecdotal reports in the popular press notwithstanding, controlled trials of testosterone therapy in older men have not revealed dramatic or life-altering changes in mood, energy, vitality, or sexual function. Testosterone treatment may increase libido in some men. Older men with testosterone levels below 300 ng/dL may perceive some improvement in their sense of physical function.

Aging, Testosterone, and Hematopoiesis

Testosterone stimulates erythropoiesis and young hypogonadal men have lower hemoglobin levels that increase with testosterone therapy. Hemoglobin levels also tend to be slightly lower in older men compared to young men.

Randomized, controlled trials of testosterone therapy in older men have uniformly shown increases in hemoglobin levels with testosterone treatment. The increases are modest, and most men maintain hemoglobin levels within the normal range. However, in these trials between 6% and 24% of testosterone-treated men developed hemoglobin or hematocrit values above the normal range, necessitating in some cases discontinuation of therapy or phlebotomy. Erythrocytosis is arguably the most common adverse effect that has been observed when testosterone is given to older men.

Aging, Testosterone, and the Prostate

The prostate is the one target organ where the analogy between hypogonadal men and aging men appears to break down. Hypogonadal young men have small, undeveloped prostates and do not develop prostatic hypertrophy or prostate cancer. On the other hand, benign prostatic hypertrophy and prostate cancer are conditions of aging that only occur in the presence of testosterone. Despite the fact that a direct association between endogenous testosterone levels and risk of prostate cancer has not been shown, the greatest concerns regarding testosterone supplementation in older men have centered on the possibility of fueling an occult or clinically insignificant prostate cancer to create a clinical neoplasm.

Reassuringly, trials of testosterone therapy in older men have so far found little evidence of significant adverse prostatic events. The most consistent finding has been significant, but small increases in PSA levels in testosterone-treated men. PSA levels have typically remained within the normal range. Other assessments such as prostate volume, postvoid residual, urinary flow rate, and urinary symptom scores have shown no significant change when compared either to baseline or placebo.

In the 3-year clinical trial of Snyder and colleagues, PSA increased significantly in the testosterone group from baseline to 3 years (1.6±1.0 to 2.2±1.8 ng/mL). PSA values did not change in the placebo group. No differences were seen in urinary flow rate, postvoid residual, or voiding symptom scores between the two groups. Only 1 of 108 men was diagnosed with prostate cancer during the trial; that subject was in the testosterone treatment arm.

Randomized, controlled trials of testosterone therapy in older men have to date involved few patients (probably less than 300 overall) and have been of short duration. Only one trial has extended beyond 1 year. Men participating in testosterone treatment trials are carefully screened at baseline for preexisting prostate disease. These men may represent a particularly low-risk group for testosterone therapy. Although the results so far are reassuring, long-term effects of testosterone supplementation on the prostate are unknown.

Clinical Clues of Male Menopause

The clinical history that should prompt a clinician to consider male menopause is shown in Tables 19–1 and 19–3.

Therapy

Testosterone Therapy

When testosterone therapy is given, the most commonly used preparations are testosterone enanthate, testosterone cypionate, and testosterone propionate for intramuscular injection. Injections are typically given at doses of 200 mg every 2 weeks to 300 mg every 3 weeks. At these doses and duration, peak levels within a day or two after injection are at the upper end of the normal testosterone range, and trough levels just before the next injection are at the lower end of normal. Some patients may report fluctuations in mood and libido between injection times. Many men learn to give the injections themselves and find them quite acceptable. When self-administered, testosterone ester therapy is relatively inexpensive.

Transdermal testosterone patches are also available. They provide stable, physiologic blood levels of testosterone. Patches are placed either on the scrotal skin or on nonscrotal skin, depending on the particular patch. Patches are changed daily. Skin irritation and allergic skin reactions are the primary side effects experienced with the transdermal testosterone patch. Implantable testosterone pellets, testosterone transdermal creams, and various other testosterone formulations for oral or parenteral therapy are under investigation or are used in some countries.

Hemoglobin, lipid levels, digital prostate examination, and PSA should probably be obtained at baseline and within 3 to 4 months of initiation of testosterone therapy in older men. After that, frequency of follow-up appropriate to the individual's age and clinical situation is probably sufficient, but should be done at least yearly. Hepatic toxicity appears to be rare with injectable testosterone esters, but many physicians check liver function tests at baseline and as part of routine follow-up. Patients should be routinely questioned about symptoms of sleep apnea.

Other Concerns Regarding Testosterone Therapy for Older Men

In addition to concerns regarding effects on the prostate and possible excess stimulation of red blood cell production, other areas of concern when older men are given testosterone include effects on blood lipids and on development or exacerbation of sleep apnea. HDL cholesterol levels are higher in hypogonadal young men compared to young controls, and HDL levels fall when testosterone therapy is initiated. On the other hand, some epidemiologic studies have found a direct association in men between testosterone

levels and HDL cholesterol. In controlled trials of testosterone therapy in older men, effects on the lipid profile have essentially been neutral. Total cholesterol, LDL cholesterol, and HDL cholesterol have tended to remain the same or fall slightly with no change in LDL:HDL ratios or triglyceride levels. Possible beneficial or adverse long-term effects, if any, on cardiovascular risk are unknown.

There have been case reports of development or exacerbation of sleep apnea with testosterone therapy; however, sleep apnea has not been reported in controlled trials. Snyder and colleagues performed sleep studies and found no difference between testosterone treatment and placebo on number of apneic and hypopneic episodes during sleep.

Concerns regarding hepatotoxicity with oral 17-alkylated derivatives of testosterone have led to recommendations that testosterone replacement be given only through periodic injection of testosterone esters or daily application of a transdermal testosterone patch.

Aging, Testosterone, and Male Menopause

Menopause is a well-defined physiologic event in the aging process of females. Reproductive function ceases and female sex hormone values fall to prepubertal levels, leading to predictable changes in bone and lipid metabolism, atrophic changes in skin and reproductive organs, and vasomotor instability. Whether estrogen deficiency is an important factor in age-related changes in cognitive function or memory in women remains to be determined.

When considered in this light, the concept of an analogous male menopause attributable to testosterone deficiency seems unlikely. Male reproductive potential is maintained throughout life and testosterone levels remain well above prepubertal values. That is not to say that hypogonadism does not occur in older men, and hypogonadal men may not come to medical attention until middle age. These men generally benefit from testosterone replacement therapy and should be offered therapy unless there are contraindications. However, the idea espoused by some, usually in the popular press, that routine testosterone therapy for older men will cure all manner of constitutional, sexual, and psychological ills is simply not supported by existing data.

Based on currently available data from controlled, blinded trials, older men with testosterone levels greater than 300 ng/dL probably have little clinically significant benefit to gain from testosterone supplementation. Older men with testosterone levels between 200 and 300 ng/dL given testosterone will probably realize small increases in muscle mass and bone density in the spine, have increased sexual interest, and feel their level of physical function is improved. Their PSA and hemoglobin levels will probably rise slightly. Whether any of these changes are clinically significant or will have long-term beneficial or adverse effects on their overall health, functional status, or longevity remains to be determined.

Bibliography

1. Tenover JS: Androgen administration to aging men. *Endocrinol Metab Clin North Am* 23:877–892, 1994.
2. Kaufman JM, Vermeulen A: Androgens in male senescence. In Nieschlag E, Behre HM (eds): *Testosterone: Action, Deficiency, Substitution*. Berlin, Springer, 1998, 437–460.
3. Schow DA, Redmon JB, Pryor JL: Male menopause, how to define it, how to treat it. *Postgraduate Med* 101:62–74, 1997.
4. Morley JE, Kaiser FE, Sih R, et al: Testosterone and frailty. *Clin Geriatr Med* 13:685–695, 1997.
5. Bagatell CJ, Bremner WJ: Androgens in men—uses and abuses. *N Engl J Med* 334:707–714, 1996.
6. Sternbach H: Age-associated testosterone decline in men: Clinical issues for psychiatry. *Am J Psychiatry* 155:1310–1318, 1998.
7. Gray A, Feldman HA, McKinlay JB, Longcope C: Age, disease, and changing sex hormone levels in middle-aged men: Results of the Massachusetts male aging study. *J Clin Endocrinol Metab* 73:1016–1025, 1991.
8. Feldman HA, Goldstein I, Hatzichristou DG, et al: Impotence and its medical and psychosocial correlates: Results of the Massachusetts male aging study. *J Urol* 151:54–61, 1994.
9. Korenman SG, Morley JE, Mooradian AD, et al: Secondary hypogonadism in older men: Its relation to impotence. *J Clin Endocrinol Metab* 71:963–969, 1990.
10. Tenover JS: Effects of testosterone supplementation in the aging male. *J Clin Endocrinol Metab* 75:1092–1098, 1992.
11. Sih R, Morley JE, Kaiser FE, et al: Testosterone replacement in older hypogonadal men: A 12-month randomized controlled trial. *J Clin Endocrinol* 82:1661–1667, 1997.
12. Snyder PJ, Peachey H, Hannoush P, et al: Effect of testosterone treatment on body composition and muscle strength in men over 65 years of age. *J Clin Endocrinol Metab* 84:2647–2653, 1999.
13. Snyder PJ, Peachey H, Hannoush P, et al: Effect of testosterone treatment on bone mineral density in men over 65 years of age. *J Clin Endocrinol Metab* 84:1966–1972, 1999.

Part

3

Miscellaneous

Christopher K. Schreiber
Roger K. Low
C. Darryl Jones
Sakti Das

Imaging Studies

Introduction

Diagnostic imaging plays an integral role in the evaluation and treatment of urologic disorders. The genitourinary system includes the kidneys, upper tract collecting system (calyces, renal pelvis, ureters), bladder, urethra, prostate, and male and female genitalia. In addition to being anatomically and functionally unique, these structures are susceptible to a number of pathologic processes. In this chapter we will describe salient points about the diagnostic studies employed most frequently when evaluating patients with urologic disorders (Table 20–1). Algorithms will be used to discuss common genitourinary disease processes presenting to the clinician with an emphasis on diagnostic radiologic evaluation.

Intravenous Urogram

The intravenous urogram, also known as the intravenous pyelogram (IVP), is considered a his-

torical cornerstone in urologic imaging and remains an integral tool for assessing the urinary tract. Intravenous urography is frequently the initial study obtained to evaluate patients presenting with hematuria, flank pain, and urinary tract infections. This study provides important information on both the anatomic and functional status of the urinary tract. The IVP offers a detailed view of the anatomy of the upper tract collecting system.

Typically, patients receive a light bowel preparation prior to the study to minimize intestinal gas and stool that may obscure details of the study. An initial "scout film" (kidney, ureters, and bladder—KUB) is obtained prior to administration of intravenous contrast (Fig. 20–1). Contraindications to using IV contrast include renal insufficiency and a

Figure 20–1

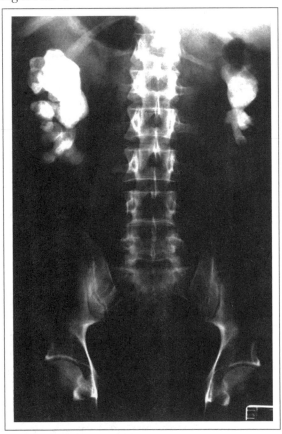

KUB (no contrast has been given). Bilateral staghorn calculi.

Table 20–1

Common Urologic Imaging Studies

- Intravenous urogram (IVU/IVP)
- Retrograde pyelogram (RPG)
- Voiding cystourethrogram (VCUG)/cystogram
- Retrograde urethrogram (RUG)
- Computed tomogram (CT)
    Noncontrast helical/spiral
    Contrast abdomen/pelvis
- Ultrasound
    Kidney
    Bladder
    Prostate
    Scrotum
- Magnetic resonance imaging (MRI)
- Renal angiogram

prior history of contrast-related allergy. Additional risk factors include dehydration, multiple myeloma, and diabetes mellitus.[1] The KUB offers valuable information about soft tissues, skeletal anatomy, and abnormal calcifications, which would be difficult to interpret after contrast administration. Tomographic views provide information on renal contour, size, and position (Fig. 20–2). The kidneys should be symmetrical in size, approximately 3 to 4 vertebral bodies in height, with the upper pole just beneath the eleventh or twelfth rib. The right kidney usually will be lower than the left because of downward displacement by the liver.

Once intravenous contrast is administered, x-rays are obtained, at 0, 5, and 10-minute intervals and as needed to visualize the entire collecting system from the kidneys to the bladder. The 0-minute film demonstrates the renal cortical anatomy. As contrast is excreted, subsequent films show progressive filling of the collecting system. Hydronephrosis is defined as dilation of the collecting system but does not necessarily imply obstruction. For example, a patient with vesicoureteral reflux may have pronounced hydronephrosis as a result of chronic reflux of urine into the upper tract but not obstruction. The sine qua non of obstruction by IVP is dilation of the collecting system accompanied by delayed excretion of contrast. If these findings are present, an obstructive process (e.g., stones, ureteropelvic junction obstruction, stricture) must be considered (Fig. 20–3).

"Delayed views" often aid in visualizing the level of obstruction in the collecting system (Fig. 20–4). The three narrowest points in the collecting system and typical locations for obstruction by urinary stones are the ureteropelvic junction, the portion of the ureter passing over the iliac vessels, and the ureterovesical junction. Acute obstruction by a distal ureteral calculus often causes hilar or perirenal extravasation of contrast during an IVP (Fig. 20–5). Urinary extravasation in itself is not an absolute indication for surgical intervention if the patient's symptoms are well controlled and passage of the stone is still feasible.

Filling defects within the pelvis, ureter, or bladder may be caused by a number of processes

Figure 20–2

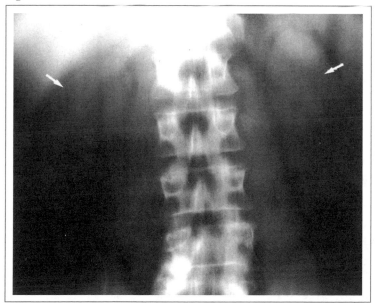

IVP. Nephrotomograms showing normal renal contour and position. (Arrows show lateral renal margins.)

Figure 20–3

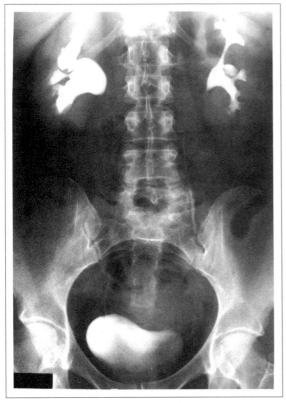

IVP. Right ureteropelvic junction obstruction.

(Fig. 20–6). Considerations include stones, tumor, blood clot, papillary necrosis, and fungal balls. The postvoid film helps determine bladder-emptying capability and also aids visualizing the distal ureter. Although the IVP is integral in evaluating the upper tracts in a patient with hematuria, it is not sufficient to fully evaluate the bladder (Fig. 20–7). Cystoscopy is required to rule out lower urinary tract pathology.

Retrograde Pyelogram

Retrograde pyelography (RPG) is performed by urologists during cystoscopy. It provides excellent definition of the upper tract anatomy. Indications for retrograde pyelography include patients with poor renal function who might not tolerate intravenous contrast, patients at high risk for contrast reactions, and poor visualization or equivocal findings on an IVU or spiral CT. Generally, a small acorn tip or open-ended catheter is placed into the ureteral orifice under cystoscopic guidance. Five to 10 mL of diluted Renograffin contrast is then instilled retrograde through the catheter. Fluoroscopic images as well x-rays are obtained allowing visualization of the entire collecting system (Fig. 20–8). Drainage films are obtained after removing the catheter.

Voiding Cystourethrogram/ Cystogram

An essential part of the diagnostic evaluation for infants and children with urinary tract infections is to detect underlying anatomic (e.g., ureteropelvic junction obstruction, posterior urethral valves, reflux) or functional (e.g., neurogenic bladder) abnormalities.[2] The voiding cystourethrogram (VCUG) is used primarily to evaluate for vesicoureteral reflux disease (Fig. 20–9). In addition to providing information on the integrity of the ureterovesical valve mechanism, the study is also used to illustrate the bladder neck, prostatic urethra, and antegrade voiding.

After a precontrast KUB is obtained, the bladder is filled with contrast by gravity through a Foley catheter. The catheter is then removed and the patient voids. The procedure is carried out under fluoroscopic monitoring with intermittent spot films obtained during filling and voiding phases. On filling, the bladder should appear smooth and ovoid with an adequate capacity (bladder capacity in children can be estimated by the formula: age in years + 2 = capacity in ounces).

Reflux of urine into the upper tracts may appear during the filling and/or voiding phase. The

Figure 20–4

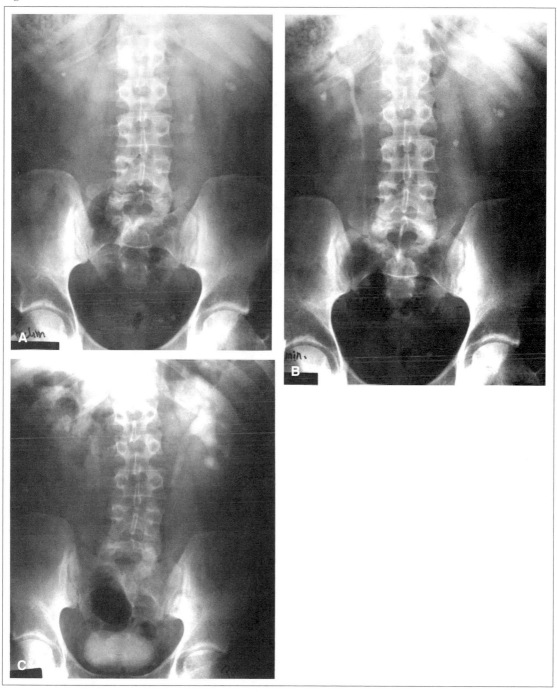

A. IVP. Scout film showing a number of calcifications overlying both kidneys. **B**. IVP. Delayed excretion from left collecting system secondary to obstructing proximal ureteral stone. **C**. IVP. Delayed view confirming obstructing stone in left proximal ureter.

Figure 20–5

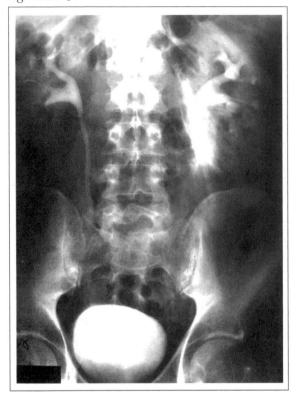

IVP. Extravasation from a small obstructing left ureterovesical junction stone.

severity of reflux is graded from I to IV depending on the degree of distortion and dilation of the ureter, renal pelvis, and calyces (Fig. 20–10). Postvoid views may unmask low-grade reflux hidden behind a full bladder. In neonates and young male children, the cystogram phase is often supplemented by antegrade voiding films to help delineate posterior urethral valves with characteristic dilation of the prostatic urethra and bladder neck (Fig. 20–11).

In contrast to a VCUG, a cystogram is performed primarily to evaluate the integrity of the bladder following trauma or surgery (Fig. 20–12). After placing a catheter into the bladder, approximately 300 to 400 mL of contrast is instilled by gravity to ensure bladder filling (this is important for demonstrating subtle intra- or extraperitoneal perforations). Films obtained after emptying the

bladder will help visualize small posterior extraperitoneal perforations that would otherwise be missed with the bladder full.

Retrograde Urethrogram

Retrograde urethrography (RUG) is an important study used by urologists for evaluation of the male urethral anatomy. It is able to delineate the location and extent of stricture disease within the anterior and posterior urethra. Retrograde urethrography is also helpful for evaluating patients with suspected pelvic and genitourinary trauma prior to attempting urethral catheterization (e.g., in patients with blood at the urethral meatus).

To perform the study, a small Foley catheter is placed into the distal urethra and the balloon inflated in the fossa navicularis with 1 to 2 mL of water. Thirty to 60 mL of contrast medium is gently injected through the catheter and films obtained in oblique and lateral views to visualize the entire length of the urethra. Voiding films can also be obtained to help delineate the proximal urethra and bladder neck. Urethral strictures appear as areas of narrowing with or without proximal dilation (Fig. 20–13).

Computed Tomogram

Computed tomography (CT) constitutes one of the most definitive diagnostic modalities available to evaluate the urinary tract. It can illustrate the anatomy of the urinary tract and retroperitoneum in exquisite detail. With dynamic scanning using intravenous contrast agents, renal vascular anatomy as well as parenchymal enhancement is appreciated. For the patient found

Figure 20–6

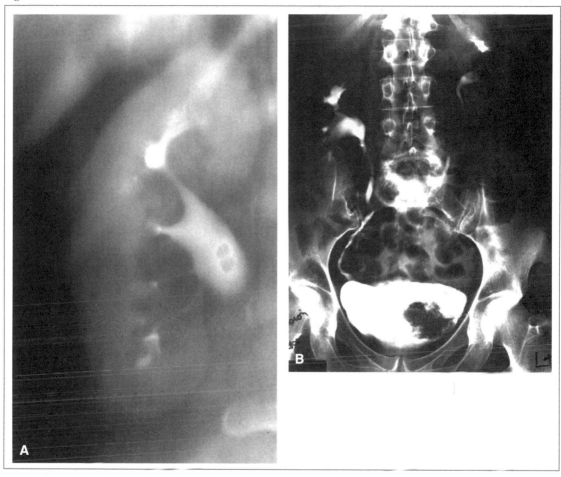

A. IVP. Filling defect right renal pelvis (radiolucent stones). **B**. IVP. Large filling defect within bladder secondary to transitional-cell carcinoma.

to have a suspicious mass in the kidney on ultrasound or intravenous pyelogram, the abdominal CT scan is the study of choice for its evaluation (Fig. 20–14). Solid renal tumors may have a homogenous or heterogeneous appearance (Fig. 20–15). On postcontrast views, renal tumors and complex cysts will typically enhance, as opposed to simple cysts, parenchymal scarring, and old hemorrhage, which will not (Fig. 20–16).

The abdominal/pelvic CT scan has remained a crucial tool to the urologist for staging genitourinary malignancies. For the patient with a renal tumor, the CT scan offers information not only on the size of the mass, which may dictate surgical exposure, but also illustrates potential involvement of adjacent structures, renal vessels, and intraperitoneal organs. Twenty-five to 70% of men with a primary testicular tumor will have regional (retroperitoneal) or distant metastatic disease on presentation (Fig. 20–17). CT will help dictate in this population whether retroperitoneal lymph node dissection or chemotherapy will be the most effective first-line therapy. Similarly, for patients with muscle invasive bladder cancer, it is important to know extent of local invasion as

Figure 20–7

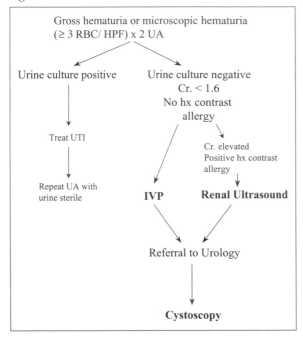

Gross hematuria or microscopic hematuria
(≥ 3 RBC/ HPF) x 2 UA

Urine culture positive   Urine culture negative
                                Cr. < 1.6
                                No hx contrast
                                allergy

                                          Cr. elevated
                                          Positive hx contrast
                                          allergy

Treat UTI

                                IVP   **Renal Ultrasound**

Repeat UA with
urine sterile

                        Referral to Urology

                              Cystoscopy

Algorithm: Hematuria.

Figure 20–8

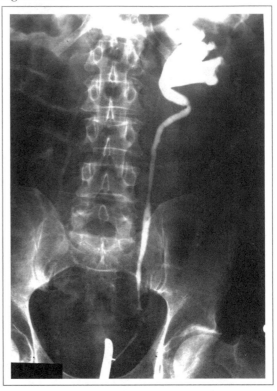

Retrograde pyelogram. Filling defect in left distal ureter found to be transitional-cell carcinoma.

well as intraperitoneal spread of disease. In contrast, CT scans typically offer little information to the urologist when evaluating patients with prostate cancer.

Within the last few years, the helical or spiral CT scan has been introduced in many centers. Several studies have shown that the unenhanced spiral CT is a safe and highly accurate technique for imaging patients with acute flank pain.[3] It has all but replaced the IVP as the diagnostic modality of choice for evaluating patients with presumed renal colic in the acute care setting (Fig. 20–18).

By gathering images in a continuous helical fashion, rather than a stepwise fashion, the examination can be performed over 30 to 45 seconds with only 1 or 2 breath holds. Sections 5 mm thick are obtained using a helical data acquisition, and image clusters are obtained from the tops of the kidneys through the bladder. Cuts of

1 to 2 mm as well as three-dimensional images can be obtained as needed. Contrast is not administered when the spiral CT is performed for renal colic, thus eliminating potential allergic reactions (incidence of 5% to 10% in general population). A recent report demonstrates a 98% sensitivity, 100% specificity, 100% positive predictive value, and 97% negative predictive value for diagnosing ureteral stones and/or obstruction with spiral CT, which matches or exceeds similar parameters for intravenous pyelogram.[4]

In addition to direct stone visualization (Fig. 20–19), secondary CT signs of ureteral obstruction are often present and useful when a stone is not readily seen. These include perinephric fat soft-tissue stranding, nephromegaly, hydroureter-

Figure 20–9

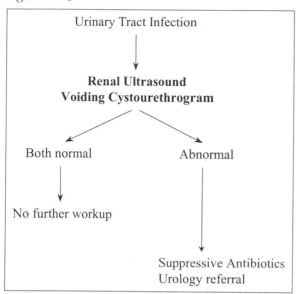

Algorithm: Pediatric urinary tract infection.

Figure 20–11

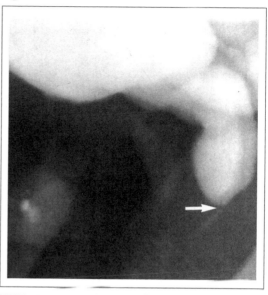

VCUG. Posterior urethral valve (*arrow*) with proximal dilation of prostatic urethra.

Figure 20–10

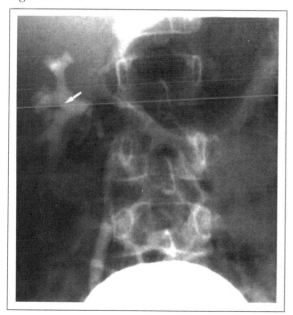

VCUG. Right ureteral reflux with contrast outlining collection system (arrow).

onephrosis, and the soft-tissue "rim sign" (visualization of a rim of soft-tissue attenuation surrounding ureteral stones; Fig. 20–20). Potential pitfalls include pelvic phleboliths, which can be seen along the normal course of the ureter and can mimic ureteral stones. Additionally, the helical CT scan is effective at diagnosing other causes of acute flank pain unrelated to the urinary tract such as appendicitis, ovarian pathology, etc.

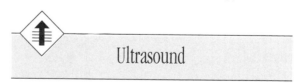

Ultrasound

Ultrasonography is probably the most commonly used imaging technique in the evaluation of the genitourinary tract. High-frequency sound waves interact with tissues of varying densities and are reflected back to a transducer creating real-time images. Advantages of ultrasound include safety, noninvasiveness, lack of radiation exposure, no need

Figure 20–12

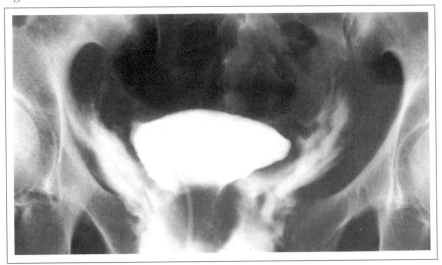

Cystogram. Extraperitoneal bladder perforation with characteristic flame appearance of contrast extravasation in the retroperitoneum.

Figure 20–13

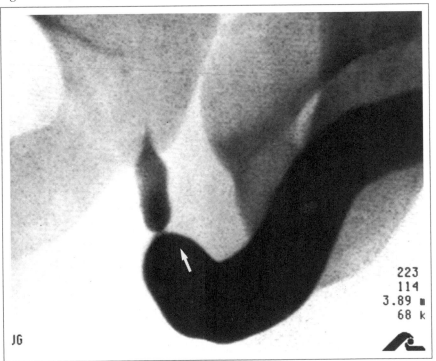

RUG. Bulbar urethral stricture (arrow). Contrast in this image appears black.

Figure 20–14

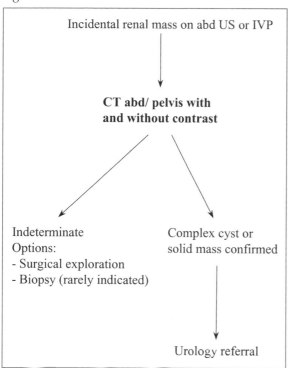

Algorithm: Renal mass.

for contrast agents, and speed of obtaining images. Additionally, ultrasound is inexpensive, widely available, and can be performed in the clinic or at the bedside. Disadvantages include poor image quality secondary to bowel gas, overlying bone, or body habitus. A number of applications currently exist for ultrasonography in urology.

Renal Ultrasound

Ultrasound is able to detect dilation of the renal pelvis, calyces, and ureter with a sensitivity of 98% and a specificity of 78%. False-negative results are possible, however, due to the fact that there may be a delay of 24 hours or more after the onset of obstruction for dilation of the collecting system to develop. Ultrasound is capable of detecting both radiopaque and radiolucent stones but is limited to evaluating only the pyelocalyceal system and proximal and distal ureters. Stones are characterized by a strong echogenic focus with posterior acoustic shadowing (Fig. 20–21).

Simple renal cysts are seen as echo-free smooth-walled structures (Fig. 20–22). These lesions are

Figure 20–15

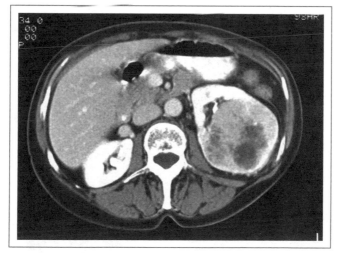

CT. Large left renal tumor.

Figure 20–16

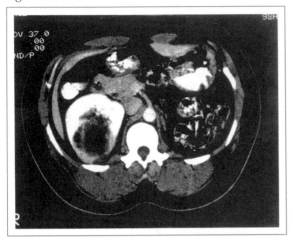

CT. Complex renal cyst (surgical pathology revealed renal-cell carcinoma).

considered benign and do not require urologic evaluation.

A renal abscess may have complex septations with debris and low-level internal echoes. Renal cell carcinoma typically appears as a hetero-geneous solid mass within the kidney (Fig. 20–23). Angiomyolipomas have a characteristic bright echogenic appearance due to the high reflectivity of the fat component of the lesion.

Figure 20–17

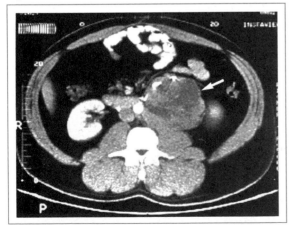

CT. Retroperitoneal lymphadenopathy (arrow) in a pa-tient with testicular cancer.

Figure 20–18

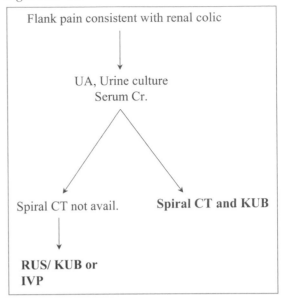

Flank pain consistent with renal colic

↓

UA, Urine culture
Serum Cr.

Spiral CT not avail.   **Spiral CT and KUB**

**RUS/ KUB or
IVP**

Algorithm: Acute flank pain. (RUS = renal ultrasound)

With the routine use of prenatal ultrasound, fetal hydronephrosis is a frequent finding. Up to 30% of hydronephrosis in this setting will be phys-iologic and will resolve on follow-up antenatal ultrasound (obtained at 4 to 7 days after birth).

Figure 20–19

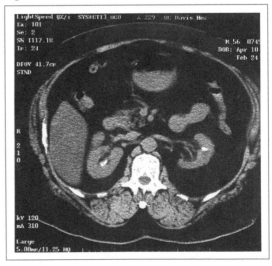

Spiral CT. Bilateral renal stones.

Figure 20–20

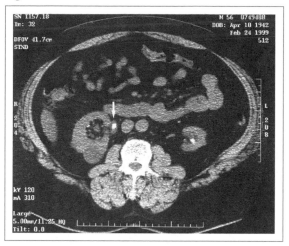

Spiral CT. Soft-tissue "rim sign" (arrow) surrounding ureteral stone.

Pathologic causes of neonatal hydronephrosis include ureteropelvic junction obstruction, vesicoureteral reflux, and a distended bladder (as seen with posterior urethral valves) (Fig. 20–24). Fetal hydronephrosis is discussed in detail in Chapter 1.

Figure 20–21

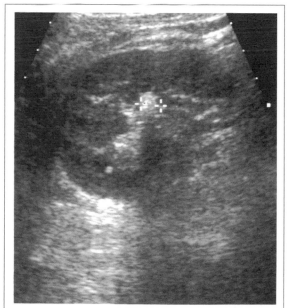

Renal US. Stone with posterior shadowing.

Figure 20–22

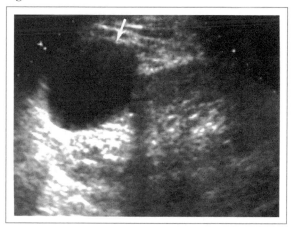

Renal US. Large simple cyst (arrow).

Bladder Ultrasound

Ultrasonographic evaluation of the bladder as part of pelvic ultrasound studies may reveal intravesical lesions such as carcinoma, calculi, or ureteroceles. It is most commonly used as a noninvasive method for determining postvoid residual urine volume (PVR), and thus replaces catheterization to determine PVR.

Figure 20–23

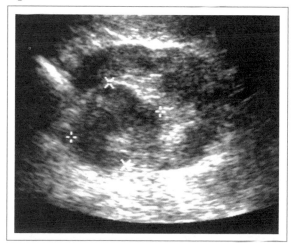

Renal US. Tumor.

Figure 20–24

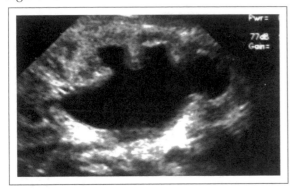

Renal US. Hydronephrosis (renal pelvis and calyces are easily seen).

Prostate Ultrasound

Transrectal ultrasonography is an important tool when evaluating men for prostate cancer. It aids in detection and delineation of abnormal masses within the prostate and directs needle placement during biopsy. Benign prostatic hyperplasia often appears as a symmetrical homogeneous enlargement as opposed to carcinoma, which may appear as hypoechoic areas within the peripheral zone (Fig. 20–25). In azoospermic patients, prostatic ultrasound may reveal cystic dilation of the ejaculatory duct, indicating ductal obstruction (see Chapter 18A).

Scrotal Ultrasound

Ultrasound is considered the primary imaging modality for evaluation of the scrotum. The normal testicle will be homogeneous with low to medium echogenicity.[5] The head and body of the epididymis should be well visualized with a similar echogenic pattern as the testicle. For patients with suspected cryptorchidism and a nonpalpable testicle, ultrasound may demonstrate the testicle along the inguinal canal, although the sensitivity is too low to warrant routine use.

When a scrotal mass is clearly intratesticular, usually no imaging study is required, and radical orchiectomy is appropriate (see Chapter 14). Some

Figure 20–25

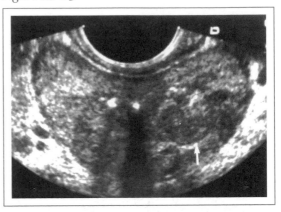

TRUS. Transverse view of prostate with heterogeneous area (*arrow*) found to be prostate cancer on biopsy. Note prostatic calcifications with posterior shadowing.

scrotal masses found on physical examination may require further evaluation with an ultrasound (Fig. 20–26) particularly when the mass cannot clearly be localized to within the testing. Ultrasound will further characterize the lesion by demonstrating whether the mass is intratesticular or extratesticular and whether it is solid or fluid filled.

Figure 20–26

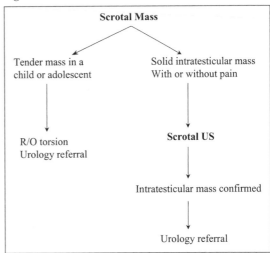

Algorithm: Scrotal mass. When physical exam shows an unequivocal intratesticular mass, testis cancer may be presumed, and scrotal imaging studies are typically not required.

CANCER

Testicular cancer typically develops in young men prior to the age of 40. Most testicular neoplasms are germ-cell tumors in this population. A cancerous lesion in the testicle of an older patient will more commonly be lymphoma. Patients typically present with an enlarged, nontender intratesticular mass. Calcifications as well as extension of the tumor beyond tunica may be seen on ultrasound (Fig. 20–27).

HYDROCELES AND SPERMATOCELES

Fluid collections within the scrotum include hydroceles and spermatoceles, both of which will transilluminate on physical examination and appear anechoic on ultrasound (Fig. 20–28). Varicoceles represent dilation of the pampiniform plexus venous drainage of the testicle. These typically occur on the left side and may be associated with atrophic changes of the testicle and/or infertility (see Chapter 18A)..

EPIDIDYMO-ORCHITIS

Inflammatory processes of the scrotum include epididymitis and orchitis. The patient presents with a painful, enlarged hemiscrotum, which may make examination of the scrotum difficult. Urinalysis will demonstrate pyuria. Dysuria and fever may be present. Occasionally, testicular cancer may mimic an inflammatory process secondary to hemorrhage within the tumor. The acutely inflamed epididymis produces a decreased echogenicity with a heterogeneous pattern on ultrasound.

TORSION

Torsion of the spermatic cord will present as acute onset testicular pain and swelling in a young or adolescent boy. Urinalysis will be normal. The diagnosis is typically a clinical one; however, ultrasound may be beneficial in equivocal cases. Acutely, the testicle will be enlarged with altered echogenicity. Doppler examination reveals no arterial or venous blood flow within the testicle.

Magnetic Resonance Imaging

By placing the body within a strong magnetic field, the magnetic resonance imaging (MRI)

Figure 20–27

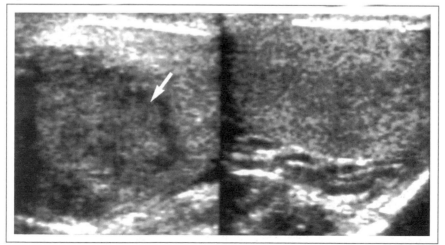

Scrotal US. Hypoechoic tumor (*arrow*) replacing parenchyma of right testicle (compare appearance to normal left testicle).

Figure 20–28

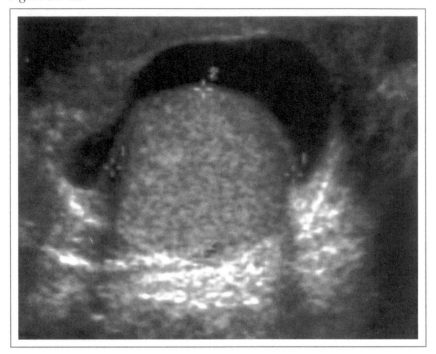

Scrotal ultrasound. Hydrocele.

device creates images by altering the natural alignment of hydrogen atoms within the body. With the additional application of short pulses of radiowaves, hydrogen nuclei will absorb energy and invert their orientation with respect to the magnetic field. When the radioenergy pulse is terminated, the hydrogen atoms will return to a resting state and release energy. The emitted energies are collected and transformed by computer analysis into cross-sectional images.

Advantages of MRI include high-resolution images in multiple planes and no exposure to ionizing radiation. Disadvantages include slow scan times, sensitivity of images to motion, and patient intolerance (claustrophobia). MRI is useful in evaluating the extent of renal vein and IVC involvement in locally invasive renal-cell cancer (Fig. 20–29). It is also helpful in evaluating for renal vein thrombosis, and in situations when contrast CT is not appropriate (renal insuffi-

ciency). MRI is excellent for imaging adrenal lesions. Hyperintense T2-weighted adrenal masses are highly suggestive of pheochromocytoma.

Renal Angiogram

With the advent of CT and MRI studies, the more invasive angiographic studies are now rarely used in urology. This study does provide helpful information on equivocal space-occupying lesions, renal artery lesions, arteriovenous malformations, and occasionally to define the vascular anatomy prior to nephron-sparing surgery (Fig. 20–30). Renal angiography and embolization are sometimes used for angioinfarction of renal cancers or to control refractory renal hemorrhage.

Figure 20–29

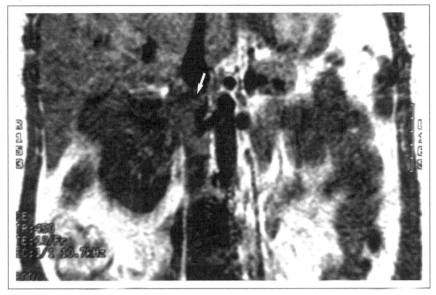

MRI. Right renal-cell carcinoma with IVC tumor thrombus (*arrow*).

Figure 20–30

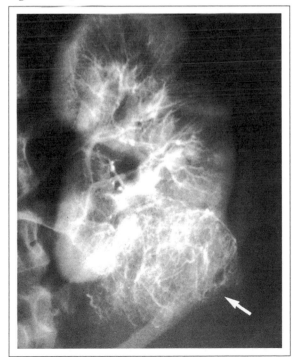

Renal angiogram showing exophytic lower-pole renal tumor (arrow) prior to partial nephrectomy.

Captopril Renal Scan

The captopril renal scan may be used to screen for renovascular hypertension. In renal artery stenosis, angiotensin II compensates for the decreased perfusion, by causing a selective vasoconstriction of efferent renal arterioles, thus maintaining glomerular filtration. The administration of captopril, an angiotension-converting enzyme inhibitor, will block the release of angiotensin II, potentiating decreased glomerular filtration. The captopril renal scan characterizes the appearance of radionuclide before and after the administration of captopril. The contralateral (normal) kidney remains normal. The ipsilateral affected kidney shows delayed uptake of radionuclide, delay in time to maximum activity, and delayed cortical retention. The test may be limited when renal function is severely compromised, or when bilateral renal artery disease precludes comparison between contralateral and ipsilateral kidneys.

References

1. Curry NS: Renal imaging and congenital lesions. In Sutton D, Young J (eds): *A Concise Textbook of Clinical Imaging,* ed 2. St. Louis, Mosby, 1995, p. 621.
2. Leonidas JC: Urinary tract infection in children. In Eisenberg RL (ed): *Diagnostic Imaging: An Algorithmic Approach.* Philadelphia, Lippincott, 1988, p. 348.
3. Smith RC, Rosenfield AT, Choe KA, et al: Acute flank pain: Comparison of non-contrast-enhanced CT and intravenous urography. *Radiology* 194:789, 1995.
4. Fielding JR, Steele G, Fox LA, Heller H: Spiral computerized tomography in the evaluation of acute flank pain: A replacement for excretory urography. *J Urol* 157:2071–2073, 1997.
5. Novelline RA: Men, women, and children. In Novelline RA (ed): *Squire's Fundamentals of Radiology,* ed 5. Cambridge, Harvard University Press, 1997, p. 425.

Index

Page numbers followed by t indicate table; those followed by f indicate figure.

A

Abdominal leak point pressure (ALPP), incontinence and, 98, 106, 107f
Adenomatoid tumors, 208
Aging. *See also* Geriatric urology
  body composition and, 297–298
  bone density and, 298–299
  cognitive function and, 299
  hematopoiesis and, 299–300
  mood and, 299
  prostate and, 300
  prostate cancer and, 168–169, 169f, 170
  sexual function and, 297
Alarm devices, for nocturnal enuresis, 56, 56t
Alpha-adrenergic blockade, for benign prostatic hyperplasia, 194–195, 194t, 195t
Alpha-antagonists, for incontinence, 138
Alprostadil
  intracavernosal medication, 267t, 269–270
  intraurethral therapy, 267t, 270
Alzheimer's patients, incontinence and, 139–140
Aminopenicillins, for urinary tract infections (UTI), 70t
Amoxicillin, for urinary tract infections, 25

Anabolic steroids, male infertility and, 276
Analgesia, for urinary calculi, 239
Androgen
  for erectile dysfunction, 267t, 269
  prostate cancer prevention, 176
Anejaculation, 284
Angiokeratomas, 227–228, 227f, 228f
Antibiotic resistance, sexually transmitted diseases and, 93
Antibiotics, for urinary tract infections, 24–25, 70t
Anticholinergics, for incontinence, 112–114, 139
Antimicrobial resistance, gonorrhea and, 83
Antisperm antibodies, male infertility and, 282
Aspermia, defined, 278t
Assisted reproductive techniques (ART), male infertility and, 282–283
Asthenospermia, defined, 278t
Asthenozoospermia, defined, 278t
Asymptomatic bacteriuria (ABU), 24
Azoospermia
  defined, 278t
  vasectomy and, 288

B

Bacteriuria, urinary tract infections and, 22
Balanitis, 223

  anaerobic erosive, 223
  circinata, 91
  erosive, 223
  syphilitic, 223
Bed wetting. *See* Nocturnal enuresis
Behavioral modification, for incontinence, 110
Behavioral therapy
  for incontinence, 109, 139–140
  nocturnal enuresis and, 56–57
Benign prostatic hyperplasia (BPH), 186–198
  diagnosis, 188–192
    cystoscopy, 190, 191t
    differential, 192
    history taking, 188
    imaging, 190
    physical examination, 188, 190
    postvoid residual urine measurement (PVR), 191
    pressure-flow studies, 191–192
    prostate-specific antigen (PSA), 190
    serum creatinine, 190
    urinalysis, 190
    uroflowmetry, 190–191
  epidemiology, 186
  etiology, 186
  hematuria and, 155–156
  medical therapy, 194–195
    alpha-adrenergic blockade, 194–195, 194t, 195t
    5-alpha-reductase inhibitor, 195